Critical Approaches to the History of Western Herbal Medicine

Critical Approaches to the History of Western Herbal Medicine

From Classical Antiquity to the Early Modern Period

Edited by Susan Francia and Anne Stobart

Bloomsbury Academic
An imprint of Bloomsbury Publishing Plc

BLOOMSBURY
LONDON · OXFORD · NEW YORK · NEW DELHI · SYDNEY

Bloomsbury Academic
An imprint of Bloomsbury Publishing Plc

50 Bedford Square 1385 Broadway
London New York
WC1B 3DP NY 10018
UK USA

www.bloomsbury.com

BLOOMSBURY and the Diana logo are trademarks of Bloomsbury Publishing Plc

First published 2014
Paperback edition first published 2015

© Susan Francia, Anne Stobart and Contributors, 2014

Susan Francia, Anne Stobart and Contributors have asserted their right under the Copyright, Designs and Patents Act, 1988, to be identified as Authors of this work.

All rights reserved. No part of this publication may be reproduced or transmitted in any form or by any means, electronic or mechanical, including photocopying, recording, or any information storage or retrieval system, without prior permission in writing from the publishers.

No responsibility for loss caused to any individual or organization acting on or refraining from action as a result of the material in this publication can be accepted by Bloomsbury or the author.

British Library Cataloguing-in-Publication Data
A catalogue record for this book is available from the British Library.

ISBN: HB: 978-1-4411-8418-4
PB: 978-1-4742-5504-2
ePub: 978-1-4411-8580-8
ePDF: 978-1-4411-4357-0

Library of Congress Cataloging-in-Publication Data
A catalog record for this book is available from the Library of Congress.

Typeset by Fakenham Prepress Solutions, Fakenham, Norfolk NR21 8NN

Contents

List of Figures and Tables	vii
Notice to Readers	viii
Acknowledgements	ix
List of Contributors	x
Foreword	xiv

1   The Fragmentation of Herbal History: The Way Forward   1
   Anne Stobart and Susan Francia

Part 1   Revisiting Original Texts: Comparative Textual Analysis and New Perspectives on Original Sources

  Introduction   23
  Susan Francia and Anne Stobart

2   Early Greek Medicine: Evidence of Models, Methods and *materia medica*   27
   Vicki Pitman

3   Evaluating the Content of Medieval Herbals   47
   Anne Van Arsdall

4   Early-modern Midwifery Manuals and Herbal Practice   67
   Elaine Hobby

5   An Anatomy of *The English Physitian*   87
   Graeme Tobyn

Part 2   Using Archival Sources: Extending the Evidence Available

  Introduction   107
  Susan Francia and Anne Stobart

6   The Use of Trade Accounts to Uncover the Importance of Cumin as a Medicinal Plant in Medieval England   111
   Susan Francia

7	Early Modern Childbirth and Herbs – The Challenge of Finding the Sources *Nicky Wesson*	131
8	Testamentary Records of the Sixteenth to Eighteenth Centuries as a Source for the History of Herbal Medicine in England *Richard Aspin*	149

Part 3   Focusing on One Individual: Biographical and Other Textual Sources

	Introduction *Susan Francia and Anne Stobart*	169
9	Galen's Simple Medicines: Problems in Ancient Herbal Medicine *John Wilkins*	173
10	Deciphering Dioscorides: Mountains and Molehills? *Alison Denham and Midge Whitelegg*	191
11	William Turner: A Milestone in Botanical Medicine *Marie Addyman*	211
12	John Parkinson: Gardener and Apothecary of London *Jill Francis*	229

Part 4   The Multi-disciplinary Nature of the History of Herbal Medicine, and Contributions from Archaeology and Ethnobotany

	Introduction *Susan Francia and Anne Stobart*	249
13	Archaeological Sources for the History of Herbal Medicine Practice: The Case Study of St John's Wort with Valerian at Soutra Medieval Hospital *Brian Moffat*	253
14	How Can Ethnobotany Contribute to the History of Western Herbal Medicine? A Mesoamerican Answer *Anna Waldstein*	271
15	Conclusion: The History of Herbal Medicine as a Developing Field *Anne Stobart and Susan Francia*	289

Select Glossary	299
Bibliography	303
Index	337

List of Figures and Tables

Figures

1.1	A framework for the history of herbal medicine	4
2.1	Diagram showing the four humours and associated concepts	31
2.2	Sitz baths at the site of an Asclepion at Gortys, Peloponnese, Greece	35
2.3	Squirting cucumber (*Ecballium elaterium*)	39
3.1	Original drawing of a nettle plant (*Urtica* spp.)	54
3.2	Original drawing of a plantain plant (*Plantago* spp.)	60
4.1	Illustration of a woman with foetus in utero: 'Dissection to expose child in the womb'	70
4.2	Lying-in room showing attendant, child being bathed and a midwife drinking her beer	74
6.1	The use of cumin (*Cuminum cyminum*) to pay rents in medieval Oxfordshire	113
6.2	Cumin (*Cuminum cyminum*)	116
8.1	Bronze mortar dated 1607, made in England	155
8.2	Illustration of a woman using a still	158
12.1	Portrait of John Parkinson	233
12.2	Crowne Imperiall (*Fritillaria imperialis*)	241
13.1	Map of medieval South-east Scotland	255
13.2	Reconstruction of the drain blocked with 'medical waste' at Soutra	256

Tables

10.1	Items in *De materia medica*	193
10.2	Places given in *De materia medica*	195
13.1	Seed count of sample (Soutra Aisle (SA) 735; 1996/7)	258
13.2	Medieval names for St John's wort and valerian according to the *Sinonomiae*	260

Notice to Readers

This book is not intended to offer treatment with herbal medicine. No herbs, recipes or other advice that may be described or considered in this book should be used without professional guidance from a medical or herbal practitioner. The publishers, editors and contributors assume no liability for any injury or damage to persons or property resulting from any use of the remedies or methods contained in this book.

Acknowledgements

A number of organizations have played a key role in bringing together our contributors and we thank the National Institute of Medical Herbalists Education Fund, Middlesex University and Wellcome Trust for funding and support.

Our grateful thanks go to our colleagues in the Herbal History Research Network for their support: Barbara Lewis, Vicki Pitman, Christina Stapley and Nicky Wesson. Sadly, a founder member of the group, Annie Hood, museum curator and herbal practitioner, passed away in 2012: she would have been delighted to see the publication of this book. Particular thanks are due to our contributors and to those who have supported the development of links between researchers in the history of herbal medicine, including Celia Bell, Claire Bowditch, Ross MacFarlane, Mark Nesbitt, Kay Piercy, Jose Prieto, Liz Williamson and Alun Withey. We are grateful to Jill Baines and Linda Lever for assistance in checking the text. Finally, a special thanks to Elaine Hobby, Jane Whittle and John Wilkins for their help and advice.

List of Contributors

Marie Addyman is an independent scholar with a focus on Tudor and Elizabethan culture. Arising out of these interests and her passion for practical gardening, she has researched and taught material relating to early plant and garden history. She helped set up and deliver the Morpeth celebrations for Turner's 500th anniversary, with publication of a short book on his life and work for that event, *William Turner: The Father of English Botany* (Friends of Carlisle Park, 2008). She contributes to the annual Morpeth William Turner Symposium, is engaged in producing a short book on William Turner's son, the London physician Peter Turner, and is in the middle of a longer study of William Turner's botanical medicine.

Richard Aspin is Head of Research and Scholarship at the Wellcome Library, and formerly Curator of Western Manuscripts and Head of Special Collections at the Wellcome Library. He has a keen interest in researching medical history, and has contributed a number of articles on items in the Wellcome collections. His publications in *Medical History* include: 'The papers of Sir Thomas Barlow (1845–1945)', 'John Evelyn's tables of veins and arteries: A rediscovered letter', 'Seeking Lister in the Wellcome collections' and 'Who was Elizabeth Okeover?'.

Alison Denham has practised as a medical herbalist since 1984. She is a Senior Lecturer at the University of Central Lancashire in Preston, and has a special interest in the quality, safety, cultivation and conservation of medicinal plants. In 2006 she was appointed to the Herbal Medicines Advisory Committee of the Medicines and Healthcare products Regulatory Agency. As a past President of the National Institute of Medical Herbalists she took an active role in the preparation of the recommendations on the regulation of herbal practitioners. Alison has contributed to *The Western Herbal Tradition* (Elsevier, 2010) and is currently researching John Skelton who was a prominent herbal practitioner in the nineteenth century.

Susan Francia has Masters degrees from both Oxford and Harvard universities, and has taught and carried out research at Harvard. Her background is in the history of medicine and in comparisons between European and Islamic medical history. She is a qualified medical herbalist and was in practice for 12 years. She has extensive experience in teaching herbal medicine, and has taught the history of herbal medicine at Middlesex University. She now works as an independent researcher. Susan has published on Islamic history and on social and medical history in England. She is currently working on the history of medicine in medieval Devon.

Jill Francis completed her PhD, working under the supervision of Professor Richard Cust, at the University of Birmingham. Her area of research was an investigation into the gardening practices of Elizabethan and early Stuart England, exploring how the inherently ephemeral activity of gardening can offer a new perspective on defining status and identity within early-modern gentry society. Her research has included a detailed examination of early-modern gardening manuals, as well as trawling through seventeenth-century gentry manuscript collections archived as far afield as the Huntington Library in California. She has had two articles published in *Garden History*, the journal of the Garden History Society, and one in the *Midland History* journal.

Elaine Hobby is Professor of Seventeenth-Century Studies in the English and Drama Department at Loughborough University. Her interest in early-modern herbal remedies grows from her experience of editing two midwifery manuals, Jane Sharp, *The Midwives Book*, 1671 (Oxford University Press, 1999), and Thomas Raynalde and others, *The Birth of Mankind*, 1540–1654 (Ashgate, 2009). Her academic training is as a literary historian.

Brian Moffat is an archaeo-ethnopharmacologist and Director of Investigations for the Soutra Hospital Archaeo-ethnopharmacological Research Project, Scotland (SHARP). The project is funded by the Soutra Archeo-Medicine Charitable Trust and by many other medical, historical and archaeological trusts and societies, as well as individual supporters. The work involves over 2,000 participating researchers, and various reports on work in progress have been published. Public outreach is achieved through open days and Dr Moffat has given lectures worldwide over a number of years.

Vicki Pitman is a practising medical herbalist and a member of the Unified Register of Herbal Practitioners and International Federation of Aromatherapists. She also holds an MPhil in Complementary Health Studies from the University of Exeter. She has published four books – on herbal medicine, reflexology, aromatherapy and on holism in ancient Greek and Indian medicine; and an article in *HerbalGram*. She is an editor of, and contributor to, *The Herbalist*, the journal of the Association of Master Herbalists and the Unified Register of Herbal Practitioners. She now works as an independent scholar.

Anne Stobart is trained as a medical herbalist and completed her PhD at Middlesex University in 2009. Her thesis focused on seventeenth-century domestic medicine in south-west England. Based at Middlesex University in London from 2000, Anne held the post of Director of Programmes for Complementary Health Sciences until 2010. She has research interests in the historical and present-day supply of herbal medicines, and has published a chapter on domestic medicine and the King's Evil in *Reading and Writing Recipe Books, 1600–1800* (edited by Michelle DiMeo and Sara Pennell, Manchester University Press, 2013). Anne is a member of the Advisory Board of the *Journal of Herbal Medicine* (Elsevier/Churchill Livingstone).

Graeme Tobyn is a Senior Lecturer in Herbal Medicine at the University of Central Lancashire. He is a fellow of the National Institute of Medical Herbalists, author of *Culpeper's Medicine* (Element, 1997/Singing Dragon, 2013) and, in collaboration with Alison Denham and Midge Whitelegg at UCLAN, *The Western Herbal Tradition* (Elsevier, 2010). He is currently undertaking a PhD at Lancaster University on 'English herbs for English bodies' in the sixteenth and seventeenth centuries.

Anne Van Arsdall's academic home is the University of New Mexico, in a region of the United States where herbalism and folk medicine are both very much alive and have influenced her work with early medieval medicine. She has published on medieval medicine, including the Anglo-Saxon period, on the mandrake plant and legends about it, and on the transmission of knowledge through texts and unrecorded deeds. She is currently working on a biography of Oswald Cockayne, a nineteenth-century scholar who was the first person to translate the Anglo-Saxon medical texts into modern English. One of her long-range projects is to publish a translation and study of an Anglo-Saxon physicians' manual called the *Leechbook of Bald*.

Anna Waldstein is a Lecturer in Medical Anthropology and Ethnobotany in the School of Anthropology and Conservation at the University of Kent. She holds a PhD in Ecological and Environmental Anthropology from the University of Georgia, and a BA in Medical Anthropology from Hampshire College. She has done fieldwork on the popular use of herbal medicines in Zimbabwe, Mexico and the United States and has published work on the role of traditional medical beliefs and practices in maintaining health among Mexican migrants. Anna's current research interests include self-medication and patient empowerment, the use of traditional medical knowledge as an adaptive strategy among migrants, biological citizenship and sovereignty and the Rastafari Way of Life.

Nicky Wesson holds a Masters degree from the Centre for Editing Lives and Letters, University of London, where her dissertation was on 'Childbed and the Use of Herbs in Early Modern England'. She also holds a BSc (Hons) in Herbal Medicine from the University of Westminster, and has studied medieval history at St Mary's University College, Strawberry Hill. Nicky was for ten years founder-member of the West London Home Birth Support Group, Chair of a Maternity Services Liaison Committee for five years, and a National Childbirth Trust ante-natal teacher for seven years. She has published several books on pregnancy, maternity, home birth and labour, and infertility and her published articles include one on the experience of childbirth for early modern women and two on the global and practical use of galactagogue herbs.

Midge Whitelegg has a first degree in Latin. Much later she studied for a PhD in the Centre for Science Studies and Science Policy in Lancaster University. She has been in practice as a medical herbalist since 1988 and more recently as a biographical counsellor. She is a past President of the National Institute of Medical Herbalists and erstwhile member of the Research and Development Committee of the Foundation for

Integrated Health. She was a senior lecturer in the University of Central Lancashire for 13 years from which post she retired. She still pursues an interest in Goethean Science. Midge contributed to *The Western Herbal Tradition* (Elsevier, 2010).

John Wilkins is Professor of Greek Culture at the University of Exeter. He has been working on food and medicine in the ancient world for the past 20 years, with various jointly edited publications including *Food in Antiquity* (University of Exeter Press, 1995), *Food in the Ancient World* (Blackwell Publishing, 2006), *Athenaeus and his World* (University of Exeter Press, 2000) and *Galen and the World of Knowledge* (Cambridge University Press, 2009). He finished an edition of Galen's treatise on nutrition in January 2010 and is currently working on a translation of Galen's *Simple Medicines*, books 1–5, and a monograph on Galen's *Maintaining Good Health*.

Foreword

The history of herbal medicine is, up until the eighteenth century, largely the history of medicine itself. Even though herbs would be mixed with animal parts and minerals, most *materia medica* came from the plant kingdom, and herbs were for everyday use.

The use of metals and minerals in medicine was made widely popular by Paracelsus (1493–1541), who burned the books of Avicenna (c. 980–1037 CE), Galen (c. 130–c. 200 CE) and Hippocrates (c. 460–c. 357 BCE) in the early sixteenth century. Many metals were toxic, but these were more likely to be used by physicians, and it was often said jokingly that well-off patients – who were able to afford a doctor – were more likely to die than poor people who could not. In many cases, the treatment was more dangerous than the disease and, since treatments included arsenic, lead and mercury salts, this is not surprising. Some were so harsh that it led Samuel Hahnemann (1755–1843) to create homoeopathy in 1790, but herbal medicine remained widespread in both lay and professional practice, and was probably much safer. Many consider this still to be the case.

Although there are very many 'herbals', there are few scholarly books dealing specifically with the history of herbal medicine and many books on the history of medicine soon divert their efforts into the branch of study which leads to modern medicine, that is, the isolation of naturally occurring highly potent chemicals and the development of synthetic drugs. Aspirin, based on the active principle of meadowsweet (*Filipendula ulmaria*) and willow bark (*Salix* spp.), was first synthesized in 1897, and Erlich's manufacture of the first totally synthetic chemotherapeutic drug, arsphenamine (Salvarsan), occurred in 1907. After this time, most texts neglect advances made in the study of herbal medicine, which rather implies that herbal medicine has remained static, despite the evidence that it is evolving and has even experienced a renaissance in the late twentieth and early twenty-first centuries.

New forms of traditional herbal medicine from China, India and other parts of Asia have been introduced into the West, and herbs from foreign lands have always formed part of the pharmacopoeia and become integrated into each country's medicine system, both conventional and otherwise. Clinical studies have been carried out on some herbal medicines and found them to be effective, and herbal medicine is as relevant today as it ever has been, occupying a special place in the treatment, and particularly the prevention, of certain types of disease. Nutritional therapies, always a part of medical herbalism, are also now very popular with consumers, and form part of the modern array of supplements available to patients to select for themselves. The European Union is now supporting and funding scientific studies into the efficacy and mechanisms of action of long-standing herbal drugs, and since many of our current drugs were originally derived from plant medicines used in a traditional manner, we can hope – or even assume – that more may follow, which makes the study of the history of herbal medicine highly relevant today, and this book shows how herbal medicine has been viewed and studied over the years.

The history of herbal medicine has been described many times, but rarely in a critical or scholarly way, and even more rarely using new and revised primary sources which are discussed by social, medical and other historians, medical scientists, herbal practitioners, language experts, anthropologists, ethnobotanists and even an archaeo-ethnopharmacologist. Their scholarly contribution and analysis of the sources has produced a fascinating and reliable account of this long-neglected subject, which is unique in my experience. As the editors explain, herbal history is fragmented, and they provide a way forward for the unification and regeneration of this branch of social and medical history which has been enthusiastically welcomed. The story starts with early Greek medicine and progresses to medieval herbals, with an emphasis on early-modern midwifery manuals, since midwives were likely experts on herbs and 'women's troubles' and their treatment. New archival sources are also described, including trade and probate accounts. Some of the most important herbal sources are described, including texts relating to Dioscorides (c. 40–90 CE), William Turner (c. 1508–68) and John Parkinson (c. 1567–1650), as well as other significant figures and their works. Finally, to the future: how ethnobotany can inform the study of the history of herbal medicine, which may then inform the future too.

Anne Stobart and Susan Francia have brought contributors together who possess a wide spectrum of expertise, and in many cases were previously unknown to each other. They are certainly to be congratulated, but may find they have started something...

Elizabeth M. Williamson, BSc(Pharm), PhD, MRPharmS, FLS, Professor of Pharmacy, University of Reading, UK

1

The Fragmentation of Herbal History: The Way Forward

Anne Stobart and Susan Francia

Overview

The history of Western herbal medicine has been little researched in any systematic and authoritative way, even though herbal medicine has been a significant element of both lay and learned health care of the past.[1] Sadly, although there is a considerable range of published material on herbal history, much of the literature is based on repeated or embellished sources and, for serious researchers, there seems to be a dearth of reliable studies from which to draw. The history of herbal medicine lacks a coherent identity and, consequently, much relevant scholarly research has been hidden from view. Yet there are scholars in various academic disciplines covering both the distant and recent past who are researching topics which have considerable relevance to the history of herbal medicine. When a number of seminars were organized in London in 2010 and 2011 in order to bring researchers in the history of herbal medicine together, there was an enthusiastic response from the contributors of papers and from all who attended. This book arises out of further work and refinement carried out by the original contributors to seminars and other researchers.

The initial inspiration for this book came from a desire to make the research topics from the London seminars on the history of herbal medicine more widely known, and from the realization of the need to support researchers and encourage further scholarly historical investigation into herbal medicine. With this book, our aim is to reach historical researchers, herbal practitioners, health professionals, lecturers, students and other interested readers wanting more detail and depth in relation to the history of herbal medicine. Alongside raising awareness of existing and potential sources, methodologies and key issues or debates, we wish to support and stimulate those interested in pursuing further research studies.

The editors are both historians of herbal medicine and herbal medicine practitioners with varied motivations for researching the history of herbal medicine: to satisfy curiosity about the past; to extend historical knowledge; to inform clinical practice today; to teach students of herbal medicine; and to support the research endeavour of both clinical and non-clinical researchers. Both editors view history as a systematic endeavour to interpret the past, albeit carried out by investigators with varied standpoints. Our experiences in gaining skills needed for historical study have been instructive in enabling us to perceive gaps in training for research in the history of herbal medicine. While training for practitioners of Western herbal medicine in the UK has recently developed at degree level, alongside Chinese, Ayurvedic and other traditional systems, and is based on a coherent core curriculum,[2] historical elements of training for the herbal practitioner are often limited, and may reflect an uncertain tradition. Current professional training in the UK for clinical Western herbal medicine practitioners provides a significant appreciation of scientific method, both in botanical and medical sciences, and herbal practitioners are able to draw on knowledge of medicinal plants based on modern research.[3] This research knowledge has to be carefully evaluated alongside knowledge of traditional *materia medica* and past practice. However, experience in using historical methods is not extensive amongst herbal practitioners. Thus, as editors, we are aware of a need for more support and training for those herbal practitioners and others interested in research, particularly if the aim is to realize a more significant body of rigorous historical research.

Due to our respective specialist historical interests, both of us have also encountered historians and other scholars, from art, classics and literature to economic, medical and social history, who wish to be better informed about historical aspects of herbal medicine and to have access to more reliable sources. Such encounters with colleagues have alerted us to a need for further investigation into matters including: the plants historically used as medicines; the contributions to herbal medicine of key people in historical context; and the nature of past beliefs and practice involving herbal medicine. Further needs are evident in specific requests, for example, for technical advice on issues such as plant identification and the correction of potential errors in the context of transcriptions of manuscripts relevant to the history of herbal medicine.[4] Thus, gaps exist in the knowledge and understanding of the history of herbal medicine amongst a range of scholars, from archivists to historians to museum curators and others. Clearly, there is a demand for more accessible and reliable research in the history of herbal medicine to be made available.

In this book, a variety of researchers have come together to share their knowledge and experience in research areas ranging from the past identification and use of medicinal plants, to the people involved in herbal medicine, and their therapeutic beliefs and practices. Our contributors come from many academic research contexts: some are herbal medicine and health care practitioners, others are specialists in archaeology, classical studies, English literature, ethnobotany, historical archives and other specific aspects of history. All have expressed support for encouraging further scholarly research through making their studies available and being explicit in terms of their approach, methodology and sources, as well as providing suggestions for reading in their respective fields of interest.

The chapters in this book are intended to inform readers about selected aspects of the history of herbal medicine. Recognizing that herbal history can incorporate a vast area in terms of chronology and geographical location, there are some limitations in scope. The primary focus is on Western herbal medicine, drawing on classical sources through to medieval and early modern texts and manuscript archives. There has not been space for consideration of other aspects of herbal history, such as herbal medicine in the context of the development of modern medicine after 1800 CE, nor to cover significant non-Western medical traditions with substantial herbal components, such as traditional Chinese and Ayurvedic medicine. These are all areas that deserve further exploration. Nevertheless, we hope that the variety of approaches and methodologies found here will provide models for research in a wide range of topics in the history of herbal medicine.

Setting the scene

This introductory chapter sets the scene for current and future research into the history of herbal medicine and gathers a brief overview of its historiography. In particular, we make four claims about research in the history of herbal medicine:

1. The history of herbal medicine can provide a recognizable and cohesive theme which incorporates research of interest and relevance to a wide range of people, issues and disciplines.
2. There is a range of existing research into the history of herbal medicine, although it may be fragmented, reflecting different interests and motivations of researchers, and this research should be made more widely accessible.
3. There is a need to promote further high-quality research in the history of herbal medicine, which can provide a firm basis for scholars with a variety of interests and backgrounds.
4. Interdisciplinary collaboration is of great importance for research in the history of herbal medicine, since many aspects can benefit from the sharing of specialist knowledge and techniques.

The next section of this chapter presents a framework and working definition for this field of study with an overview of key research disciplines relevant to the history of herbal medicine. Historiographical aspects of the history of herbal medicine are then considered, including relationships to other historical studies. There are a number of challenges in developing more critical studies and these are explored and, finally, a way forward is outlined.

Recognizing research in the history of herbal medicine

A framework for herbal history

Plants have been used for centuries in many contexts and, as a result, the potential scope of research into herbal history is huge. Historical studies reflecting this breadth include botanical and garden history, economic history, food history, maritime history, social and cultural history and much more. Further research areas of particular relevance to herbal history include ethnopharmacology and ethnobotany.

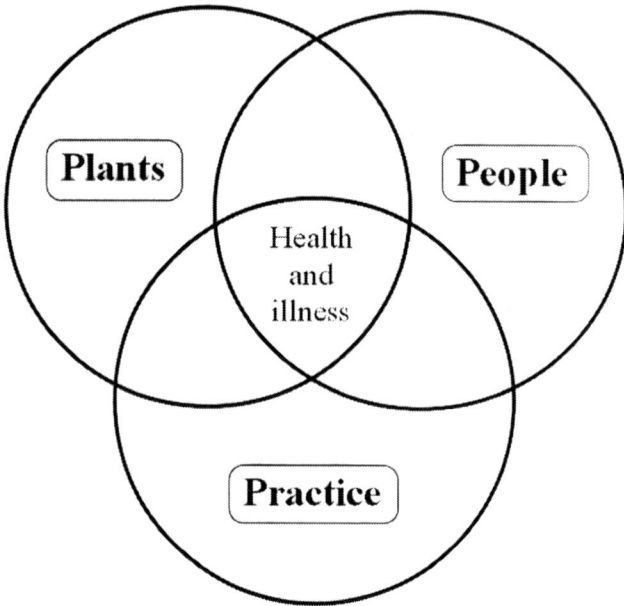

Figure 1.1 A framework for the history of herbal medicine. Illustration by Anne Stobart.

This book focuses on research into the history of herbal medicine. However, it is likely that there are at least three different understandings of the nature of herbal medicine: the phrase 'herbal medicine' may be used to describe a drug or prepared remedy based on plants, but it also may have a broader scope in referring to the activity of individuals obtaining and using plant remedies in a domestic context, or indeed to clinical practice with a therapeutic approach incorporating plant medicines alongside other treatments.[5] In order to structure our consideration of the range of areas linking to research into the history of herbal medicine, it is helpful to use these varied understandings to formulate three categories: plants, people and practice (see Figure 1.1). Whilst it is unlikely that any study will focus on one of these categories exclusively, there is a considerable range of research with which to populate this framework. Considering each part of the framework in turn, we provide an indication of contributions to the research literature.

We can also draw on the framework of categories of plants, people and practice to consider sources for studying the history of herbal medicine. For the study of plants, herbals provide a key source, and other sources include those relating to plant discovery and identification such as herbariums and writings about foreign travel; papers relating to estates and gardens including plans, seed catalogues and printed horticultural advice; and trade records including merchant records, customs and import books. For the study of people in the history of herbal medicine, sources include diaries, letters and other personal papers in cultural and social history such as domestic recipe collections, household accounts, probate records, household inventories alongside other suggestive evidence of daily life in plays, poems and prose. For the study of practice in the history of herbal medicine, sources include prescriptions, individual case histories, printed medical advice books and pharmacopoeias, medical treatises, apothecary bills and notebooks and institutional, professional and legal records. Whilst these three categories and their related sources may overlap to some extent, they provide an indication of the wide range of possibilities. Although we have outlined mainly textual sources, there are others which deserve consideration and these range from art works to artefacts. Further discussion of sources, and related studies, can be found in the introductions to the book sections and in the individual chapters.

Fragments of research in the history of herbal medicine

The following outline list of relevant areas of research is organized into the categories of plants, people and practice. In each category some examples are provided to give an indication of the nature of research and literature available.

Plants in the history of herbal medicine

Botanical history

Botanical history investigates a range of aspects of plants and has many historical links to medicine.[6] Plants and their identification, alongside qualities and medicinal indications, are described in herbals from classical to early modern times, and a comprehensive overview by Agnes Arber of early English herbals was first published in 1912.[7] Much of the history of plants as herbs is organized in lists, including original lists of herbs and their virtues in early modern herbals; past catalogue lists of garden herbs; modern lists bringing together common names for plants; or other modern lists of herbal remedies such as those recalled in oral history projects.[8] There are relatively few texts which comprehensively and systematically evaluate details of plants used as herbal medicines across historical periods. One of the most substantial listings available, *A Modern Herbal*, provides a body of evidence, organized by common plant name, amassed in the early twentieth century and citing past authorities from classical to early modern times.[9] The editor, Hilda Leyel, wrote of how 'botany and medicine came down the ages hand in hand' and then parted company in the seventeenth century.[10] More recently, Tobyn et al. have considered the textual history of a selection of medicinal plants through examination of changes in significant texts from Dioscorides through to the present day.[11]

Pharmacy history

The study of the history of drugs inevitably has a considerable focus on plants as sources, and these constitute the most significant proportion of entries in pharmacopoeia, or listings of medicinal preparations.[12] Although regarded as part of medical history, pharmaceutical history tends to be found in separate contexts specific to the pharmaceutical profession. Linked to the Royal Pharmaceutical Society in the UK, the *Pharmaceutical Historian* provides an ongoing forum for in-depth articles on specific medications, and there is an active equivalent body in the USA based on the American Institute of the History of Pharmacy.[13] Other writers provide detail of the context of pharmacy in different periods: for example, Alan Touwaide provides a detailed account of changing understandings of the nature of medications or *pharmaka* in the classical period.[14] However, Touwaide's discussion of meanings is atypical compared to other overviews of the past use of plants as drugs which make general reference to toxic medications or remedies of 'unproven worth'.[15]

Garden history

Plants in the garden context have been explored by a number of writers, ranging from the arrangements of monastery gardens to the gardens of the landed gentry.[16] Andrew Wear notes how a lack of knowledge of medicinal plants and reliance on apothecaries and 'silly Hearb-women [sic]' could result in the medical practitioner being 'out-witted'.[17] Thus, the problem of plant recognition and lack of certainty about herb supplies encouraged the printing of botanical books and establishment of botanic gardens.[18] These gardens were intended to provide plant knowledge for the practitioner rather than the lay person, one of the most familiar being the Chelsea Physic Garden, maintained to this day in London.[19]

Economic history

Detailed studies on some individual plants have been published, particularly considering exotic remedies, such as rhubarb (*Rheum palmatum*) and the quinine-containing *Cinchona* species (spp.). These, and other studies, have highlighted political and economic aspects of international trade.[20] Authors have identified a need for further studies, including research into trade routes and how the 'emergence of mass drug consumption' in the seventeenth and eighteenth centuries came about.[21]

Ethnopharmacology

Ethnopharmacology is an expanding area of research with a potentially significant relationship to herbal history.[22] Pharmaceutical discovery has been a major driving force for the exploration of natural resources for new cures. In this search, oral and other historical sources are examined for likely active remedies for particular complaints, for example studies of herbals have been carried out for malaria treatments or rheumatic disorders.[23] Traditional use of plants as an indicator for drug discovery has not been without criticism as there has also been recognition that a search for a phytochemical 'golden bullet' of plant origin may be flawed, since expectations may be unrealistic or traditional systems may have provided treatments deriving synergy, or 'multiple and mutually potentiating therapeutic effects' from combinations of plants.[24]

The exploration of historical herbal texts has been likened to 'mining' in the discovery of new drugs.[25] Much of the research reveals the interplay of medical practices between cultures, for example between South American and European countries.[26] Many ethnopharmacological studies are based on traditional societies, although Paula de Vos is significant in searching European historical texts for *materia medica* to compare with current-day usage.[27]

People and the history of herbal medicine

Culinary history

In the classical Western world, dietetics played a major role in the maintenance of health, and subsequent regimens giving advice on diet and lifestyle have provided a ready source for exploring both beliefs and practice in relation to health.[28] Thus, the study of the history of food and herbal medicines have overlapped to some extent.[29] The introduction of exotic items in diet has often been associated with health-promoting properties, and there are some studies of patterns of consumption of spices and other items.[30]

Social history

The historical study of the use of herbal medicine has benefited indirectly from developments in the social history of medicine, since increasing attention to the patient experience in historical terms has helped to draw out perceptions of therapeutic treatment and efforts at self-help, often noting the relationship between lay and learned health care.[31] Some significant contributions to historical writing related to health care use gender as a key category of analysis,[32] and a focus on medicinal recipes as a genre of women's writing reveals the importance of social networks in the compilation of recipe collections and health care.[33] Yet, an uncritical acceptance of assertions about household medicine and herbs needs to be challenged, as available evidence reveals that although hundreds of recipes were collected by households, only a limited number were made.[34]

Ethnobotany

Ethnobotanical studies of people and plants focus attention on matters of intellectual knowledge, rights and matters of biodiversity, some of which feature historical and medicinal aspects. This has been a recent and exciting area of development largely informed by anthropology and social sciences.[35] Conservation projects have also provided a motivation for gathering of data on the past medical uses of plants in many cultures, particularly aiming at safeguarding both knowledge and plants.[36]

Practice and the history of herbal medicine

Medical history

Studies of medical history up to the twentieth century tended to recount the evolution of the medical professions of physicians, surgeons and apothecaries. However, more recent studies question whether boundaries can be so readily identified, and show that the 'marketplace' of health care in the past was both more extensive and more pluralistic.[37] Other writers draw attention to historical changes in the concepts of health and disease.[38] Amongst medical personnel in history, the role of apothecaries as suppliers of herbs is discussed by Burnby.[39] Many histories of medicine refer in passing to the role of herbs in medical practice. In relation to practitioners, Barbara Griggs has compiled a readable account of herbal medicine across the ages.[40] Scholars such as Andrew Wear draw attention to the widespread use of herbal remedies in lay as well as professional contexts, discussing in detail how changes developed from the sixteenth century.[41]

Folklore studies

Folklore and magic were extensively considered by Keith Thomas as significant elements of a bygone age and, although sometimes persistent, they gave way to a modern rational perspective on medicine.[42] Considerable effort in the later nineteenth and twentieth centuries went into the recording of people's earlier beliefs about plants in folklore studies, and numerous local collections of herbal folklore from oral and other sources can be located.[43] Folklore records vary considerably in their provenance, and the difficulty of adducing beliefs from limited records requires critical appraisal of the sources, although it has been argued that this appraisal is essential to counter assumptions about the reliance of past health care on herbals largely deriving from Mediterranean areas.[44]

History of science and ideas

Many aspects of the history of science are related to the development of herbal medicine; indeed the history of medicine is usually considered as part of the history of science. The ways in which past individuals and societies understood nature influenced their beliefs about appropriate therapeutic practices. Ideas about natural history deriving from the classical period and their subsequent development in medieval and early modern times are captured by a number of studies.[45] Also of interest in recent studies are the ways in which ideas and knowledge were communicated in the past. For example, increased studies of household records including recipe collections reveal much about the form and transmission of medical knowledge, including knowledge relating to medicinal plants.[46] These studies have intersected with others on the secrets of nature.[47]

Defining research in the history of herbal medicine

As can be seen above, there are many 'fragments' of the history of herbal medicine which are located in a multitude of research areas and disciplines. To some extent, this may reflect the varied nature of herbal medicine itself. Fortunately, many researchers in these different contexts have indicated interest in reaching beyond their disciplines to link with others. A broad definition providing a framework may be helpful, drawing on the three categories of plants, people and practice used above. In the various sub-disciplines of history and other areas identified above, a common factor is the examination and appraisal of sources incorporating these categories to a greater or lesser extent, using a variety of scholarly methodologies. Thus, we suggest that research in the history of herbal medicine can be broadly defined as 'systematic enquiry to understand and explain the supply, knowledge and use of plants incorporating people's beliefs, knowledge and involvement in past therapeutic practices in the context of health and illness'. This definition is intended to support a unifying framework for elements of scholarly research that contribute to the history of herbal medicine. Following a brief overview of methods, we consider historiography, or the writing of the history of herbal medicine, and we show how this is related to the varying perspectives on history and herbal medicine of different authors.

Methods in researching the history of herbal medicine

Historical research in aspects of herbal medicine can draw on a wide range of methods: generally these depend on the nature of primary sources selected for study. Many studies are based on textual analysis, drawing on both printed or manuscript archives, and range from herbals, casebooks and medical advice books to letters and family papers. The researcher can select from biographical (extending from significant figures in medicine to patients, lay healers and practitioners) and narrative approaches (covering a variety of contexts and time periods from war to domestic scenes) through to comparative studies (especially comparisons between cultures and therapeutic approaches). The range of possible methods also encompasses the qualitative study of ideas (particularly beliefs and conflicts about health and illness, analysis of original texts such as herbals for understanding of the elemental basis of plant medicines) and more quantitative styles of analysis (such as quantities of imported herbs, frequency of mention of selected plants and complaints in herbals, accounts portraying trends and fashions in health care, analysis of inventories). Some recent approaches have adopted a style of micro-history in which a more rounded and detailed picture of past practice is sought in a particular family, parish or other location, drawing on a range of sources such as letters, accounts and household papers. Textual studies have implications in terms of the specific techniques needed to examine and interpret sources, including language and transcription skills. Linguistic studies, and detailed etymological searches, have also been developed, for example looking at medieval herbals. Further specialist techniques are necessary for sources which are non-textual, ranging from illustrations to material objects and buildings, and for the purposes of identification and interpretation. Overall, the range of methods appropriate to research in the history of herbal medicine is at least as wide as the range of methods in history as a whole.

Writing the history of herbal medicine

We have seen how research into the history of herbal medicine is fragmentary, occurring in a number of different study areas. How has this affected the way that the history of herbal medicine has been written? Since, historically, medicine has involved much reliance on plants, we might expect that there would be considerable interest in writing about herbal aspects of the past. However, although the use of medicinal herbs is frequently mentioned in passing as part of a lengthy tradition, little detail is provided and evidence of actual use is rarely considered, only efficacy or the likelihood of successful treatment. For example, Raskin et al. (2002), in their review of trends in plant research, make the general point that 'for centuries people have used plants for healing' with 'varying success'.[48]

Historiography and herbal medicine

Past writers have varied considerably in their approach to writing about herbal medicines. In medieval and early modern times, writers had a need to emphasize the status and lineage of their medical knowledge. Thus, for example, in Gerard's herbal, the 'courteous and well willing Readers' were told that 'both Kings and Princes have esteemed them [herbs] as Jewels' and this was followed by a review of a glorious history of key figures from Dioscorides onwards.[49] Gerard's preface indicates the 'professional snobbery' found amongst medical writers in claiming these high-status antecedents, as described by Barbara Griggs.[50] In the context of the development of modern medicine in the nineteenth century, later historical descriptions of herbal medicine shifted towards antiquarian and folklore studies.[51] By the twentieth century, herbal medicine came to be widely regarded by both historical and medical researchers as part of alternative medicine, quackery or folk medicine.[52]

The modern historiography of herbal medicine is marked by ambiguities and contradictions. Roberta Bivins notes the 'diversity'[53] of non-orthodox healing practices and the ambiguous position of herbal medicine:

> Herbal remedies have an ambiguous place in medical historiography. They were, of course, a mainstay of the Western pharmacopoeia and mainstream therapeutics well into the nineteenth century, and remain a crucial part of non-biomedical therapeutics globally. However, herbalism has also been conventionally regarded as the acme of European and American folk or traditional medicine, and certainly in the nineteenth and twentieth centuries modified and systematized forms of herbalism have been at the core of explicitly alternative medical systems…[54]

Bivins discusses the differing agendas of researchers, some aiming to 'debunk' and others being interested in the valuable perspective gained by studies of popular perceptions of health and the emergence of medical orthodoxy.[55] Studies published in the twenty-first century which relate to the history of herbal medicine thus reflect varying standpoints of the writers. Some remain explicitly of antiquarian interest for a medical audience. A typical example is a study by a clinical neurologist who comments on the bizarre nature of remedies used in the past in the classical *materia medica* indicated by Dioscorides for epilepsy (designated as the 'falling sickness').[56] Such studies provide an opportunity to celebrate modern medicine and to reaffirm its boundaries.

Other studies in medical history refer to 'herbalists' alongside a variety of other non-orthodox or lay practitioners. Thus, Conrad et al. in *The Western Medical Tradition: 800 BC to AD 1800* refer to 'wise-women, astrologers, herbalists, uroscopists, empirics, apothecaries, barber-surgeons, physicians, or specialists like tooth-drawers and lithotomists'.[57] Whilst this observation likely reflects contemporary accounts, it should not be taken to indicate that herbal medicine was solely associated with the empiric or lay practitioner of past health care.

Potentially contradictory observations about herbal medicine in history can be found elsewhere in the literature. For example, plants as medicines have long been associated with lower costs, even as freely available in the hedgerow. Andrew Wear notes that claims of cheaper services than physicians were characteristic of 'empirics, mountebanks, herbalists, astrologers and uroscopists'.[58] However, illustrated early herbals were extremely costly and the survival of numerous copies of printed herbals suggests that there was great care for these items, which acted as repositories of knowledge and authority in health care.[59] These apparent contradictions need further exploration to understand the complexities in the perceptions and values of people of the past.

Such further studies may have direct relevance to present-day perceptions of herbal medicine. Although a range of examples of research in the history of herbal medicine are given here, there remain many gaps which allow ambiguity and contradiction to persist in modern perceptions of herbal medicine. We suggest that research related to the history of herbal medicine has resonated with the changing position of herbal medicine in society, and consider that this has further increased the fragmentation of studies, marginalizing some aspects and neglecting others. Yet, promotion of research into the history of herbal medicine could be of value in understanding conflicting viewpoints. For example, many people today believe 'natural' products to be safe and effective, judging by the way that this perception is widely exploited in advertising for health and cosmetic products. Meanwhile, there is vocal opposition to herbal medicine and other complementary therapies, based on claims of a lack of sufficient evidence.[60] Further investigation of the history of herbal medicine could help to explain the development of these contrasting views. The quality of historiography of herbal medicine would benefit from greater awareness of the standpoint of writers and researchers.

Science, the history of medicine and herbal history

The content of writing on the history of medicine has changed considerably in recent decades. Mark Jackson effectively outlines the turn away, in medical history, from accounts of triumphant discovery towards interest in 'the relationship of medicine to society', although noting something of an 'identity crisis' in present-day research.[61] Roger Cooter further notes an increased focus on cultural history and a lack of theoretical underpinning of studies in the history of medicine, and argues that there is a need for more critical awareness of values, perspectives and aims.[62] Other writers have discussed a trend in the history of medicine which has effectively excluded the medicinal aspects.[63]

Some similarities can be noted between studies of the history of medicine and herbal history. In both we can see a varied set of 'producers' of history, from clinical practitioners to social scientists. John Burnham has ably described the 'complex, nuanced and even ragged accounts' which are inevitable in medical history because of different perspectives amongst the producers.[64] Likewise there are variations in the interested audience. Yet there are significant differences between the history of medicine and herbal history, especially when considering the historical development of herbal knowledge and professional standing. The particularly interesting area of epistemology and herbal medicine deserves further exploration regarding issues in the control of herbal knowledge. Ludmilla Jordanova argues that the history of medicine cannot be treated purely as the history of science, and claims that a science focus is problematic as it marginalizes many healing practices and behaviours. Rather, she suggests, medicine might be considered more akin to technology in that matters of health and illness are generally far more commonplace and immediate, involving people in a very direct sense.[65] Such an approach fits well with our framework of plants, people and practice, allowing for the inclusion of both scientific knowledge and practical experience.

The practice of herbal medicine in the past was inseparable from knowledge about the actions of plants, then embodied in the herbals which provided indications for use. Although generally known for a 'chemical' style of distillation, Paracelsus was as much in favour of plants as other natural remedies.[66] Today there is a rapid accumulation of knowledge about the constituents of plants and efforts to sift this knowledge for the 'active' chemicals which may be useful in pharmaceutical terms.[67] The accumulation of this knowledge is not primarily intended to validate past uses, but the dominance of bio-medicine and science infuses our view of herbal history – and it becomes hard to put aside such knowledge. Thus, a kind of comparative history underlies many investigations in which herbal treatments of the past are examined. Indeed, as herbal practitioners and historical researchers, a question we encounter in relation to the history of herbal medicine is concerned with efficacy, and we are often asked 'Did it work?'. As practitioners and researchers, we need to be able to consider such questions in a rigorous way, without undue influence arising from today's knowledge.

Interdisciplinary approaches

Philip Curtin describes the explosion of knowledge in science and history and claims that it is no longer possible to investigate everything at once as scholars are deprived of 'the breadth of span they need in order to ask the most pertinent new questions', or are separated by institutional definitions and boundaries from rephrasing those questions.⁶⁸ However, approaches to research in the history of herbal medicine which draw on different disciplines to solve problems can bring enhanced understandings of the past. For example, drug discovery strategies have drawn attention to Anglo-Saxon sources.⁶⁹ There is a problem of identification of particular plants in this context: for example, the same common name can be used for more than one plant – as in the case of *brynwort* or brownwort – and interdisciplinary collaboration of chemists and herbal practitioners (not to mention botanists, linguists, pharmacists) is needed in effectively deciphering the nature of the plants involved.⁷⁰

In an interdisciplinary approach, both historically-trained and science-based scholars may come together. Herein lies another problem, in that it is not readily accepted by historians (particularly in cultural and social history) that today's knowledge and understanding should impose on the past. Writers who attempt to bridge the gap can suffer criticism for assumptions about past practices.⁷¹ This creates a potential obstacle for the study of the history of herbal medicine, if modern understandings provide a perspective on the past that can make researchers unable to be objective. However, such knowledge can also enhance understanding of the past if used with sensitivity in an interdisciplinary context.

The way forward

In this introduction we have outlined many fragmented elements of research in the history of herbal medicine and considered various historiographical aspects. Continuing interest in the history of herbal medicine presents further challenges beyond those of bringing together researchers and making studies more accessible. As discussed above, one challenge is to find approaches which can integrate present understandings of herbal medicine with traditional findings and usage. Another challenge is to develop explicit standards for research, and our view is that there needs to be recognition of the varied skills and knowledge required to effectively research the history of herbal medicine. Yet another challenge is to encourage interdisciplinary approaches which may be critical to the success of future research. This book represents a significant step in responding to these challenges, by bringing together research studies and providing details of a range of sources and examples of methodologies, and we hope it will encourage and illuminate further investigations in the history of herbal medicine.

Structure of this book

This book is arranged in four main sections, each consisting of between two and four chapters. Each section has a short introduction which identifies some key aspects of the context for research into the history of herbal medicine, and introduces the subsequent chapters. The chapters in Part 1 revisit some of the texts which are well known in the history of herbal medicine and provide some fresh perspectives on those texts. Chapters in Part 2 introduce further historical sources which may be examined for their contribution to the history of herbal medicine. Part 3 contains chapters which focus on selected individuals and their contributions to the history of herbal medicine. The chapters in Part 4 outline several disciplines beyond history, specifically archaeology and ethnobotany, providing studies of relevance to the history of herbal medicine. Suggestions for further reading can be found at the end of each chapter. Our conclusion briefly considers the history of herbal medicine as a developing research field.

Some technical notes

Dating. Where dates are given these are in the BCE/CE (Before Common Era/Common Era) format rather than BC/AD (Before Christ/Anno Domini). Otherwise, dates have not been altered and readers should note that prior to 1752, the start of each year was in March. Details of known dates of birth and death of individuals are provided where appropriate and where details differ, or may be subject to ongoing debate, those of the *Oxford Dictionary of National Biography* or from Oxford Reference Online are given.[72]

Terminology. Terminology has to be carefully considered when considering past medicinal and botanical knowledge and, wherever possible, we have used terms consistently. The use of general terms like 'traditional' medicine has been avoided unless they are more explicitly placed in context. For other terms, see the Select Glossary at the end of the book. The format of plant names has varied through the ages and we have indicated this as follows: (i) modern Latin binomial plant names begin with a capital letter and are in italics; (ii) modern common plant names are not capitalized (unless proper names are included) or italicized; (iii) historical binomial plant names are capitalized but not italicized; (iv) historical common plant names are capitalized if generally appearing as such in original texts.

Translations. Individual contributors have specified the sources that they have used for translated material, including available editions or translations to date. Individual original language terms are indicated in italics, for example *kosmos*.

Transcriptions. Inserted letters, words or comments from the author for clarification are indicated by the use of brackets [thus]. Original spellings have generally been preserved, using present-day format; for example, 'vv' is shown as 'w'. However, to clarify meaning, some contractions have been expanded and punctuation adjusted.

Notes

1 Suzanne Taylor and Virginia Berridge, 'Medicinal Plants and Malaria: An Historical Case Study of Research at the London School of Hygiene and Tropical Medicine in the Twentieth Century', *Transactions of the Royal Society of Tropical Medicine and Hygiene* 100, no. 8 (2006): 708.
2 An umbrella body, the European Herbal and Traditional Medicine Practitioners Association (EHTPA), represents professional associations of herbal/traditional

medicine practitioners offering Western herbal medicine, Chinese herbal medicine, Ayurveda and traditional Tibetan medicine.

3   Professional herbal practitioners in the UK train to accredited degree level with a core syllabus in botanical and medical sciences, and have to achieve a level of clinical experience in order to join the larger professional organizations such as the National Institute of Medical Herbalists. See http://www.nimh.org.uk/ (accessed 26 June 2013).

4   Anecdotal examples in the editors' experience illustrate a range of needs arising from academic scholars, archivists and others. These include an archivist at a stately home and garden seeking help in transcription of medicinal recipes, a historian requesting reliable sources for details about classically used herbs, and a museum curator wishing to correct a mistaken identification of valerian (*Valeriana officinalis*) as the source of the drug Valium.

5   A modern herbal practitioner perspective would view 'herbal medicine' as 'the use of plants, and their extracts, in a systematic and planned way to promote, sustain and restore health, drawing on traditional experience and other scientific knowledge' (our definition).

6   For example, see Douglas Guthrie, 'Plants as Remedies: The Debt of Medicine to Botany', *Transactions of the Botanical Society of Edinburgh* 39, no. 2 (1961): 184–95; Karen M. Reeds, *Botany in Medieval and Renaissance Universities* (New York: Garland, 1991).

7   See Agnes Arber, *Herbals, Their Origin and Evolution: A Chapter in the History of Botany, 1470–1670*, 3rd ed. (Cambridge: Cambridge University Press, 1986); Eleanor S. Rohde, *The Old English Herbals*, reprint of the 1922 ed. (New York: Dover Publications, 1971).

8   For example, a 1648 transcript of plants in the Oxford Botanical Garden is reproduced in *A Catalogue of the Plants Growing in the University of Oxford Botanic Garden and Harcourt Arboretum* (Oxford: University of Oxford Botanic Garden, 1999). Lists of names for plants include Tony Hunt, *Plant Names of Medieval England* (Cambridge: D. S. Brewer, 1989) and Geoffrey Grigson, *The Englishman's Flora*, facsimile of 1955 ed. (London: Phoenix House, 1987). For an example of a modern listing of orally remembered plant remedies, see Gabrielle Hatfield, *Country Remedies: Traditional East Anglian Plant Remedies of the Twentieth Century* (Woodbridge: Boydell Press, 1994).

9   Maud Grieve, *A Modern Herbal: The Medicinal, Culinary, Cosmetic and Economic Properties, Cultivation and Folklore of Herbs, Grasses, Fungi, Shrubs and Trees with All Their Modern Scientific Uses*, ed. C. F. Leyel, reprint of the 1931 ed. (London: Peregrine Books, 1976).

10 Grieve, *Modern Herbal*, editor's introduction, xiii.

11 Graeme Tobyn, Alison Denham and Margaret Whitelegg, *The Western Herbal Tradition: 2000 Years of Medicinal Plant Knowledge* (Edinburgh: Churchill Livingstone/Elsevier, 2011).

12 Friedrich A. Fluckiger and Daniel Hanbury, *Pharmacographia: A History of the Principal Drugs of Vegetable Origin, Met with in Great Britain and British India* (London: Macmillan, 1874).

13 These organizations have regular publications. A further body links numerous country-based interest groups, the International Society for the History of Pharmacy, http://www.histpharm.org/iggp.htm (accessed 17 June 2013).

14 Alain Touwaide, 'Therapeutic Strategies: Drugs', in *Western Medical Thought from*

Antiquity to the Middle Ages, ed. Mirko D. Grmek (Cambridge, MA: Harvard University Press, 1998), 259-73. For classical medicine, see John Scarborough, *Roman Medicine* (Ithaca, NY: Cornell University Press, 1969); Jerry Stannard, 'Hippocratic Pharmacology', *Bulletin of the History of Medicine* 35 (Nov.-Dec. 1961): 497-518.

15 Miles Weatherall, 'Drug Treatment and the Rise in Pharmacology', in *The Cambridge Illustrated History of Medicine*, ed. Roy Porter (Cambridge: Cambridge University Press, 1996), 277; Ilya Raskin et al., 'Plants and Human Health in the Twenty-First Century', *Trends in Biotechnology* 20, no. 12 (2002): 522-31.

16 For example, see Teresa McLean, *Medieval English Gardens* (London: Barrie and Jenkins, 1989); Carole Rawcliffe, '"Delectable Sightes and Fragrant Smelles": Gardens and Health in Late Medieval and Early Modern England', *Garden History* 36, no. 1 (2008): 3-21.

17 Andrew Wear, *Knowledge and Practice in English Medicine, 1550-1680* (Cambridge: Cambridge University Press, 2000), 62-3.

18 Leah Knight, *Of Books and Botany in Early Modern England: Sixteenth-Century Plants and Print Culture* (Farnham: Ashgate, 2009); Charles Webster, 'The Medical Faculty and the Physic Garden', in *The History of the University of Oxford, Vol. V: The Eighteenth Century*, ed. Lucy S. Sutherland and Leslie G. Mitchell (Oxford: Clarendon Press, 1986), 683-723.

19 See, for example, Sue Minter, *The Apothecaries Garden: A History of Chelsea Physic Garden* (Stroud: Sutton, 2000).

20 For example, Clifford M. Foust, *Rhubarb: The Wondrous Drug* (Princeton, NJ: Princeton University Press, 1992); Fiametta Rocco, *The Miraculous Fever Tree: Malaria, Medicine and the Cure That Changed the World* (New York: HarperCollins, 2003). See also the background to modern drugs arising from plants: for example, Jordan Goodman and Vivien Walsh, *The Story of Taxol: Nature and Politics in the Pursuit of an Anti-Cancer Drug* (Cambridge: Cambridge University Press, 2001). For studies relating to colonial trade, see Londa Schiebinger, ed., *Plants and Empire: Colonial Bioprospecting in the Atlantic World* (Cambridge, MA: Harvard University Press, 2004).

21 David B. Haycock and Patrick Wallis, *Quackery and Commerce in Seventeenth-Century London: The Proprietary Medicine Business of Anthony Daffy* (London: The Wellcome Trust Centre for the History of Medicine at UCL, 2005); Steven King, 'Accessing Drugs in the Eighteenth-Century Regions', in *From Physick to Pharmacology: Five Hundred Years of British Drug Retailing*, ed. Louise H. Curth (Aldershot: Ashgate, 2006), 49-78; Patrick Wallis, 'Exotic Drugs and English Medicine: England's Drug Trade, c. 1550-c. 1800' (Working Paper No. 143/10: London School of Economics, July 2010), 26.

22 A brief survey using keywords of 'herbal'+'medicine' in a search of the PubMed journal article database (http://www.ncbi.nlm.nih.gov/pubmed [accessed 6 June 2011]) suggested that new research publications between 2000 and 2010 increased from less than 1,000 to upwards of 3,000 articles per annum. Many of these publications were ethnopharmacological in nature. For a view on history from ethnopharmacologists, see Michael Heinrich et al., 'Ethnobotany and Ethnopharmacology - Interdisciplinary Links with the Historical Sciences', *Journal of Ethnopharmacology* 107, no. 2 (2006): 157-60.

23 Michael Adams et al., 'Malaria in the Renaissance: Remedies from European Herbals from the 16th and 17th Century', *Journal of Ethnopharmacology* 133, no. 2 (2011):

278–88; Michael Adams et al., 'Medicinal Herbs for the Treatment of Rheumatic Disorders – a Survey of European Herbals From the 16th and 17th Century', *Journal of Ethnopharmacology* 121, no. 3 (2009): 343–59; Melina G. Giorgetti and Eliana Rodrigues, 'Brazilian Plants with Possible Action on the Central Nervous System – a Study of Historical Sources from the 16th to 19th Century', *Journal of Ethnopharmacology* 109, no. 19 (2007): 338–47.

24 Jürg Gertsch, 'How Scientific Is the Science of Ethnopharmacology? Historical Perspectives and Epistemological Problems', *Journal of Ethnopharmacology* 122, no. 2 (2009): 177; Elizabeth M. Williamson, 'Synergy and Other Interactions in Phytomedicines', *Phytomedicine* 8, no. 5 (2001): 401–9; Raskin et al., 'Plants and Human Health', 529.

25 Eric J. Buenz et al., 'Searching Historical Herbal Texts for Potential New Drugs', *British Medical Journal* 333, no. 7582 (2006): 1314–15.

26 Joao B. Calixto, 'Twenty-Five Years of Research on Medicinal Plants in Latin America: A Personal View', *Journal of Ethnopharmacology* 100, nos 1–2 (2005): 131–4; Andreas-Holger Maehle, 'Peruvian Bark: From Specific Febrifuge to Universal Remedy', *Clio Medica* 87 (1999): 223–309.

27 Paula De Vos, 'European Materia Medica in Historical Texts: Longevity of a Tradition and Implications for Future Use', *Journal of Ethnopharmacology* 132, no. 1 (2010): 28–47.

28 For example, see Klaus Bergdolt, *Wellbeing: A Cultural History of Healthy Living*, trans. Jane Dewhurst (Cambridge: Polity, 2008).

29 Jane O'Hara-May, 'Foods or Medicines? A Study in the Relationship between Foodstuffs and Materia Medica from the Sixteenth to the Nineteenth Century', *Transactions of the British Society for the History of Pharmacy* 1, no. 2 (1971): 61–97.

30 Paul H. Freedman, *Out of the East: Spices and the Medieval Imagination* (New Haven, CT: Yale University Press, 2008).

31 Mary E. Fissell, *Patients, Power, and the Poor in Eighteenth-Century Bristol* (Cambridge: Cambridge University Press, 1991), 27. See also Joan Lane, *A Social History of Medicine: Health, Healing and Disease in England, 1750–1950* (London: Routledge, 2001). For more on patient–practitioner relationships, see Roy Porter, ed., *Patients and Practitioners: Lay Perceptions of Medicine in Pre-Industrial Society* (Cambridge: Cambridge University Press, 1985).

32 Rebecca Flemming, *Medicine and the Making of Roman Women: Gender, Nature, and Authority from Celsus to Galen* (Oxford: Oxford University Press, 2000); Monica H. Green, *Women's Healthcare in the Medieval West: Texts and Contexts* (Aldershot: Ashgate, 2000); Monica H. Green, 'Gendering the History of Women's Healthcare', *Gender and History* 20, no. 3 (2008): 487–518; Lisa W. Smith, 'The Relative Duties of a Man: Domestic Medicine in England and France, c. 1685–1740', *Journal of Family History* 31, no. 3 (2006): 237–56.

33 Elaine Leong and Sara Pennell, 'Recipe Collections and the Currency of Medical Knowledge in the Early Modern "Medical Marketplace"', in *Medicine and the Market in England and Its Colonies, c. 1450–c. 1850*, ed. Mark S. R. Jenner and Patrick Wallis (Basingstoke: Palgrave Macmillan, 2007), 133–52.

34 Anne Stobart, 'The Making of Domestic Medicine: Gender, Self-Help and Therapeutic Determination in Household Healthcare in South-West England in the Late Seventeenth Century' (Unpublished PhD thesis, Middlesex University, 2008).

35 Nina L. Etkin, ed., *Eating on the Wild Side: The Pharmacologic, Ecologic, and Social Implications of Using Noncultigens* (Tucson, AZ: University of Arizona Press, 1994).

36 Anthony B. Cunningham, *Applied Ethnobotany: People, Wild Plant Use and Conservation* (London: Earthscan, 2001).
37 For discussion of the concept of a 'medical marketplace', see Mark S. R. Jenner and Patrick Wallis, 'The Medical Marketplace', in Jenner and Wallis, *Medicine and the Market*, 1–23. For upwards revised estimates of numbers of medical practitioners, see also Ian Mortimer, *The Dying and the Doctors: The Medical Revolution in Seventeenth-Century England* (Woodbridge: Royal Historical Society/Boydell, 2009).
38 Jacalyn Duffin, *Lovers and Livers: Disease Concepts in History* (Toronto: University of Toronto Press, 2005); Nancy G. Siraisi, *Medieval and Early Renaissance Medicine: An Introduction to Knowledge and Practice* (Chicago: University of Chicago Press, 1990).
39 Juanita G. L. Burnby, *A Study of the English Apothecary from 1660–1760*, Medical History Supplement, vol. 3 (London: Wellcome Institute for the History of Medicine, 1983).
40 Barbara Griggs, *Green Pharmacy: A History of Herbal Medicine* (London: Jill Norman and Hobhouse, 1981).
41 Wear, *Knowledge and Practice*, see ch. 2, 'Remedies'.
42 Keith Thomas, *Religion and the Decline of Magic: Studies in Popular Beliefs in Sixteenth- and Seventeenth-Century England* (London: Weidenfeld and Nicolson, 1971); Keith Thomas, *Man and the Natural World: Changing Attitudes in England 1500–1800* (Harmondsworth: Penguin, 1984).
43 For example, Oswald Cockayne, *Spoon and Sparrow, Spendien and Psar, Fundere and Passer: Or, English Roots in the Greek, Latin, and Hebrew* (London: Parker, Son, and Bourn, 1861); Gabrielle Hatfield, *Hatfield's Herbal: The Secret History of British Plants* (London: Allen Lane, 2007); Enid Porter, *Cambridgeshire Customs and Folklore: With Fenland Material Provided by W. H. Barrett* (London: Routledge and Kegan Paul, 1969); T. F. Thiselton-Dyer, *The Folk-Lore of Plants*, facsimile of 1889 ed. (Felinfach: Llanerch Publishers, 1994); Roy Vickery, *Garlands, Conkers and Mother-Die: British and Irish Plant-Lore* (London: Continuum, 2010).
44 David E. Allen and Gabrielle Hatfield, *Medicinal Plants in Folk Tradition: An Ethnobotany of Britain and Ireland* (Portland: Timber Press, 2004), 15–19.
45 For example, see Alix Cooper, *Inventing the Indigenous: Local Knowledge and Natural History in Early Modern Europe* (Cambridge: Cambridge University Press, 2007); Lorraine Daston and Katherine Park, *Wonders and the Order of Nature 1150–1750* (New York: Zone Books, 1998).
46 See Leong and Pennell, 'Recipe Collections'.
47 See William Eamon, *Science and the Secrets of Nature: Books of Secrets in Medieval and Early Modern Culture* (Princeton, NJ: Princeton University Press, 1994); William R. Newman and Anthony Grafton, *Secrets of Nature: Astrology and Alchemy in Early Modern Europe* (Cambridge, MA: MIT Press, 2001).
48 Raskin et al., 'Plants and Human Health', 522.
49 John Gerard, *The Herball or Generall Historie of Plantes... Very Much Enlarged and Amended by Thomas Iohnson Citizen and Apothecarye of London* (London: Printed by Adam Islip, Ioice Norton and Richard Whitakers, 1633), 4.
50 Griggs, *Green Pharmacy*, 57–8.
51 Allen and Hatfield, *Medicinal Plants*, 46. For discussion about earlier antiquarian-style historical approaches in relation to science, see Eileen K. Cheng, *Historiography: An Introductory Guide* (London: Continuum, 2012), 19–22.
52 Keith Bakx, 'The "Eclipse" of Folk Medicine in Western Society', *Sociology of Health and Illness* 13, no. 1 (1991): 21; Roger Cooter, 'Alternative Medicine, Alternative

Cosmology', in *Studies in the History of Alternative Medicine*, ed. Roger Cooter (Basingstoke: Macmillan in association with St Antony's College, Oxford, 1988), 63–78.
53 Roberta Bivins, 'Histories of Heterodoxy', in *The Oxford Handbook of the History of Medicine*, ed. Mark Jackson (Oxford: Oxford University Press, 2011), 578.
54 Ibid., 580.
55 Ibid., 579.
56 Mervyn J. Eadie, 'The Antiepileptic Materia Medica of Pediacus Dioscorides', *Journal of Clinical Neurosciences* 11, no. 7 (2004): 697–701.
57 Lawrence I. Conrad et al., *The Western Medical Tradition: 800 BC to AD 1800* (Cambridge: Cambridge University Press, 1995), 165, 232.
58 Wear, *Knowledge and Practice*, 22.
59 Rebecca Laroche, *Medical Authority and Englishwomen's Herbal Texts, 1550–1650* (Farnham: Ashgate, 2009).
60 There are methodological and other difficulties in assessing such therapies in the form of randomized controlled trials, although the quality of research designs is not necessarily less than in drug trials. See L. Nartey et al., 'Matched-Pair Study Showed Higher Quality of Placebo-Controlled Trials in Western Phytotherapy Than Conventional Medicine', *Journal of Clinical Epidemiology* 60, no. 8 (2007), 787–94.
61 Mark Jackson, introduction to Jackson, *Oxford Handbook*, 6, 13. See also Frank Huisman and John H. Warner, 'Medical Histories', in *Locating Medical History: The Stories and Their Meanings* (Baltimore, MD: Johns Hopkins University Press, 2004), ed. Frank Huisman and John H. Warner, 1–30.
62 Roger Cooter, '"Framing" the End of the Social History of Medicine', in Huisman and Warner, *Locating Medical History*, 310–37.
63 Susan M. Reverby and David Rosner, 'Beyond the Great Doctors Revisited: A Generation of the "New" Social History of Medicine', in Huisman and Warner, *Locating Medical History*, 167–93.
64 John C. Burnham, *What Is Medical History?* (Cambridge: Polity, 2005), 141.
65 Ludmilla Jordanova, 'The Social Construction of Medical Knowledge', in Huisman and Warner, *Locating Medical History*, 338, 352.
66 David B. Troy, ed., *Remington: The Science and Practice of Pharmacy*, 21st ed. (Philadelphia, PA: Lippincott, Williams and Wilkins, 2006), 9. On Paracelsus, see also Allen G. Debus, 'The Medico-Chemical World of the Paracelsians', in *Changing Perspectives in the History of Science: Essays in Honour of Joseph Needham* (London: Heinemann, 1973), ed. Mikulas Teich and Robert Young, 85–99; Charles Webster, 'Alchemical and Paracelsian Medicine', in *Health, Medicine and Mortality in the Sixteenth Century*, ed. Charles Webster (Cambridge: Cambridge University Press, 1979), 301–34.
67 For authoritative guides on known constituents and potential interactions of herbal medicines, see Simon Mills and Kerry Bone, *The Essential Guide to Herbal Safety* (St Louis, MO: Elsevier/ Churchill Livingstone, 2005); Elizabeth Williamson, Samuel Driver and Karen Baxter, *Stockley's Herbal Medicines Interactions* (London: Pharmaceutical Press, 2009).
68 Philip D. Curtin, 'Overspecialization and Remedies', in *The Backbone of History: Health and Nutrition in the Western Hemisphere*, ed. Richard H. Steckel and Jerome C. Rose (Cambridge: Cambridge University Press, 2002), 603–8.
69 Frances Watkins et al., 'Anglo-Saxon Pharmacopoeia Revisited: A Potential Treasure in Drug Discovery', *Drug Discovery Today* 16, nos 23/24 (2011): 1069–75.
70 Ibid., 1070.

71 An example of a text which has been much debated is John M. Riddle, *Goddesses, Elixirs, and Witches: Plants and Sexuality Throughout Human History* (New York: Palgrave Macmillan, 2010). See the discussion in John K. Crellin, 'Revisiting Eve's Herbs: Reflections on Therapeutic Uncertainties', in *Herbs and Healers from the Ancient Mediterranean through the Medieval West: Essays in Honor of John M. Riddle*, ed. Anne Van Arsdall and Timothy Graham (Farnham: Ashgate, 2012), 307–28.

72 H. C. G. Matthew and Brian Harrison, eds., *Oxford Dictionary of National Biography* (Oxford: Oxford University Press, 2004). The online reference source is at http://www.oxfordreference.com/ (accessed 2 September 2013).

Part One

Revisiting Original Texts: Comparative Textual Analysis and New Perspectives on Original Sources

Introduction

Susan Francia and Anne Stobart

In this first section we bring together contributors who have a starting point in revisiting original texts, some using comparative textual analysis to examine the changes in subsequent versions and editions, and all providing new perspectives on original sources. Some of the texts considered have been cited through the ages as authorities in various medical and health contexts. Thus, their provenance, authorship, alterations and reception can all provide us with valuable insight into beliefs and activities of their time. Although the analysis of textual sources is a traditional method of researching medical history, there is still much more scope for researchers interested in the history of herbal medicine to revisit well-known texts, as well as to discover new ones, and to discuss them from a perspective of how plants were understood and used as medicines in history.

Historical studies of medicine are often divided into time periods, for ease of description, although there are obviously overlaps in many areas. Sources for the study of classical medicine range from texts to artefacts. Greco-Roman treatments were characterized by plant remedies, diet and lifestyle advice and a belief in the healing power of nature, *vis medicatrix naturae*.[1] Classical writers about medicine flagged up the important and longstanding role of herbs as remedies in health care, and Celsus noted the ubiquity of such knowledge:

> Just as agriculture promises nourishment to healthy bodies, so does the Art of Medicine promise health to the sick. Nowhere is this art wanting, for the most uncivilized nations have had knowledge of herbs, and other things to hand for the aiding of wounds and diseases.[2]

Alongside details of plants, we have writers providing a context of theory and belief for ancient medicine, such as Rebecca Flemming and Helen King who examine perspectives on disease, particularly of women's complaints.[3] We should also note that past descriptions of medicinal plants in ancient texts can be economical on detail, and that botanical identification is an area requiring considerable skill.

Throughout the medieval period, medicinal information was eagerly sought and repeatedly copied. Scholars have sought to transcribe medieval manuscripts, many described as herbals, and interpret their meaning.[4] Medieval texts sometimes based information on that found in the classical Greek texts, but also on texts which had been adapted and substantially added to in the Islamic world.[5] In the late medieval period there was a rapidly growing popular interest in medical learning and in the use of remedies, as opposed to having a focus on the regulation of lifestyle and diet laid down by the classical medical writers.[6] Further overviews of the development of the English herbal were produced, in the 1920s and 1930s.[7]

The early modern period, usually considered as from 1500 to 1800 CE, saw some major shifts in thinking about medicine, although theory and knowledge were not always immediately reflected in changes in practice. Significant developments, aside from advances in scientific understanding, included further voyages of discovery, the development of botany, the establishment of gardens, a great increase in trade in medicines, the origins of professionalization, a widespread demand for printed texts and dissemination of changing perceptions of nature.[8]

Many of the original texts under discussion have now been made available online.[9] In addition, research aids such as online dictionaries for Greek and Latin are also readily available.[10]

In this section, Vicki Pitman provides a firm grounding in early Greek medicine, considering evidence of models, methods and *materia medica* in the texts of the Hippocratic corpus to provide new perspectives. Her study informs the understanding of subsequent scholars and practitioners, and she argues that the survival of many aspects of holism can still be appreciated today, so that continuity with some ancient practices is not entirely broken. Anne Van Arsdall considers scholarly approaches and medieval herbal texts with a view to evaluating the contents of texts for information on practices concerning medicinal plants. Her chapter raises interesting possibilities of further interpretation drawing on the knowledge and experience of modern-day practitioners. Moving forward to the printed text and the early modern period, Elaine Hobby uses literary analysis to consider early-modern midwifery manuals for evidence of changes in perspectives and practice involving herbal medicine. Her study includes advice for those interested in using literary criticism, including the pitfalls and problems which may occur. Another study of changes in the detail in texts comes from Graeme Tobyn, who has examined the way in which the widely acclaimed publication of Nicholas Culpeper was compiled, revealing the influences and intentions of the originator. His research leads him to dispute beliefs that Culpeper's *English Physitian* is original and he argues that it draws largely from the work of John Parkinson.

Notes

1 Jacalyn Duffin, *History of Medicine: A Scandalously Short Introduction* (Toronto: University of Toronto Press, 1999), 93–6.
2 Cited in Mirko D. Grmek, ed., *Western Medical Thought from Antiquity to the Middle Ages* (Cambridge, MA: Harvard University Press, 1998), 3.
3 Rebecca Flemming, *Medicine and the Making of Roman Women: Gender, Nature, and Authority from Celsus to Galen* (Oxford: Oxford University Press, 2000); Helen King, *Hippocrates' Woman: Reading the Female Body in Ancient Greece* (London: Routledge, 1998).
4 George Henslow, *Medical Works of the Fourteenth Century: Together with a List of Plants Recorded in Contemporary Writings, with Their Identifications* (London:

Chapman and Hall, 1899); F. W. T. Hunger, ed., *The Herbal of Pseudo-Apuleius: From the Ninth-Century Manuscript in the Abbey of Monte Cassino (Codex Casinensis 97)* (Leiden: Brill, 1935); Jerry Stannard and Richard Kay, eds., *Herbs and Herbalism in the Middle Ages and Renaissance* (Aldershot: Ashgate, 1999); Anne Van Arsdall, *Medieval Herbal Remedies: The Old English Herbarium and Anglo-Saxon Medicine* (New York: Routledge, 2002).

5   For more on the unsung contribution of Islamic writers to the history of Western medicine, see ch. 4 in this book.
6   Faye M. Getz, ed., *Healing and Society in Medieval England: A Middle English Translation of the Pharmaceutical Writings of Gilbertus Anglicus* (Madison, WI: University of Wisconsin Press, 1991), xxii.
7   Agnes Arber, *Herbals, Their Origin and Evolution: A Chapter in the History of Botany, 1470–1670*, 3rd ed. (Cambridge: Cambridge University Press, 1986); Eleanour S. Rohde, *The Old English Herbals*, reprint of the 1922 ed. (New York: Dover Publications, 1971).
8   An excellent overview is provided by Andrew Wear, *Knowledge and Practice in English Medicine, 1550–1680* (Cambridge: Cambridge University Press, 2000).
9   The databases can be accessed through organizations such as Gallica in France (http://gallica.bnf.fr), the Wellcome Library in the UK (http://wellcomelibrary.org/), the Gutenberg Project in the USA (http://www.gutenberg.org/) and the National Library of Medicine in the USA (http://www.nlm.nih.gov) (all accessed 28 October 2013). Subscription-based organizations providing databases of digitized texts, such as Early English Books Online, offer further detailed access to complete sets of images of original texts, often with accompanying transcriptions (http://eebo.chadwyck.com).
10 For example: Perseus Search Tools, http://www.perseus.tufts.edu/hopper/search (accessed 28 October 2013).

2

Early Greek Medicine: Evidence of Models, Methods and *materia medica*

Vicki Pitman

Introduction and methodology

This chapter discusses the philosophy behind, and the evidence of, herbal medicines in the practice of ancient Greek physicians; the Hippocratic physicians. It also explores such concepts and practices that may have survived into the modern-day practice of Western herbal medicine in the UK. Today one can still hear the phrase 'Hippocrates says, you are what you eat', and learn that Hippocrates is held as the 'father of medicine',[1] and so one is prompted to ask what else may be found in the practice of Hippocratic physicians which would be of interest to a modern herbalist.

The basic methodology is a textual analysis of elements of ancient Greek medical treatises, primarily found in the Hippocratic corpus. In addition, some related philosophical writings of the sixth and fifth centuries BCE were consulted. Two further texts were also consulted: *De materia medica* of Dioscorides, first century CE, is the earliest extant pharmacological text; *The Medical Writings of Anonymus Londinensis*, a text, probably fourth century BCE, that preserves different medical practices and concepts of the period.[2] As the author of this chapter is not a classical scholar but a herbal medicine practitioner, these works have been studied in their English translations.[3] While classical scholars have substantially investigated the corpus and continue to do so, few if any are medical practitioners. According to Wesley Smith, the last scholar who found the corpus of practical medical interest was M. P. E. Littré (1801–81) in the nineteenth century, 'for whom Hippocrates was alive and meaningful in day to day medical practice'.[4] In contrast to the modern medical practitioner, for a clinical herbalist the approach and practices of ancient Greek physicians, being largely based on herbal and dietary therapeutics, may be of clinical interest.

Initially, significant features of ancient thought relevant to the Hippocratic physician-writers will be discussed, with examples of how these are reflected in the approach of physicians as recorded in the treatises. The basic features of the model for understanding health and the origins of disease are presented before evidence for treatment methods and *materia medica* is considered. An evaluation of some of the challenges faced in interpreting the evidence and using sources follows. Finally, aspects of Hippocratic thought and practice discernible in the approach and practice of modern herbal medicine or phytotherapy are explored.

The Hippocratic corpus comprises the earliest extant texts of the Western medical tradition. The treatises were attributed to Hippocrates, a famous physician in his own time and thereafter. However, the treatises, some 60 in all, are by different physician-writers spanning the period roughly 450–230 BCE, a seminal time in the development of Western thought and civilization. The corpus was chosen for study because these texts had enormous influence on subsequent medical thought and practice, particularly influencing Galen who himself was held in high esteem for centuries.

Each writer has his own voice and purpose, and the treatises vary in intention, content, methods and style. The treatises by some physicians are characterized by careful clinical observation of disease conditions and the symptoms of their patients, or by an explicit break with the widely held Greek view that disease is ultimately caused by the gods.[5] Other treatises are considered to be of a rhetorical nature, perhaps not even written by a physician, and aim at arguing for the need for medicine as a separate 'profession' in society. Some treatises focus on environmental aspects of health and disease, others on the centrality of food, digestion and exercise, and others are a collection of helpful aphorisms or discuss guiding principles of the medical art.[6]

The philosophy underpinning Greek medicine

Holism and cosmic nature: *Holos, kosmos* and *phusis*

Herbalists today use the term holistic, referring to a concept that, long before it was recoined by Smutts in the early twentieth century,[7] was fundamental to Hippocratic and later Galenic medicine (second century CE). It is today a widely used Western cultural term, although not always readily defined. For early Greek thinkers, *to holon* or *to pan*[8] contained the idea of a divine wholeness of the *kosmos* – the goodness, order and beauty of the universe – of which mankind and nature are the microcosm.[9] This view is reflected in several Hippocratic treatises. One treatise, *Breaths*, links the behaviour of air in the environment and in the human body with the cosmic, vital air.[10] Another treatise, *Airs, Waters, and Places*, relates local diseases to prevailing local environmental and seasonal conditions.[11] Numerous passages in Hippocratic treatises reflect this view, linking the wholeness of the body to health, emphasizing the relationship between nature and human health, between the wholeness of body and its parts, the need to treat both an individual part, where the symptoms are manifest, and the whole body. Also, many treatises include the need for due regard to what today would be termed psychological and/or spiritual aspects of the patient.[12] Important also was for the physician to know 'what a man is in relation to foods, drinks and habits generally', that is, to understand the individual patient.[13] The author of the treatise *Regimen I* states: 'Wholes are divided into parts and from union of the parts wholes are formed.... In other respects too Nature is the same as the physician's art'.[14] An external observer, the philosopher Plato in his dialogue in *Charmides*, describes the physicians' method as applying 'their regimens to the entire body and [attempting] to heal the part in conjunction with the whole'.[15] Galen, writing some 500 years later, also subscribes to this outlook.[16]

Divine and individual nature

The vision of the universe as a cosmic *holos* derives from the ideas of sixth- and fifth-century BCE nature philosophers, some of whom were also physicians. Such thinkers as Empedocles (c. 492–c. 432 BCE), Alcmaeon (fl. 450 BCE), Heracleitus (c. 540–c. 480 BCE) and Pythagoras (died c. 500 BCE) held views that radically shifted Greek thought away from an exclusively magico-religious understanding of mankind's place in the cosmos towards what is today sometimes termed a 'rational' one.[17] For example, Empedocles, who may also have been a physician, conceives of the cosmos as a 'Sphere' which, through 'Love', binds together all things.[18] The phenomena of the natural world, including living things, derive ultimately from 'root elements' (earth, water, fire and air).[19] Life-forms are created by a 'blending' and 'mingling' of these elements, so that no single element separates, thereby becoming much stronger than the others.[20] Separation does happen during periods when the creation comes under the influence of 'Strife', Love's opposite power. Within the Sphere, at periods in time, under the influence of Strife, separation can initiate a destructive tendency.[21] In such mingling and separation, the created world alternates between greater or lesser harmony.[22]

We find a very similar understanding in the context of the body eloquently expressed by the physician Eryximachus in a dialogue from Plato. Medicine, Eryximachus says, is the:

> knowledge of the principles of love at work in the body in regard to repletion and evacuation. The most skilful doctor is the doctor who can... implant love in a body which lacks but needs it.... He must be able to bring elements in the body which are most hostile to one another into mutual affection and love.[23]

A similar view is found in the treatise *Ancient Medicine*, in which the Hippocratic physician observes:

> But all the other components of man become milder and better the greater the number of other components with which they are mixed. A man is in the best possible condition when there is complete coction [digestion-mingling] and rest, with no particular power displayed.[24]

Greek physicians practised and wrote about their medical *techne*, their 'art', in a milieu in which such ideas were being advanced and debated. It seems they used or adopted some of these ideas in their medical models and practice,[25] and reflected contributors to the philosophical revolution in Greek thought who preferred an empirical-rational explanation of natural phenomena.[26] Wholeness was seen as inherent in nature, *phusis*. For physicians, nature itself had the creative and life sustaining force of the *kosmos*.[27] Nature was an intelligent and healing power, which, given proper study, man's own intelligence and reason could comprehend and harness. For example, the author of the treatise *Epidemics 6* writes: 'The body's nature is the physician in disease. Nature finds the way for herself, not from thought. Well trained, readily and without instruction, nature does what is needed'.[28] For the author of the treatise *Nutriment*, 'Nature is sufficient in all for all'.[29]

As a microcosm of cosmic nature, each person's individual *phusis* was of central concern for ancient physicians. A patient's nature was also called the constitution, *katastasis*, being the individual blend of constituting elements. In particular, physicians enquired about what elements constituted this human nature and how such constituent parts behaved when influenced by a range of factors.[30] The fundamental model of health was founded on Greek concepts of harmony and balance (*harmonia* and *metria*), maintained among constituent parts and achieved through their mingling or blending (*krasis*).[31] A disposition towards disease occurred when one or more constituents 'separated' and became too strong, destabilizing the balance. Examples of the constitutional approach include passages such as the following:

> This [the patient's habitual regimen] one should learn and change and carry out treatment only after examination of the patient's constitution, age, physique, the season of the year and the fashion of the disease, sometimes taking away and sometimes adding... and so making changes in drugging or in regimen to suit the several conditions of age, season, physique, and disease.[32]

> he who aspires to treat correctly of human regimen must first acquire knowledge and discernment of the nature of man in general, knowledge of its primary constituents and discernment of the components by which it is controlled [fire and water].... And further the power possessed severally by all the foods, and drinks of our regimen, both the power of each of them possessed by nature and the power given them by the constraint of human art. For it is necessary to know both how one ought to lessen the power of these when they are strong by nature, and when they are weak to add by art strength to them, seizing each opportunity as it occurs.[33]

Overlying this constitutional model, we find disagreement or variety among the physician-writers as to the details. In this early period the exact number and nature of these constituent parts was in flux. Some authors used a model of elements – air, fire, earth, water, or some just fire and water – primarily acting in the body via their powers, *dynameis*, properties or qualities, for example the hot, the moist, the dry, the cold, or through their tastes.[34] The author of the treatise *Fleshes* spoke of three constituents: *aither* (a distinct heat associated with the heavens), earth and water. Each contained corresponding qualities: aither – heat; earth – cold and dryness; and water – moisture and thickness.[35] Others viewed constituents as vital fluids, the humours, *chumoi*. Some physicians worked on the basis of two humours, phlegm and bile, some a fourfold model of blood, bile, phlegm and water. The author of *Nature of Man* used a model of four humours: bile, phlegm, blood and *melanchole* or black bile. These body fluids were the somatic vehicles of the vital principles, those elements of nature operating in the body and necessary to its health.[36] Like the author of *Airs, Waters and Places*, and writers of several clinical treatises, the author of *Nature of Man* associated each humour with the prevailing qualities of one of the four seasons. Blood, for example, was associated with the warming and moistening qualities of spring. Disruption to the functioning of the humours was viewed as the originating cause of disease. Such a view is found both in what are considered the more rhetorical treatises and also in more clinical texts such as *Epidemics, Affections* and *Regimen in Acute Diseases*.[37]

Along with the healing power of nature, and the individual's nature or constitution as influenced both by its internal and external environment, the concept of qualities and humours has had lasting influence. The four-humour model of *Nature of Man* was also used by Galen and became the archetype for subsequent generations of physicians and also lay herbalists.[38]

A schematic representation first published by Schöner,[39] shows the possible evolution of the humoral model through the centuries, from *Nature of Man* through Galen's development of it to its adaptation into Christian and later astrological cosmic schemes (see Figure 2.1).

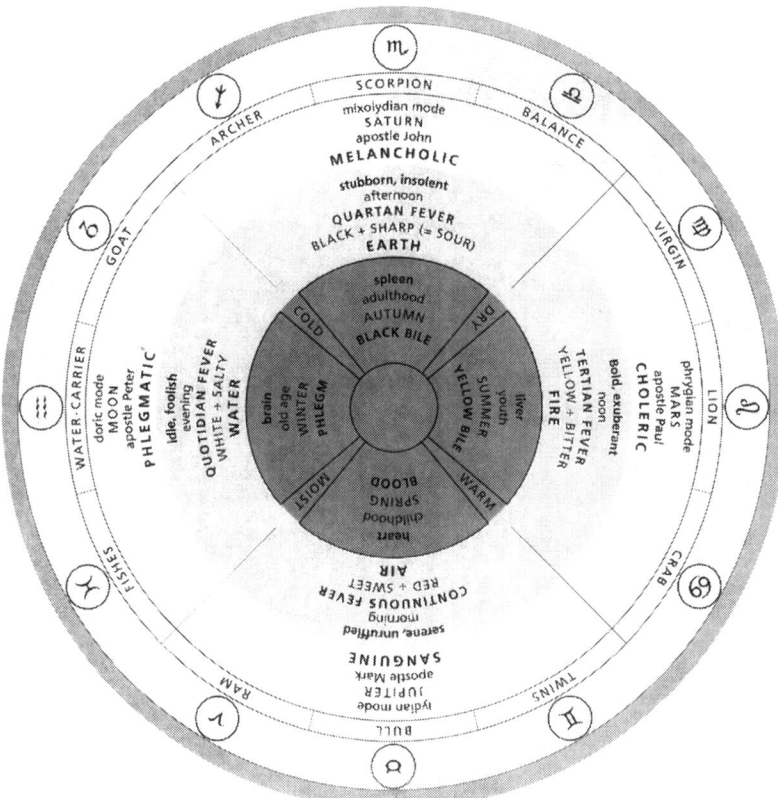

Figure 2.1 Diagram showing the four humours and associated concepts. Original diagram in Erich Schöner, *Das Viererschema in der Antiken Humoralpathologie* (Wiesbaden: F. Steiner, 1964) and adapted and published in Paul Cartledge, ed., *The Cambridge Illustrated History of Ancient Greece*, revised ed. (Cambridge: Cambridge University Press, 2002), 314. Image courtesy of F. Steiner and Cambridge University Press.

As a concomitant of understanding that the patient's nature or constitution needed individualized therapy, the physicians established the practice of taking and recording a detailed individual case history and noting how an illness developed. This included identifying a range of influencing factors: important aspects of symptoms (heat, cold, dryness, moisture, swelling) and factors that worsen or improve them (sleep or mental disturbance, critical days). In *Epidemics I*, the physician also noted the 'constitution' of the time, place and climate, any sudden changes in weather, or to the patient's occupation, mode of life (*diaita*) and relevant emotional factors or crises.[40] In the *Epidemics* treatises as a whole, all manner of folk are found: individuals of different social and economic standing and gender, identified by name, or sometimes by a specific address or location.[41] This precedent of recording individual histories through careful observation is itself an extremely important legacy of the holism of Hippocratic medicine.

Causal factors of disease

We have seen that discerning how the constitutional humours become unblended and separated, creating the conditions for disease to occur, was the crucial concern of Hippocratic physicians. In many treatises the emphasis was on regimen as the primary or fundamental cause for the disruption of the humours and their balanced, healthy mixture. A diet which was wrong for a particular individual and/or poor digestion of his foods and drinks could lead to a lack of complete digestion, *pepsis*, and thus poor assimilation. This state then affected the *eukrasia*, the healthy mixing together of humours. In other works, a disturbance in the vital breath, *pneuma*, was the underlying cause of all imbalance.[42] An example is found in *Breaths* where the condition of excess phlegm was ascribed to the body becoming too full of food and consequently full of wind. If then the food remained in the digestive tract too long, because its quantity kept it from passing through, the lower intestine became blocked so that breaths, *phusai*, rushed through the whole body and fell on the parts that were 'full of blood' and chilled them.[43]

In fact all such factors, that is, the healthy blending or not of one's humours, the state of one's digestion, the healthy flow of the vital breath, were interlinked. While some physicians cited poor functioning in diet and digestion as creating an excess, plethora, of one humour, for other writers it created 'residues'. These are the acid, bitter or acrid secretions mentioned in the treatise *Ancient Medicine*, or the *perissomata* of *Anonymus Londinensis*, which could accumulate and then disturb the proper functioning of humours in various ways, not least disturbing the normal flow of vital air in the body.[44]

Though the diagram from Schöner is useful, it gives an impression of a definitive, comprehensive system, and tends to obscure the fact that in the ancient period there continued to be great fluidity and variety. From the fifth century BCE until Galen's time in the second century of the Christian era and beyond there were several competing medical approaches. Some followed Hippocrates but emphasized a particular interpretation of Hippocratic practice. Approaches differed among the medical 'schools' or 'sects' which emerged, known as Empiricists, Methodists, Pneumatists and

Dogmatists. In addition, there was the distinct tradition of healing and cures in the cult of Asclepius, the healing god.[45]

Evidence of methods and *materia medica* in ancient practice

Medicinal agents and methods used by ancient physicians were quite varied, a fact which reflects both the variety of factors that might trigger imbalance and disharmony, and probably the physician's own training and experience. While imbalances of the humours were seen to affect all or part of the body and cause disease, the course and nature of the condition was individual to the case and treatment was adapted accordingly.

Maintaining the patient's health was basic to the approach, with emphasis on prevention against disease, which involved adjustments to diet, exercise and life habits. Such adjustments were also part of treating disease. While disease conditions were often discussed in terms of disturbed humours, such disturbances, whether from contagion, wounds or other factors, did lead to specifically named disease entities. Treatises such as *Affections*, *Diseases I* and *Diseases II*[46] detail treatment for specific diseases or conditions such as sciatica, strangury, gout, jaundice, angina, consumption and pleurisy. From the descriptions, certain conditions may possibly be recognized as corresponding to the modern disease. In other descriptions, the condition cannot be equated in modern biomedical terms. Plagues of contagious infections occurred but we do not know the cause nor can we match them to those of modern times.

Treatment was given not only for the symptoms, for example the pain of gout, but was also focused on the digestive tract: stomach and bowel function, sometimes the 'upper' or 'lower' 'belly' or simply 'the belly', or 'cavity'. Treatment included herbs and foods as well as lifestyle changes to modify and restore digestive and bowel function by removing excesses of humours or residues. A common treatment was 'evacuation', 'cleaning' or 'purging' the belly or cavity, sometimes 'upwards' through emesis therapy but more often 'downwards' using purging herbs or herbal enema.[47] Examples of herbs used include white hellebore (*Veratrum album*), black hellebore (*Helleborus cyclophyllus*),[48] scammony (*Convolvulus scammonia*),[49] Cnidian berry (*Daphne cnidium*),[50] squirting cucumber (*Ecballium elaterium*)[51] and also barley gruel.[52] Each substance would be used for a slightly different effect.[53] As needed, additional herbs and therapeutic foods were prescribed for the particular organs involved, such as the head, liver, lungs and joints.[54] An important adjunctive method used by Hippocratic physicians, especially in cases of fevers, was what some modern herbalists may recognize as therapeutic fasting: the use of a therapeutic food, most often the barley *ptisane* or gruel.[55] Such gruel, prepared with great care in a variety of ways particular to the case, was aimed at eliminating residues and restoring the digestive balance while sustaining the patient. Within this context, further dietary prescriptions, and the use of specific herbs, together with lifestyle and exercise advice tailored for the individual, would be given. This treatment focus on the digestive tract in order to restore healthy balance and blending of humours was the fundamental approach.

An example of how a physician might treat a particular disease while allowing for the individualities of the case is found in *Internal Affections*. The author recorded variations of each disease in different patients, each one calling for a different treatment. In chapters 39–41, different forms of typhus were recorded. One occurred in summer, another was observed to occur in any season, another when putrid bile became mixed with blood in vessels and joints. The symptoms of each type varied with the individual, and treatment varied as well. For one patient the treatment included thin gruel with honey and some dark wine, abstention from cereals for a time, boiled polyp [octopus or cuttlefish], turnips and cleansing with Cnidian berry followed by a rich boiled meal.[56] For another, the physician employed a fomentation (probably herbal) to the site of pain, massage, vapour-baths to the whole body, the hellebore cleanse, followed by a therapeutic diet of goat's whey, honey and salt, lentil soup, boiled beets and barley meal, and also, as symptoms indicated, various meats, fish, wine, whey, milk and ass's milk.[57]

That the physicians had a view as to what such fomentations could achieve, using various herbs for specific outcomes, we learn from a detail in the later classical text *Anonymus Londinensis*:

> And that certain accretions, perceived by the eye of the reason, will penetrate into us, we may first illustrate from the strong qualities of drugs, of mints or of fumitories and of plasters, which being placed on the surface sometimes dissolve what lies under it, sometimes dissipate it in perspiration, and sometimes draw it to themselves. What happens to cause this? The strong quality of the drug not only settles on the surface but also penetrates down to a certain depth through the passages of the body.[58]

Having considered the various approaches to treatment, the discussion moves on to review the herbal and other treatments found in the Hippocratic corpus. Approximately 130 medicinal substances are mentioned in the Hippocratic corpus, the majority of them herbs. In selecting, the physician considered a herb or food's *dynameis* or qualities of heating, cooling, moistening, drying, sharpness and mildness (not a neutral but a positive virtue). Such qualities would have been ascertained by the senses directly, for example by tasting or by observation of the effect on the body.[59] Thus the quality indicated its physiological effect. This approach, that of reasoning from observation as a means of informing the selection of the medicine, is clearly present in these earliest medical writings, though not in the form of a comprehensive explanation by any particular writer. Examples may be found in *Epidemics 2*,[60] *Regimen in Acute Diseases*,[61] *Regimen II*,[62] *Affections*[63] and *Nature of Man*.[64]

At a later period, the time of Dioscorides in the first century CE, such understanding was more codified. While Dioscorides largely ignores humoral theory in his *De materia medica*, his perception that a substance's quality was indicative of its action was the work's organizing principle. Each plant has a chapter, and those plants with similar actions are grouped together: for example, several strongly cooling plants are so grouped – henbanes (*Hyoscyamus* spp.), opium poppy (*Papaver somniferum*) and the poisonous hemlock (*Conium maculatum*). Today's understanding of their properties confirms their similar physiological action on the central nervous system.[65]

By comparison to a modern pharmacopoeia or herbal textbook, explicit details as to methods of preparation are scarce or generalized in the corpus.[66] The author of *Affections* refers the reader several times to the now lost 'Medication Book' for more treatment options.[67] An example of specified herbs and preparations is found in *Regimen in Acute Diseases (Appendix)*:

> Lozenge for pneumonia: all-heal juice and pine cone in Attic honey; also have the patient drink southernwood in oxymel [vinegar-honey] and pepper. Boil off black hellebore, and give it to the patient with pleurisy, at the beginning when he is in great pain. It is also good to boil up all-heal in oxymel and, sieving it, to give it to drink both to patients with liver complaints and to those with severe pains arising from the diaphragm.[68]

The passage omits details of preparation and dosage but illustrates a variety of preparations: a lozenge made with honey, an oxymel with infused herbs, boiling and sieving. Hippocratic physicians would have used herbs in the form of liquids, pressed to obtain the juice or boiled, or the parts crushed and blended[69] with a particular wine, honey or vinegar, sometimes itself chosen to add a specific effect to the whole.[70] Herbs were also made into salves and pessaries. Aromatic herbs would have been used in oil-based applications (anointing), fomentations, vapour baths and fumigations.[71] The herbs used were not limited to those found in the Mediterranean area: there was already in the fifth century BCE a trade in exotics such as black pepper (*Piper nigrum*) and cardamom (*Elettaria* spp.) from India.[72]

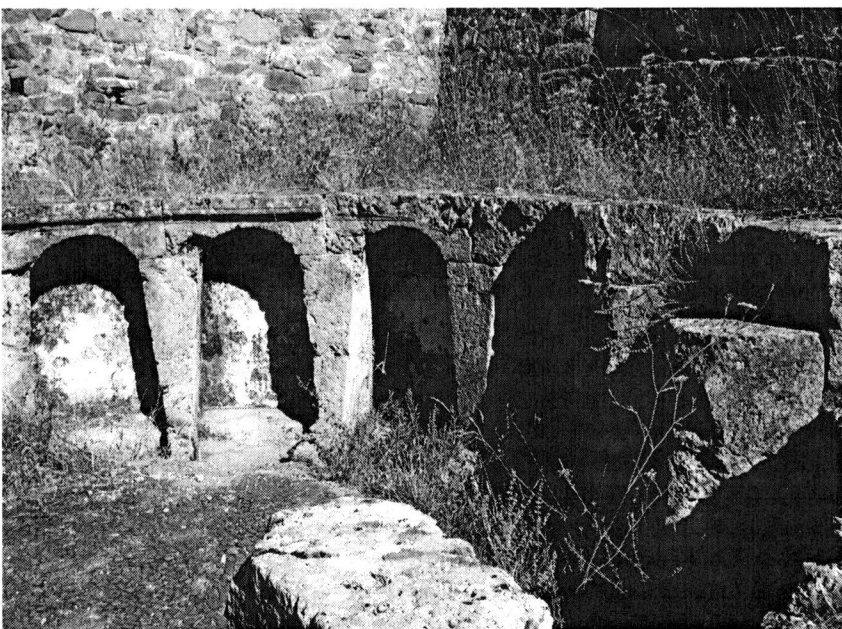

Figure 2.2 Sitz baths at the site of an Asclepion at Gortys, Peloponnese, Greece. Photo courtesy of A. R. Pitman.

In addition to herbs, the use of soda, wines, animal parts, minerals, clays, cupping, bloodletting, cautery, even possibly moxibustion, were part of the physicians' repertory.[73] Physicians attended to the emotional side of a patient's condition, as in a prescription given to contemplate comic things, an early instance of laughter therapy.[74] Physicians prescribed massage with oil and therapeutic bathing.[75] A group of sitz baths has been identified at the site of an Asclepion at Gortys, in the Peloponnese, Greece (see Figure 2.2).[76] It is likely that at such religious healing centres some treatments offered by priest-physicians were similar to those of Hippocratic physicians.[77]

Holism, ancient and modern

An important mark of much modern herbal practice in the UK is the concept of holism. By this is meant that the patient is assessed by taking into account not only physical factors but also mental-emotional, social, environmental and spiritual factors. In addition, the herbal medicine itself is subject to minimal processing in order to retain its inherent complex pharmacology (in contrast to biomedicine's use of single active ingredients used to treat a large population with the same condition).[78]

Features of modern holism

Herbal medicine practice today exhibits a range of salient features of modern holism, to which many herbalists would be committed. These could include:

- the 'vital force' as the healing power of nature;
- the wisdom of the body;
- the body–mind–spirit connection;
- the relationship of health and disease (the degrading of health predisposing to disease);
- treatment to support healing processes, and to balance the body's functions;
- treatment of the individual as a whole, not solely the disease entity;
- the partnership of the patient with the practitioner.[79]

In this chapter I have noted that several of these features were also fundamental to the practice of physician-writers of the Hippocratic corpus: the healing power of nature, the relationship of health and disease, the aim of treatment to support the healing process and restore healthy functions and harmony among the humours, the understanding and treatment of the individual *phusis*.[80] With possible exceptions, today most Western herbalists do not primarily use the model of the Hippocratic physicians, or much of the language – that is, that of the *phusis* of the patient, the assessment and treatment of the four humours, or the regulation of a vital *pneuma*.[81] However, important still is the commitment for some herbalists, in precept and in practice, to concepts of a vital force and the healing power of nature. In practice, many herbalists 'follow nature', as the Hippocratic physicians sought to do, both by understanding the individual aspects of the patient's symptoms and imbalances and the influencing factors, and by choosing whole, close-to-nature medicines (herbs and therapeutic foods) as a positive means to enhance the body's innate healing, cleansing and corrective functions.[82] Herbs are prescribed for specific symptoms in a context of prescriptions to restore healthy function. Thus 'balance' and 'harmony' of function are still signallers of health. An important difference is that the level of understanding of the biological and physiological mechanisms underlying health and disease is far greater today. The role of the practitioner, also discussed among Hippocratic writers,[83] is held to be not only that of a prescriber but also that of partner and guide in preventative healthy living, acting in harmony with nature in the wider sense and with the individual patient's own nature or constitution. Herbalists also continue to view the accumulation of non-vital substances as a source of imbalance which can lead to disease. The imperative to take and record the patient's case history, to assess and consider in depth the individual patient, rather than only the disease condition, and to vary treatment accordingly, is again something that is retained in modern herbal medicine practice. Indeed, professional clinical practice in the United Kingdom requires a private, face-to-face consultation before a prescription may be given.[84]

As has been noted, the language of the four humours – blood, yellow bile, phlegm and black bile – is largely absent from the modern terminology of phytotherapy. There are issues around the changes in the language of medical knowledge and practice over time, how and why these changed, and how they continue to change. This may make it difficult to trace a consistent view or practice. However, there may be more continuity than is at first obvious. For example, the concept of the blood humour may survive into modern practice in a different guise. In Western herbalism today, importance is given to the health of blood. This shows itself in an emphasis on treatment strategies, with terms such as 'blood cleansing', 'alterative', 'antidyscratic' or 'depurative'. These are all different terms for essentially the same therapeutic approach,[85] and suggest an under-recognized survival of the sanguine or blood humour. This attention to treating the blood may retain the thought of Empedocles that the four roots are most evenly proportioned in the blood,[86] so that if the blood is well-balanced, the health is good.

Sources of evidence

There are many challenges in comparing modern herbal medicine with ancient Greek medicine. First, for the researcher without a classics background, the textual evidence is not readily available, unless one has access to a university library with a classics department and translated texts. This situation is improving with the digitizing of material available on the Internet. Unlike the Chinese or Ayurvedic physician, the herbal medicine practitioner in the West is no longer in direct touch with the classical languages. Additionally, there are many texts as yet untranslated which would be useful to study. It is fortunate that with the current renewed interest in ancient medicine among classical scholars, new and updated editions and translations of many texts are becoming more available. Researchers are under an obligation to judiciously interpret the meaning of translated texts and, if without the appropriate background, to seek advice from specialists with a knowledge of the cultural and historical context. Conversely, for the researcher without training in herbal medicine, the expertise of practising clinical herbalists could offer insights based on actual experience of working with patients and *materia medica* in a way comparable to that of ancient physicians.

Novel evaluations of textual evidence are needed. Assessments of the efficacy of *materia medica* and methods of historical herbal treatment would greatly benefit from collaboration between herbalists, botanists and pharmacologists. Majno and Riddle have made a welcome beginning. A surgeon himself, Majno explored ancient surgical methods to discover if they could possibly have worked.[87] Taking examples from different cultures, including Egyptian, Greek, Indian and Chinese, he compared or re-created the therapies with modern methods and pharmacological knowledge to investigate their effectiveness and safety. Successful ones included a Hippocratic surgeon's wound salves with anti-bacterial and haemostatic effects; a correctly performed surgical drainage of the lungs; and use of zinc oxide for antisepsis, along with wine and vinegar.[88] Riddle opened up a new approach when he used modern pharmacology and chemistry to demonstrate the substantial therapeutic effects of many of the plant medicines in Dioscorides' pharmacopoeia. He found that Dioscorides correctly recorded uses of plants containing pharmacologically active volatile oils and alkaloids for physiological effects, uses substantiated by modern chemistry. Examples include ginger (*Zingiber officinale*), peppers (*Piper nigrum* and *P. longum*), henbane (*Hyoscyamus niger*) and black nightshade (*Solanum nigrum*).[89] Such interdisciplinary exploration needs to be continued and developed.

Other methods of study are possible. Textual evidence can also be augmented with archaeological evidence. This carries its own problems,[90] but can bring rewards.[91] For example, cupping was once part of the Western tradition. Its use is recorded in texts and in archaeological finds. Jackson has researched many aspects of medical practice gleaned not only from texts but also from archaeology: stone reliefs, gems, vase and wall paintings, surgical and cupping instruments, medical apparatus, plant remains (some as traces in containers), animal and human skeletal remains and micro-organism remains.[92] He found stone stamps, with 'product information' of how eye ointments were created from specific herbs.[93] A medieval monastic hospital in Scotland has been investigated with novel ethno-archaeological methods which might be of use in an ancient context.[94]

Jashemski, a classicist and archaeologist specializing in Roman gardens, discovered that the local workmen helping her at Pompeii were using local plants to treat their own ailments. Jashemski identified the plants as the same or closely related species to those in ancient texts, and also found their modern use was consistent with ancient usage. Similarly, certain implements used by the workmen were identical to ancient ones uncovered at the site.[95] It might be possible to develop Jashemski's experience, that is, to interview or exchange information with contemporary Mediterranean professional and lay herbalists and botanists to discover other plants and methods of use which may have managed to survive, unknown to us in the English-speaking world. Some of these may then be investigated for potential uses and reincorporation into the modern *materia medica*.

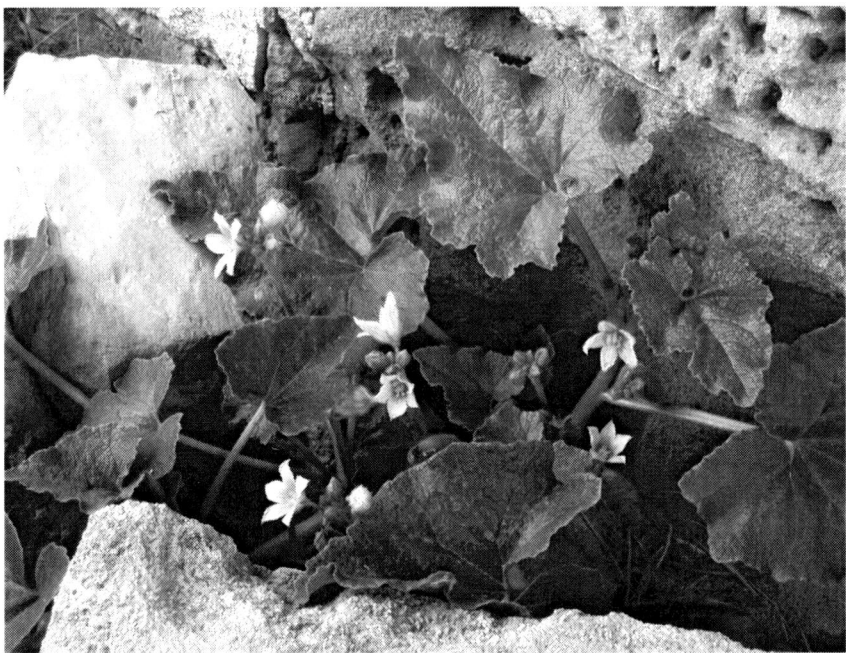

Figure 2.3 Squirting cucumber (*Ecballium elaterium*). Photo by the author, V. Pitman.

Researchers need to exercise caution in the question of identification of species of herbs mentioned in ancient texts as they may not be those we recognize by the same or similar names today.[96] Botanical identification is problematic, yet some certainty is achievable. Manniche, Farrar and Jashemski have made important contributions in this area.[97] They have used carbonized remains, root cavities, seeds from storage jars, material from waste areas, pollen and pictorial and sculptural evidence. Any research that elucidates this issue is greatly welcomed. As Jashemski showed, it is possible that many species are the same or closely related.[98] Such plants as the squirting cucumber (*Ecballium elaterium*), used by Hippocratic physicians, still grow in the Mediterranean area (see Figure 2.3). This is a plant so distinctive as to suggest it is the same or very similar to the ancient variety.

For the researcher who must often rely on the translations of scholars who may be working from a cultural viewpoint at odds with that of herbal medicine, a final caution is offered: one person's 'starvation diet' is another's 'therapeutic fast' or mono-diet.[99] Some scholars' interpretations of what ancient practice could achieve may hold a cultural bias in favour of biomedicine, as for example the idea that the ancient physician's main role was one of watching and waiting, implying he did not have access to any effective medicines and thus could do little else,[100] or modern assumptions that treatments were most often ineffectual, or sometimes more dangerous than the condition and fell short of cure.[101] In fact, several herbs in the repertory were capable of strong effects: for example, anaesthetic (e.g. black nightshade)[102] and anti-microbial (e.g. myrrh, *Commiphora* spp.) effects.[103] Though, as Riddle has shown, with regard to later practice, ancient physicians knew well the effects of different 'dangerous' herbs and at what dose they should be used for a safe effect.[104] Jackson finds evidence of scurvy, a condition of vitamin deficiency, being successfully treated with dock root (*Rumex* spp.).[105] Using the ancient pharmacopoeia, parasitic infection, or infection following wounds, or the exposure of eyes to pathogens, could have been controlled with herbs such as myrrh, frankincense (*Boswellia* spp.) and thyme (*Thymus* spp.). Physicians would also use surgery and other very 'active' interventions.[106]

Another challenge may be to reconsider some assumptions about the validity of ancient medicine in the light of current medical knowledge. For example, the humoral model – with its focus on the importance of the quality and functioning of bodily fluids – may not be merely a useless superstition from a medically primitive age. Nutton and others have highlighted that this ancient model contained the idea that some substances, for example what we now recognize as informational peptides and hormones, are transported in the body via the vital fluids. The integrity of the fluids, for example blood and lymph, as well as the abundance or deficiencies of the informational substances and their receptors on cells, influence health and the organism's reaction to pathological challenges.[107] This integrity of fluids and the healthful balance of hormonal communications constitute a form of 'balance' that is maintained (or not maintained). In this sense, modern medicine may be said to have confirmed with detail the practical experience and insights of ancient physicians that the health of bodily fluids is critical to health.

A clean break?

In contrast to practitioners of traditional medicine in China and India, whose training combines science and the study of traditional texts, Western herbalists' training is often science-based but containing little of substance about the practices and clinical wisdom from 500 or 2,000 years ago.[108] Western herbalists do not reference in detail our predecessors: we cannot know them directly through a shared language, unless we become proficient in classical tongues. The clinical insights of Galen and the Hippocratic authors, or the pharmacology of Dioscorides, are difficult to access. Although herbalists may acknowledge such a tradition, they know comparatively little detail about it, and some feel themselves to be cut off from it. The possible reasons for this disconnection with the past are many and complex, ranging from cultural to linguistic and technological: they deserve further exploration.

No matter at which time or place, the practice of healing and medicine uses a knowledge system or model with which, and through which, observations and experience about nature, health and disease are rendered coherent and of practical use. This is no less true in our own time than it was in the early centuries of Western culture. Today, terms such as elements, humours, temperaments, *krasis* and *pneuma* have largely disappeared from the language and discourse of Western herbalists, and are largely forgotten, though, ironically, biomedical terms derive from the ancient Greek and Latin. Herbalists have responded to ever-changing scientific discoveries in anatomy, physiology and pathology, and to models and theories of disease: germ theory, autoimmunity, hormones, peptides, genetics, molecular and cell biology and evolution. Over the past 300 years, it would seem that herbalists have constantly adjusted their language in order to stay 'modern' and current within their own culture. Perhaps to have insisted on the language of the humours in such a context would have invited more marginalization. The contemporary herbalist learns and employs the current understanding of physiology, pathology and phytochemistry in diagnosis and treatment. The herbal repertory and methods have changed and evolved, and continue to evolve.[109]

Yet this chapter has revealed that several key ideas, precepts and practices of ancient physicians are still present in contemporary herbal medicine. Albeit in different guises, ancient holism is at the heart of modern practice and therapeutics. Continuity with the past may have been seriously frayed, but is not broken. Surviving aspects of the ancient Western model include the philosophical grounding in a cosmic holism and vital principle; the intention to understand and to treat the individual in a multi-dimensional way; and the complex use of herbs and allied treatments to support and harmonize normal functions while addressing pathological conditions. Alongside current knowledge of biomedical physiology and pharmacological phytochemistry, ancient holistic principles are expressed in a constellation of language that speaks of vital force, harmony and balance, restoration of function, alterative properties, and of cleansing and healing crises. Combined with methodology and *materia medica*, these form the core of the Western herbal tradition, at least as practised in the UK. Whereas medical science has removed a unifying metaphysical vital force from its model and employs a reductionist approach, many clinical herbalists remain committed to a fundamental principle first articulated by ancient physicians: the healing power of nature.

Recommended reading

Dioscorides, Pedanius. *Pedanius Dioscorides of Anazarbus De materia medica*, translated by Lily Y. Beck. Altertumswissenschaftliche Texte und Studien. 2nd revised and enlarged ed. Vol. 38. Hildesheim: Olms, 2011.

Nutton, Vivian. *Ancient Medicine*. London: Routledge, 2004.

Riddle, John M. *Dioscorides on Pharmacy and Medicine*. Austin, TX: University of Texas Press, 1985.

Singer, P. N., ed., *Galen: Selected Works*. Oxford: Oxford University Press, 1997.

Totelin, Laurence M. V. *Hippocratic Recipes, Oral and Written Transmission of Pharmacological Knowledge in Fifth- and Fourth-Century Greece*. Leiden: Brill, 2008.

Notes

1   Judy Pearsall, ed., *The New Oxford Dictionary of English* (Oxford: Oxford University Press, 1998), 867; Henry E. Sigerist, *A History of Medicine, Vol. 2., Early Greek Hindu*

and *Persian Medicine* (New York: Oxford University Press, 1961), 267; Wesley D. Smith, *The Hippocratic Tradition* (Ithaca, NY: Cornell University Press, 1979), 177.
2. Vivian Nutton, *Ancient Medicine* (London: Routledge, 2004), 59.
3. The translations of the works attributed to Hippocrates used here are those of W. H. S. Jones, Paul Potter and Wesley D. Smith, published by William Heinemann Ltd and Harvard University Press, the most complete English translations of the works together to date. Also used are W. H. S. Jones, ed., *The Medical Writings of Anonymus Londinensis* (Cambridge: Cambridge University Press, 1947) and Dioscorides, *Pedanius Dioscorides of Anazarbus: 'De materia medica'*, trans. Lily Y. Beck (Hildesheim: Olms, 2005). The English words given here for Greek terms are based on these works and where it may be helpful to the reader, the author has put a more modern term in brackets. The reader may wish to consult Henry G. Liddell and Robert Scott, *An Intermediate Greek-English Lexicon Founded Upon the Seventh Edition of Liddell and Scott's Greek-English Lexicon* (Oxford: Clarendon Press, 1991).
4. Smith, *The Hippocratic Tradition*, 31.
5. *Hippocrates, Vol. I*, trans. W. H. S. Jones (London: William Heinemann, 1972), x, xi. See also Nutton, *Ancient Medicine*, 30–40.
6. See *Hippocrates, Vol. I*, General introduction; Nutton, *Ancient Medicine*, 53–102.
7. Jan C. Smutts, *Holism and Evolution* (London: Macmillan, 1927).
8. Liddell and Scott, *Intermediate Greek-English Lexicon*, 553; M. R. Wright, ed., *Empedocles, the Extant Fragments* (London: Bristol Classical Press, 1995), 183.
9. Geoffrey S. Kirk and John E. Raven, *The Presocratic Philosophers: A Critical History with a Selection of Texts* (Cambridge: Cambridge University Press, 1962), 228; William K. C. Guthrie, *A History of Greek Philosophy: The Earlier Presocratics and the Pythagoreans*, Vol. 1 (London: Cambridge University Press, 1962), 208, n. 1.
10. *Hippocrates, Vol. II*, trans. W. H. S. Jones (Cambridge, MA: Harvard University Press, 1981), *Breaths*, 231.
11. *Hippocrates, Vol. I, Airs, Waters, Places*, 71–137.
12. Vicki Pitman, *The Nature of the Whole: Holism in Ancient Greek and Indian Medicine* (Delhi: Motilal Barnasidass, 2006), 48–62.
13. *Hippocrates, Vol. I, Ancient Medicine*, 54–5.
14. *Hippocrates, Vol. IV*, trans. W. H. S. Jones (Cambridge, MA: Harvard University Press, 1979), *Regimen I*, 253. See also chs VI, VIII and XVII of *Regimen III* in the same volume.
15. Plato, *Charmides* in *Early Socratic Dialogues*, ed. Trevor J. Saunders (Harmondsworth: Penguin, 1987), 156b–c, 187.
16. For a summary of Galen's therapeutic method, see Smith, *Hippocratic Tradition*, 101–4.
17. Guthrie, *History of Greek Philosophy*, 208–12.
18. Wright, *Empedocles*, 166–7, 181, 205–6. See also pages 31–56. This is but the barest rendering of Empedocles' ideas which are difficult and complex. Several of his terms are echoed in the Hippocratic works, e.g. the mingling and separation of constituent elements as factors in health and disease.
19. Wright, *Empedocles*, 164–6, 181–4.
20. Ibid., 182.
21. Ibid., 181–2.
22. Ibid., 55–6, 142, 208.
23. Plato, *The Symposium*, trans. Walter Hamilton, repr.; first published 1951 (Harmondsworth: Penguin, 1972), 54.

24 *Hippocrates, Vol. I, Ancient Medicine*, 53.
25 For example, *Nutriment*, in *Hippocrates, Vol. I*, Introduction, 337-40.
26 Although the author of the treatise *Ancient Medicine* specifically rejects the intrusion of philosophy and 'postulates' into medicine, his position is that medicine does not need to learn from philosophy about natural science, health, disease and man's nature, as this can all be learned through the study of medicine. *Hippocrates, Vol. I, Ancient Medicine*, 53.
27 Owsei Temkin, *Hippocrates in a World of Pagans and Christians* (Baltimore, MD: Johns Hopkins University Press, 1995), 188-90.
28 *Hippocrates, Vol. VII*, trans. Wesley D. Smith (London: William Heinemann, 1994), *Epidemics*, 255.
29 *Hippocrates, Vol. I, Nutriment*, 347.
30 Pedro Laín Entralgo, *The Therapy of the Word in Classical Antiquity* (New Haven, CT: Yale University Press, 1970), 145-7; *Hippocrates, Vol. IV, Regimen I*, 227.
31 *Hippocrates, Vol. I, Ancient Medicine*, 38, 53-7; *Hippocrates, Vol. VI*, trans. Paul Potter (Cambridge, MA: Harvard University Press, 1988), *Hippocrates, Vol. IV, Nature of Man*, 9-11; *Regimen I*, 227-31, 243-5, 255-7.
32 Ibid., *Nature of Man*, 27.
33 Ibid., *Regimen I*, 227.
34 Ibid., *Nature of Man*, 3; *Regimen I*, 231. See also ch. 9 in which John Wilkins discusses *dynameis* or 'powers' of drugs.
35 *Hippocrates, Vol. VIII*, trans. Paul Potter (Cambridge, MA: Harvard University Press, 1995), *Fleshes*, 133, 135. Although not discussed in the treatise, *aither* is likely to be used in the sense that Empedocles used it, as that elemental form of air associated with heat and residing in the heavens (the author here calls it 'immortal') and also around us so that we breathe it. There is another word for air, *aer*, indicating air of the lower atmosphere which is always moist, as discussed in Peter Kingsley, *Ancient Philosophy, Mystery, and Magic: Empedocles and Pythagorean Tradition* (Oxford: Clarendon Press, 1995), 28-35.
36 *Hippocrates, Vol. IV, Nature of Man*, 11. 'The body of man has in itself blood, phlegm, yellow bile and black bile; these make up the nature of his body, and through these he feels pain or enjoys health'.
37 For example, see *Epidemics I*, 155; *Epidemics III*, 255, in *Hippocrates, Vol. I*.
38 For example, Hildegard of Bingen (1098-1179) retains aspects of Hippocratic humours and qualities (warmth, moisture, cold, dryness). She considers good and bad humours, conditions of phlegm and melancholy, and a herb's qualities as indicating how it helps the condition – its warmth, coldness, dryness or moisture. Wormwood prepared in wine and honey 'checks… melancholy, warms the stomach, purges the intestines, and makes good digestion possible'. See Bruce W. Hozeski, ed., *Hildegard's Healing Plants: From Her Medieval Classic Physica* (Boston: Beacon Press, 2001), 1-3, 58, 65, 101.
39 Erich Schöner, *Das Viererschema in der Antiken Humoralpathologie*, Archiv für Geschichte der Medizin und der Naturwissenschaften, Supp. 4 (Wiesbaden: F. Steiner, 1964).
40 *Hippocrates, Vol. I, Epidemics I*, 181.
41 Ibid., *Epidemics I*, 143, 187; *Hippocrates, Vol. VII, Epidemics*, 5, 183.
42 Ibid., General introduction, li; *Hippocrates, Vol. IV, Regimen I*; *Hippocrates, Vol. II, Breaths* and *The Sacred Disease*.
43 Ibid., *Breaths*, 237.

44 *Hippocrates, Vol. I, Ancient Medicine*, 39; Jones, *The Medical Writings of Anonymus Londinensis*, ch. V, 35-7.
45 Nutton, *Ancient Medicine*, 147, 187, 202-15. See Smith, *The Hippocratic Tradition*, 204-15, 222-33; and for Asclepius, see Emma J. Edelstein and Ludwig Edelstein, eds, *Asclepius: A Collection and Interpretation of the Testimonies* (Baltimore, MD: Johns Hopkins University Press, 1998); Nutton, *Ancient Medicine*, 103-4, 274-5.
46 *Hippocrates, Vol. V, Affections, Diseases I, Diseases, II*, trans. Paul Potter (Cambridge, MA: Harvard University Press, 1988).
47 *Hippocrates, Vol. I, Ancient Medicine*, 51; *Hippocrates. Vol. IV, Aphorisms*, 107, 137; *Hippocrates, Vol. VI, Diseases III*, 17, 23, 29.
48 *Hippocrates, Vol. II, Regimen In Acute Diseases*, 81, 83.
49 *Hippocrates, Vol. VI, Internal Affections*, 125, 131.
50 Ibid., 147, 199.
51 Ibid., 131, 165, 227.
52 *Hippocrates, Vol. II, Regimen In Acute Diseases*, 71.
53 *Hippocrates, Vol. V, Affections*, 59.
54 Ibid., 7-13, 47-51; *Diseases I*, 153, 165; *Diseases II*, 243; *Hippocrates, Vol. VI, Diseases III*, 63, 83.
55 *Hippocrates, Vol. II, Regimen In Acute Diseases*, 71.
56 *Hippocrates, Vol. VI, Internal Affections*, 205-7.
57 Ibid., *Internal Affections*, 207-9, 211.
58 Jones, *Medical Writings of Anonymus Londinensis*, ch. XXXVI, 137.
59 This may be understood today by some herbalists as an 'energetic' approach, which derives from the qualities of herbs.
60 *Hippocrates, Vol. VII, Epidemics 2*, 51.
61 *Hippocrates, Vol. II, Regimen in Acute Diseases*, 111-17.
62 *Hippocrates, Vol. IV, Regimen II*, 329, 333, 341.
63 *Hippocrates, Vol. V, Affections*, 59, 83, 85.
64 *Hippocrates, Vol. IV, Nature of Man*, 17, 18.
65 John M. Riddle, *Dioscorides on Pharmacy and Medicine* (Austin, TX: University of Texas Press, 1985), 107-11. For more on Dioscorides, see also ch. 10 in this book.
66 Some centuries later, Dioscorides and Celsus occasionally give more detailed instructions for preparations and dosage amounts: Dioscorides, *De materia medica*, III, 150.2; Ralph Jackson, *Doctors and Diseases in the Roman Empire* (London: British Museum Press, 1988), 78.
67 *Hippocrates, Vol. V, Affections*, 13, 17, 29-33, 49, 51, 65.
68 *Hippocrates, Vol. VI, Regimen In Acute Diseases (Appendix)*, 299.
69 *Hippocrates, Vol. IV*, 327-9; *Hippocrates, Vol. VI, Regimen In Acute Diseases (Appendix)*, 323-5.
70 *Hippocrates, Vol. II, Regimen In Acute Diseases*, 105-17; *Hippocrates, Vol. VI, Regimen In Acute Diseases (Appendix)*, 295-7, 303.
71 *Hippocrates, Vol. IV, Regimen III*, 393, e.g. an acrid hellebore vapour bath. 'Aromatic' did not always mean pleasant. *Hippocrates, Vol. VIII, Places In Man*, 97-9.
72 *Hippocrates, Vol. VII, Epidemics 4*, 135; *Epidemics 5*, 199; *Epidemics 7*, 409.
73 *Hippocrates, Vol. VI, Internal Affections*, 133, 143; *Regimen In Acute Diseases (Appendix)*, 321, 323; *Hippocrates, Vol. VIII, Places In Man*, 45, 63, 73, 81; *Ulcers*, 365-7.
74 *Hippocrates, Vol. IV, Regimen IV*, 433.
75 Ibid., 343, 363, 407, 411.

76 See also Peter Connolly, *The Ancient City: Life in Classical Athens and Rome* (Oxford: Oxford University Press, 1998), 34, 35.
77 Nutton, *Ancient Medicine*, 109.
78 This aspect is discussed by various authors, e.g. Kerry Bone and Simon Mills, *The Principles and Practice of Phytotherapy: Modern Herbal Medicine* (Edinburgh: Churchill Livingstone, 2000), 22–3; Rudolf F. Weiss, *Herbal Medicine* (Beaconsfield: Beaconsfield Publishers, 1988), 2–3.
79 Pitman, *Nature of the Whole*, xix–xxiv; Cornelia Featherstone and Lori Forsyth, *Medical Marriage: The New Partnership between Orthodox and Complementary Medicine* (Findhorn: Findhorn Press, 1997), 24–7. See also Patrick Pietroni, *The Greening of Medicine* (London: Gollancz, 1990), one medical doctor's account of the history of the holistic concept from Jan C. Smuts to contemporary scientists such as James Lovelock on Gaia theory and Weiss and Von Bertanfly on General Systems Theory. Bone and Mills, *Principles and Practice*, 19–20, invoke complexity theory for understanding the intricacies of holism in the organism.
80 Other features are discussed in Pitman, *Nature of the Whole*.
81 For example, Simon Mills, *Out of the Earth: The Essential Book of Herbal Medicine* (London: Arkana, 1991), 54–161, traces eighteenth- and nineteenth-century herbalists' responses to prevailing contemporary conditions and knowledge as they tried to articulate new theories (using new terminology) for understanding how herbal remedies work. Bone and Mills, *Principles and Practice*, 15–20, continue this effort, in this century, to frame a modern theoretical structure and language for phytotherapy, again based on holism.
82 Albert W. Priest and Lilian R. Priest, *Herbal Medication: A Clinical and Dispensary Handbook* (Saffron Walden: C. W. Daniel Company, 2000), 2–3, 82, 98, use terms such as 'equilibrium' and 'restores balance'; Bone and Mills, *Principles and Practice*, 465, while largely avoiding such terms, do indicate that liquorice 'moderates and harmonises' in a formula.
83 *Hippocrates, Vol. I, Ancient Medicine*, 15, 17; *Hippocrates, Vol. IV, Aphorisms*, 99.
84 UK Medicines Act 1968, Part II, Section 12, http://www.legislation.gov.uk/ukpga/1968/67/section/12 (accessed 8 February 2013). See also Peter Conway, *The Consultation in Phytotherapy: The Herbal Practitioner's Approach to the Patient* (Edinburgh: Churchill Livingstone, 2010).
85 Definitions of these terms vary among practitioner-oriented texts, e.g. Thomas Bartram, *Bartram's Encyclopedia of Herbal Medicine* (London: Robinson, 1998), 16–17, 62; John R. Christopher, *School of Natural Healing* (Provo, UT: Bi-World Publishers, 1976), 50; Mills, *Out of the Earth*, 486; Alan K. Tillotson, Nai-Shing H. Tillotson and Robert Abel, *The One Earth Herbal Sourcebook: Everything You Need to Know About Chinese, Western, and Ayurvedic Herbal Treatments* (New York: Kensington Books, 2002), 68; Weiss, *Herbal Medicine*, 259–60; Donald Yance, *Herbal Medicine, Healing and Cancer: A Comprehensive Program for Prevention and Treatment* (Lincolnwood, IL: Keats Publishing, 1999), 123.
86 Kirk and Raven, *Presocratic Philosophers*, 344–5.
87 Guido Majno, *The Healing Hand: Man and Wound in the Ancient World* (Cambridge, MA: Harvard University Press, 1975), viii.
88 Ibid., 154–5, 176, 183, 185.
89 Riddle, *Dioscorides on Pharmacy and Medicine*, 104–11.
90 John Scarborough, *Roman Medicine* (Ithaca, NY: Cornell University Press, 1969), 162.
91 Jackson, *Doctors and Diseases*, 75–85.

92   Ibid., 7, 79.
93   Ibid., 83–5.
94   See ch. 13 by Brian Moffat in this book.
95   Wilhelmina F. Jashemski, *A Pompeian Herbal: Ancient and Modern Medicinal Plants* (Austin, TX: University of Texas Press, 1999), 2.
96   See ch. 3 by Anne Van Arsdall and ch. 10 by Alison Denham and Midge Whitelegg in this book for more on issues of plant identification.
97   Lise Mannish, *An Ancient Egyptian Herbal* (London: British Museum Publications, 1989); Linda Farrar, *Ancient Roman Gardens* (Stroud: Budding Books, 2000); Wilhelmina F. Jashemski, *The Gardens of Pompeii: Herculaneum and the Villas Destroyed by Vesuvius*. Vols 1 and 2 (New Rochelle, NY: Caratzas Bros, 1979, 1993).
98   Jashemski, *A Pompeian Herbal*, 19.
99   See *Hippocrates, Vol. II, Introductory Essays*, xiii.
100 *Hippocrates, Vol. I*, General introduction, xvi, xix–xx. See also Smith, *The Hippocratic Tradition*, 9.
101 Geoffrey E. R. Lloyd, *The Revolutions of Wisdom: Studies in the Claims and Practice of Ancient Greek Science* (Berkeley, CA: University of California Press, 1995), 18–21.
102 *Hippocrates, Vol. VI, Internal Affections*, 167.
103 *Hippocrates, Vol. V, Diseases II*, 213.
104 Riddle, *Dioscorides on Pharmacy and Medicine*, 97, 111, 131. For an example of knowing correct dosage, see Dioscorides, *De materia medica*, Book IV, 73, entry on thorn apple (*Datura stramonium*).
105 Jackson, *Diseases and Doctors*, 80.
106 Majno, *Healing Hand*, 156–7; Nutton, *Ancient Medicine*, 93, 148.
107 Vivian Nutton, 'Humoralism', in *Companion Encyclopedia of the History of Medicine*, ed. W. F. Bynum and Roy Porter (London: Routledge, 1993), 282; Chandler M. Brooks et al., *Humors, Hormones and Neurosecretions: The Origins and Development of Man's Present Knowledge of the Humoral Control of Body Function* (New York: State University of New York, 1962), 23. Humoral immunity is mediated through the body's blood and fluids. Weiss, *Herbal Medicine*, 257–60, discusses the importance of the state of 'humours', i.e. fluids, in relation to cell metabolism in chronic metabolic disease, and mechanisms of herbal medicines' effects.
108 See the European Herbal and Traditional Medicine Practitioners Association, 'The EHTPA Core Curriculum and Tradition Specific 8th Modules', 29–30, 99–101; http://ehtpa.eu/standards/curriculum/index.html (accessed 16 June 2013). The syllabus for Ayurveda includes study of Sanskrit and ancient texts and use of these in practical contexts. For the Western herbal medicine syllabus, students study the philosophy of health and disease and the underlying philosophies and historical traditions (along with current theory and innovations). It is left unspecified which particular texts or aspects of history are to be studied.
109 For example, St John's wort in Hippocrates was used internally in respiratory conditions, or jaundice (*Hippocrates, Vol. V, Diseases* II, 291, 313; *Hippocrates, Vol. VI, Internal Affections*, 193), and in Dioscorides for pain in the hip (sciatica probably), for burns and as a styptic (Dioscorides, *De materia medica*, 248–50), whereas today it has been found effective for mild to moderate depression and anxiety and is also used for wounds, bruises, neuralgia (including sciatica) and muscular rheumatism (Bone and Mills, *Principles and Practice*, 252).

3

Evaluating the Content of Medieval Herbals

Anne Van Arsdall

Introduction

A major challenge in evaluating the content of primary sources from a bygone age is also being able to sift through, evaluate and in many instances see beyond the mounting pages of scholarship that have been produced concerning those texts, some of them factual and informative, some interpretative and at times judgemental, though put forward as fact. Stephen Harris, one of the editors of a recent volume probing the nature of cultural biases in scholarship and the reasons for them, writes:

> In describing the past to a contemporary audience, one needs to be aware of the distorting effects of one's own convictions, concerns, and ideals. In unguarded moments, one risks projecting contemporary faults or ideals onto the data and records of the past. A past said to be teeming with fools may reveal our own intellectual insecurities; a past said to be teeming with heroes, our desire for reform. Thus do our own insecurities and desires become a part of academic history.[1]

Medieval herbals represent a very old type of medico-pharmaceutical text that has accumulated quite a bit of scholarship. We include in this study a kindred type of medical writing, the remedy book, a type popular throughout the medieval period and afterward though not as familiar to modern readers as the herbal itself. Remedy books, too, were primarily based on the use of medicinal plants and natural substances and were closely tied to herbals.[2] Whereas herbals feature plants and their uses; remedy books feature medical conditions and plant- or natural-substance-based remedies for them; however, to a person of the time, little distinction would have been made between the two genres. Examples of both types are provided further on in this chapter. It should be noted that this study focuses exclusively on texts from the Western European area.

An earlier study of mine demonstrates that for decades, both types of texts have often been misinterpreted, even maligned.[3] Most of these negative assessments are by literary scholars and historians; regarding the herbals in particular, the true purpose of the illustrations is generally ignored by art historians in favour of stylistic studies. Few consult the writings for useful information on medicine, pharmacy, medicinal plants or herbalism, but read them as curiosities from a bygone age. And most readers of these technical texts do not have the inclination or requisite training to try to understand writings intended to convey pharmaceutical and medical knowledge from one practitioner to another.

However, in recent years, a more open approach has been emerging toward the older medical literature, and this chapter joins it in advocating serious evaluations of the content of these writings.[4] Only twenty-first century hubris would dismiss as totally useless and ineffectual a more than 2,000-year-old healing tradition, and with it, its texts and its remedies.

Background and methodology

My initial research into earlier scholarship on the *Old English Herbarium* (a herbal, c. 1000 CE) and the system of medicine it represents quickly persuaded me that many studies are extremely biased. The system of medicine represented by the *Herbarium* is nearly universally condemned in the most disparaging terms, as discussed in the following section. Several writers suggest the early-medieval medical texts, such as the *Herbarium* and its plant illustrations, were useless and had been mindlessly copied. Yet hundreds of medical manuscripts exist dating from c. 500 to 1100 CE. It seems illogical to assume such effort and expense was exerted during those centuries to copy and even lavishly illustrate texts that had no value.

Questions arose as to whether these texts were actually of any practical value. Could their imprecise instructions (so maligned by scholars) in fact be followed? It occurred to me that modern herbalism, the kind that is based on use and preparation of medicinal plants (of which I knew little at the time) might hold some answers. I followed a year-long course of study on the Foundations of Herbalism at the North American College of Botanical Medicine in Albuquerque, New Mexico, USA,[5] and attended numerous workshops on herbalism and seminars with practising *curanderos*, Latino folk healers. I began to read literature on modern evaluations of traditional remedies, on herbalism, and related topics. And gradually, the content of the early-medieval herbals and remedy books began to make more sense in the context of what I was learning.

The system of early medieval medicine and that of traditional herbalists[6] and folk healers appeared to share some obvious similarities, and I began to use what I was learning from the modern healers to try to understand the writings of healers who came more than a thousand years earlier. To the extent that a literary scholar and historian is able to delve into the basics of traditional herbalism and use that knowledge to shape her method of evaluating and interpreting medieval herbals and remedy books, I did. I began to translate the medieval herbal/remedy texts from the original with the mindset that before me were texts to treat human medical conditions, outlining techniques and remedies that had been employed for centuries.

Somewhat later, I was introduced to modern theories that describe the difficulties in transmitting practical knowledge from one person to another, despite modern communication methods. To my mind, these theories applied directly to deciphering the technical medieval texts, whose purpose was to transmit practical knowledge to users. The modern theories explain how tacit knowledge is essential to fully understand many written instructions, a concept explained more fully below. In brief, tacit knowledge is knowledge that cannot be easily verbalized or written but is essential to performing tasks (how to ride a bike is a popular example). I became intrigued with the role that tacit knowledge (actually its absence in the texts) might play in interpreting medieval medical texts, a topic not commonly addressed by my colleagues who study these writings. Apprenticeship of some kind has long been assumed for classical and medieval medical practitioners, but that leaves open the role of texts in training and practice. That possessing some kind of tacit knowledge about the subject might help interpret words on the pages of a medieval medical manuscript seemed a possibility.

In sum, my training is in languages and history; I have only scratched the surface of herbalism and related systems of healing. Because of the role tacit knowledge plays in interpreting technical texts, it has become crystal clear to me that to deepen the study of older medical texts, collaboration of scholars with practising medical professionals, in particular herbalists such as those involved with the publication of this volume, is absolutely imperative. I am all too aware of the superficiality of my training in herbalism and healing. And hundreds of manuscripts and texts in Latin and various vernaculars await and deserve such collaborative study.

The medieval herbal

A herbal can be generally considered a book about herbs or plants, but more precisely for the period of interest:

> A herbal may be defined as a series of descriptions of plants (sometimes including animal and mineral substances) regarded as medicinal, accompanied by medical, pharmacological, and scientific data concerning their names, uses, habitat, and related information.... Such herbals have exhibited a basically similar pattern since the Middle Ages.[7]

Modern understanding of the term tends to emphasize plants used medicinally. Today, almost all herbals are illustrated either with drawings and/or photos, and more or less detailed scientific information is provided.[8] Medieval herbals often had beautiful plant illustrations, but many did not and contained only text about plants and their uses, including remedies and how to administer them.

Minta Collins, an expert on the illustrations in medieval herbals, describes a herbal from the viewpoint of the several disciplines to which it is of interest:

> The medieval Herbal stands in a category of its own. Although its origins date from antiquity it is seldom included in studies of antique texts which discuss history, literature and poetry. Usually classed as a medical manuscript, it is also a demonstration of natural philosophy. It is of interest to botanical historians, philologists and students of manuscripts.[9]

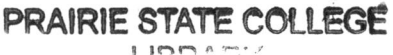

The early medieval herbals and other medico-pharmaceutical texts are for the most part derived from the classical medical tradition, and the chapters in the present volume by Vicki Pitman on Greek medicine, John Wilkins on Galen's (c. 130–c. 200 CE) pharmacy, and Alison Denham and Midge Whitelegg on Dioscorides (c. 40–90 CE) indicate the rich and ancient classical legacy that can be discerned in medieval herbals, and also some of the problems in interpreting them.[10]

The term 'medieval herbal', however, involves two terms, not one, and 'medieval' itself is a concept with various interpretations, a long-standing one being that these were the so-called Dark Ages.[11] In 1937, writing about medicine in the medieval period, historian Loren MacKinney stated:

> It is popularly known as the dark age.... We dismiss with only brief comment, the completely discredited idea that the ten centuries from 476 when the Western Empire fell, to 1453 when Constantinople was captured by the Turks, were a dreary abyss of darkness, ignorance, and superstition.[12]

Though he claimed optimistically at the time that such a tainted view of the period was eroding, 'medieval' used as a descriptor today is still nearly universally pejorative. Thus, it is not easy to sell a positive spin on the concept of medieval medicine or its texts.

My focus has been the early Middle Ages, c. 450–1100 CE. The witnesses to this period, such as manuscripts, buildings and archaeological finds, are few compared with those from the later Middle Ages. (In this volume, Brian Moffat discusses the use of archaeology in studying medieval medicine.) Yet among the manuscripts that do survive from this period are a large number of medical texts, including herbals and remedy books.[13] Almost all of them are in Latin, but unique to Great Britain are three that were written in the vernacular, Old English, before the year 1000 CE.[14]

In the early Middle Ages, monasteries kept alive the herbals and other medico-pharmaceutical texts by copying, recopying and adding to them and, we presume, using their information in infirmaries, though precious little information survives about actual practice and how the texts figured into it. A great deal of their content can be traced to identifiable classical sources – it was a fairly fixed body of information that was then increasingly augmented with information important to the copier or user. Since the classical herbals originated in the regions of southern Europe and the Levant around the Mediterranean Sea and were transmitted through the system of monasteries to northern climates, studies are being made, for example, on non-native plants mentioned in them that might have been grown in the north, perhaps in protected gardens, and on whether native varieties of these Mediterranean plants were identified in the north.[15]

The large number of medieval herbals and remedy books in libraries across Europe attests to their popularity and perceived value (remember also that an untold number of medieval manuscripts were lost over the centuries for various reasons, so the true number that existed can never be known). Though other kinds of medical and pharmaceutical texts are increasingly to be found as time went on, and the types changed and evolved, the herbal remained a constant and is still to be found in use.

Established cultural biases toward medieval medical texts

In addition to misconceptions of the Middle Ages as a dark age, other biases tend to distort modern understanding of medieval herbals and related medical texts. Some of them have to do with the modern concept of how medicine and pharmacy must or should be practised. The medical system in which most Westerners have been raised today necessarily influences their thinking, and scholars cannot be entirely exempt from this influence. The system is in general science-based, involving the ability to perform sophisticated diagnostic tests to identify illnesses and then to prescribe chemically prepared prescriptions for them.

How mainstream medicine is practised in any age tends to influence what the population expects of medicine and pharmacy, and this influences how older – and in today's world what are considered non-conventional – systems of medicine are regarded and how seriously they are taken. Today, many aspects of herbalism as it is currently practised are being increasingly scrutinized as well.[16] The scientific rigour in all areas of medicine and pharmacy that has become prevalent since at least the mid-nineteenth century cannot help but affect cultural assessments of what constitutes acceptable medical practice. In turn, all of this tends to affect the way in which early medical texts have been and often continue to be evaluated.

Important to understanding the prejudice that can be detected in modern writings about older and non-conventional systems of medicine is evidence that it began with several nineteenth- and early twentieth-century British scholars. They wrote that medieval medical texts were interesting yet ineffectual, often appalling relics from the past, and this information was handed down as gospel. In an article about pharmacy a millennium before his own time, S. W. F. Holloway contends that:

> Many pharmacists and most medical historians believe that, in such prescientific times, available therapies did more harm than good. Arthur K. Shapiro, an eminent pharmacologist, asserts that the only link between medieval and modern medicine is the placebo effect.[17]

In the same article, he quotes early twentieth-century historians' terms for early medieval medicine, including perverted, corrupted, the product of ignorance and perversion, and degraded, to name but a few.

With a flourishing new interest in the Middle Ages during the nineteenth century, a handful of scholars (many of them folklorists and linguists) also plumbed newly discovered medical texts and herbals. Their primary interest was material such as superstitions, charms, word formation, folklore motifs, herbal lore and the like, and this influenced the way they were interpreted.[18] The medieval herbals and remedy books, for example, were considered interesting and curious, but not useful in the context of medical practice. Charles Singer (1876–1960), himself a physician, offered a typical assessment:

> In fact dark age medical manuscripts are partly mere literary material and in places hardly more than scribal exercises. They are always unintelligently copied and the prescriptions are often mere elaborate displays of learning. Many of the remedies that they set forth were completely unintelligible to the leeches of the

time; others involved preparations altogether beyond their meager technical skill.[19]

Elsewhere, I have shown how nineteenth-century clergyman and Latin schoolmaster T. O. Cockayne (1807–73) brought such cultural biases toward Anglo-Saxon medicine in his translations of the Old English medical texts and prefaces to them, and how many other writers have not only followed his lead but introduced their own prejudices toward medieval and non-conventional medical practices generally.[20] Their assessments tended to stick until fairly recently.

In an issue of *Social History of Medicine* which is devoted to articles on the theory and practice of medieval medicine, Peregrine Horden provides a summary of current scholarship on medieval medicine, with emphasis on the early period:

> The medical writings of early medieval western Europe c. 700–c. 1000 have often been derided for their disorganised appearance, poor Latin, nebulous conceptual framework, admixtures of magic and folklore, and general lack of those positive features that historians attribute to ancient or later medieval medicine.[21]

Horden covers many of the issues addressed here, with different conclusions, but with an up-to-date outline of the discipline and excellent bibliography on those who are currently working on – and wrestling with – problems in medieval medicine generally. Yet Horden concludes his essay with the following assessment:

> Let us concede that early medieval medicine did not work. It is, to borrow David Wootton's title, 'bad medicine', at best a placebo. To say that is to deny the claims of the 'biological realists', for whom early medieval remedies were copied because they were efficacious. Laboratory tests on Old English remedies provide no confirmation. Instead of looking for biomedical efficacy we should perhaps think, as anthropologists do, in terms of therapeutic success: a matter of overall patient satisfaction with the therapeutic encounter rather than altered pathology. And on that score there is no reason to deny the early Middle Ages its probable successes.[22]

Though not championing here abandoning mainstream medicine and returning to the early medieval system, new evaluations of the medieval remedies and herbals might reveal valuable information, including cultural, showing that they should not be dismissed out of hand.[23]

Re-evaluating medieval herbals: The written and unwritten texts

Most remedies in medieval herbals follow a pattern – for this condition, take this plant, prepare it in a certain manner, administer it, and this is the result you can expect. Parts of the formula may be missing, and most remedies give no idea of how much of anything to use or at best indicate only the most general amounts: a pinch, a cup, a jar. Even when amounts are specified, directions on how to make the remedies are not copious or precise. Medical manuals, or remedy books, from the early medieval period offer the same kind of information. Minor surgical procedures may also be included.

To give the reader an idea of what these texts contain, three excerpts follow. Little obvious difference exists between the herbals and remedy books in Western Europe during the early medieval period because the vast majority were taken or excerpted from similar sources. A few have original entries or observations; most are derivative. Scholars today study them in great detail and can discuss minute differences, alterations, sources and borrowings; however, for the purposes of this chapter, we can say that the texts are all quite similar. Herbals begin by naming the plant (and possibly illustrating it), sometimes giving its growing conditions, and then listing uses for it. Remedy books take up medical conditions, generally in order, from head to toe, giving one or many possible treatments and remedies. As a consequence, the choice of examples here is in some ways arbitrary. One example serves as well as another.

The first example concerns uses of the nettle from a herbal that was compiled from sources in the Mediterranean area, possibly southern France, but ultimately going back to Dioscorides. It was compiled some time before the fifth century of our era, circulated in Latin throughout the West, was copied and reconfigured numerous times, and even translated into Old English before the year 1000 CE. The *Herbarium of Pseudo-Apuleius* was extremely popular from the time of its composition into the early modern period.[24] Samples from two general remedy books or medical manuals follow: first from fifth-century writer/physician Marcellus of Bordeaux (or Marcellus Empericus), second, from the anonymous Old English *Leechbook of Bald*.

Nettle [*Urtica dioica*], urtica, Netele
(1) For wounds that have cooled, take the juice of this same plant, called *urtica* or nettle, mixed with the sediment from oil with a little salt added, and put it on the wound. Within three days it will be healed. (2) For swellings, do the same thing, that is, put it on the swelling in the same manner, and it will be healed. (3) If any part of the body has been struck, take the same plant, pounded, and lay it on the wound. It will be healed. (4) For pain in the loins, if they are injured because something happened to them or because of a chill or anything else, take the juice of this plant and oil in equal quantities and simmer them together. Put this on where it hurts the most, and within three days you will heal the person. (5) For foul, putrefied wounds, take the same plant pounded and add a little salt. Fasten this to the wound, and within three days it will be healthy. (6) For a woman's menses, take the same plant, pounded thoroughly in a mortar so that it is very soft. Add to it a little honey, take some moist wool that has been teased, and then use it to smear the genitals with the medication. Then give it to the woman, so that she can lay it under her. That same day, it will stop the bleeding. (7) So that the cold will not bother you, take the same plant soaked in oil and rub it on the hands and all over the body. You will not experience cold on any of your body.[25]

See Figure 3.1 for an illustration based on medieval images of nettle (*Urtica* spp.).

Marcellus's book is titled *De medicamentis liber*; it is divided into lengthy chapters on many medical topics, with the instructions running together one after the other

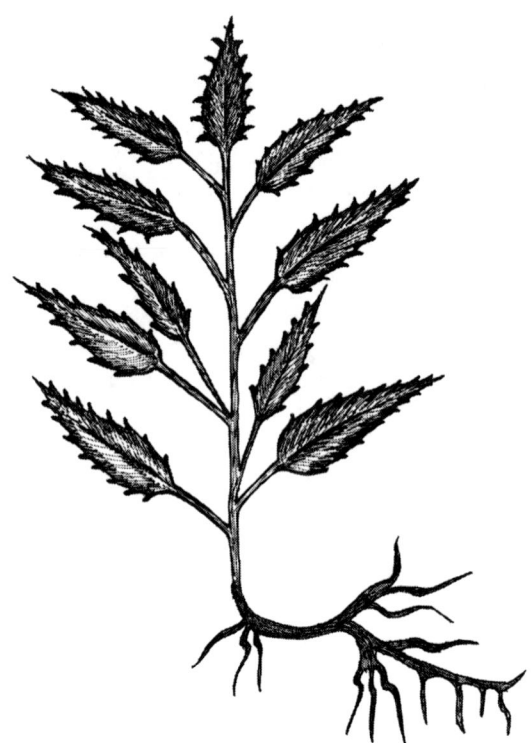

Figure 3.1 Original drawing of a nettle plant (*Urtica* spp.). Based on the illustration of 'netele' in the medieval manuscript British Museum Cotton Vitellius C III. It initially appeared in Anne Van Arsdall, *Medieval Herbal Remedies: The Old English Herbarium and Anglo-Saxon Medicine* (New York: Routledge, 2002) and is used with permission of the artist, Robby Poore, University of North Carolina at Chapel Hill.

following descriptive headings. The sample below provides the long title of his chapter 26 and a brief excerpt of his plant-based remedies. Note that Marcellus generally provides precise amounts in his remedies, something that is unusual for the time. It might be added that his work has been studied more often for its philology than its medical wisdom because Marcellus combined classical sources with his own findings on medical treatment and pharmacy, thus saving in his writings many localized terms that are of linguistic interest.[26]

> From Marcellus of Bordeaux (Marcellus Empericus)
> A Selection of Simple and Compound Remedies Gained Through Experience For Every Kind Of Pain and Afflictions of the Kidneys and Bladder, For Stones, Dysuria, that is, Bladder Pain, Pain When Urinating, and Also For Those Who are Incontinent.
> The following remedy not only heals the bladder but also completely heals internal wounds that are hidden, and abscesses. It is prepared in the following

manner: A regular nine-pint cooking pot is filled with water, which is cooked down by half; then to this is added 4 ounces of mashed asparagus [*Asparagus officinalis*], the same amount of celery root [*Apium graveolens var. rapaceum*], 2 ounces of carefully washed spikenard [*Conyza squarrosa*], half an ounce of cassia bark [*Cinnamomum cassia*], 8 pinches of amomum [*Amomum* spp., exact species unknown], 1/8 cup of parsley [*Apium petroselinum*], half an ounce of Illyric iris [probably *Iris germanica*], and 2 ounces of mastic [*Pistacia lentiscus*] from Chios; after that, fill the pot with water, cover it, taking care to simmer it so the medicine does not escape; let it cook down by half, and leave it in the pot. When needed, administer it with some wine, enough to make a good draught; give it to the patient on an empty stomach and when he goes to sleep. [Author's translation]

Some time before the year 1000 CE, an unknown physician in Anglo-Saxon England set down guidelines for medical treatment in an untitled work that is part original and part indebted to others (including Marcellus), which is now called the *Leechbook of Bald* after one of the healers named in it.[27]

From the *Leechbook of Bald*
Here are to be found salves for all kinds of wounds, and tonics, and purgatives of all sorts for external and internal use. Crushed plantain [*Plantago*, exact species unknown] mixed with aged fat, not with fresh. (2) A salve for wounds: take plantain seed, crush it finely, sprinkle it on the wound, and the wound will be better soon. (3) For old wounds: broken-up groundsel [*Senecio* spp., exact species unknown] mixed with aged fat and applied heals such wounds. To clean wounds: take purified honey, warm it over heat, put it into a clean container, add salt and stir until it is as thick as porridge, apply it to the wound so it fills it. If a bone in the head is broken, mix pulverised chamomile [*Anthemis* spp., exact species unknown] and goatweed [*Epimedium* spp., exact species unknown] thoroughly in honey, add some butter; that makes a good salve for wounds. For the same: a bunch of lady's mantle [*Alchemilla vulgaris*] is good laid on a wounded head, and also for dog bite. For a dog bite, take equal amounts of purple deadnettle [*Lamium purpureum*], cockspur grass [*Echinochloa crus-galli*], and lard; seethe this in butter; work it to make it into a salve; the bone splinters will soon come out.[28]

The samples above are fairly representative, and are provided so that anyone unfamiliar with them can see how they are written. Perhaps the first thing that strikes a modern reader is how much is *not* there. In the first example, what is meant by 'cooled wounds'? In fact, what is meant by 'wounds' (cuts?, scrapes that are infected?, perhaps wounds that are a couple of days old?). How does one obtain nettle juice and from what part of the plant? Any type of nettle? What kind of oil has sediment and how does one obtain that? In the other two samples, 'hidden internal wounds' is an interesting concept: how does a person detect them or know they are present? How exactly will one know the mixture has boiled down enough to be usable? Obviously there is a difference between pounding and crushing and chopping up a plant: does it matter? What sorts of fats are acceptable? Such questions abound as one reads the texts – all of the samples are perfectly comprehensible in terms of the words that are there, but not in terms of their meaning on all levels.

So how should we understand such texts?

The first step is to accept these texts as representing serious medico-pharmaceutical knowledge that is being presented in a written form for someone else to use. For practising herbalists trained to use medicinal plants, the information will not seem too unfamiliar: others may have to suspend judgement. The second step – the most difficult – is to determine how to follow the instructions the medieval healers have left us and how, or whether, to use any accompanying illustrations since they do not appear to us to be representative.[29] It would appear that not enough information has been provided for anyone to be able to use the instructions or illustrations. Or has it?

Since the numerous medieval herbals and remedy books read so similarly, it is not out of the question to assume that they made sense to their community of readers. History shows that these texts were sought out, borrowed and copied over and over: comments and explanations are even found in the manuscript margins. We live in an era when it seems that anything we want to know is fully documented and accessible in a written or visual form: we are accustomed to extremely detailed instructions on everything. Accustomed to such instructions, we see the medieval text as lacking.

Yet detailed as they are, many modern technical manuals and reports themselves also have proven insufficient to transmit all the knowledge needed to successfully complete tasks, such as building machines or installing equipment.[30] A burgeoning modern field of research has been formed to explore what knowledge is and how it is transmitted. Funded mainly by large companies eager to hold on to proprietary knowledge and keep competitive advantages, that which is named 'Information Technology' (IT) looks at communication effectiveness because modern corporations need to unambiguously transmit the knowledge of how they produce their products, sometimes on a global scale. It is a huge topic, far beyond the scope of this chapter, but germane to understanding the early-medieval medical writings because the problems are the same: how to follow explicit written directions for performing a task with which one may, in practice, be unfamiliar (the most popular modern example is 'how to ride a bicycle'). Kneading and shaping bread, practising carpentry, tying knots, repairing lawn mowers: all of these seemingly simple activities involve explicit knowledge that can be written down to some extent, but require a good deal of unverbalized tacit knowledge to be able to do them correctly.

A pioneer in the IT field, Harry Collins, has analyzed such communication problems in detail.[31] Collins found that something was missing in many written instructions, precluding them being complete to the point that a user could follow them and achieve the desired result. What was missing turned out to be knowledge that could not be easily put into words, what he calls 'tacit knowledge', the part that is missing from written instructions. Apropos the tacit part of knowledge, Collins and others are finding that, as Collins put it, 'we can know more than we can tell'.[32]

An intriguing modern theory about the nature of knowledge, which describes it as a spectrum, helps to explain the situation both for medieval and modern technical texts, both of which are intended to impart knowledge:

At one extreme it [knowledge] is almost completely tacit, that is semiconscious and unconscious knowledge held in people's heads and bodies. At the other end of the spectrum, knowledge is almost completely explicit, or codified, structured, and accessible to people other than the individuals originating it. Most knowledge, of course, exists in between the extremes.[33]

In his book devoted to the topic, Collins writes:

The pioneers of the idea of tacit knowledge, reacting to the enthusiasm for science and computing typical of the 1940s and '50s that made the explication of everything seem easy – no more than a technical problem on its way to being solved – had to fight to create space for the tacit, and, as a result, they made it into something mysterious.[34]

In some cases, Collins explains, the tacit involves collective knowledge, unspoken but necessary knowledge gleaned from the society to which one belongs.

It is possible then, to regard early-medieval medical texts as examples of explicit technical knowledge written for users of their time, under the assumption that the readers would have enough tacit or communal knowledge to understand what was written: in other words, a deep-seated comprehension that goes beyond understanding merely the words on the page. Contrary to the way in which modern people operate, in the early medieval period, the text or written instructions may not have been what one relied on primarily in learning and doing, but was an adjunct or an aide. If this argument holds true, it certainly helps explain why the technical texts of the past read as they do. It also helps to explain the lack of many technical documents, even from the late medieval period, as is the case with few exceptions for building medieval cathedrals, bridges, towers, carts, and so on, where documentation is largely absent.

If medieval herbals and remedy books were aimed at a community of readers who understood and could use them, and that community has long been gone and hence is unavailable to help us interpret them, what now? Modern organizations faced with problems in understanding data and machines from the past can call in retirees to help them: we cannot. In the present volume, Anna Waldstein suggests that ethnobotany can help in understanding the early texts. S. W. F. Holloway, too, maintains that anthropologists can help shed light on early pharmacy and medicine: 'It does not require subscription to unilinear theories of social evolution to recognize the potential value of anthropological insights for the study of early-medieval therapeutic practices', noting the empirically rational medical procedures and efficacious herbal remedies anthropologists have observed in African societies.[35]

So far, in this discussion on how medieval herbals and remedy books can be more objectively evaluated, the texts have been considered to be serious writings on medicine and pharmacy aimed at readers with some amount of tacit experiential knowledge of the subjects. It could be said that the medieval writers wrote down as best they could guidance and wisdom for others to use. Now it is up to us to understand and evaluate it – or, as has been done so often in the past, dismiss it as poppycock.

Text and practice

As a textual scholar engaged in translating early-medieval medical texts, I thought it important not only to translate the words of explicit medico-pharmaceutical knowledge, but to try also to understand as much as possible the tacit information behind those words. Only then could the translation be fair to the originals. As explained earlier, because the medieval texts were based on use of medicinal herbs, I studied modern herbal medicine in the hope that it could help me decipher the terse medieval medical writings. In addition, I listened to practising Hispanic *curanderos* (folk healers) to learn about their tradition and consulted related sources.[36] Partly text-based, mostly taught by apprenticeship, the *curanderos* brought their medieval healing arts with them to the New World from Spain. This situation had similarities to the transmission of medical knowledge in the late classical and early medieval periods in the West, and it seemed appropriate to study it in an attempt to understand how medical knowledge might have been transmitted when texts were few or non-existent.

What follows are a number of observations and conclusions reached after studying early-medieval medical texts, such as those provided as brief examples above, and then learning a fair amount about how two related systems of alternative healing operate: this was an attempt to bridge the gap between text and practice. In studying modern herbalism and *curanderismo*, if only in a cursory manner, in conjunction with the medieval writings, it became clear that they share many commonalities. It became equally clear that translating technical texts requires some knowledge, both explicit and tacit, of the technology: in this case medicine and pharmacy as it has been traditionally practised. Clearest of all was the certainty that only with the help and guidance of professionally-trained herbalists and/or physicians could a textual scholar understand the early-medieval medical writings in more than a superficial way.

From my observations, it seems that hands-on experience, including personally making remedies with plants, is a major goal in the training of these healers. Oral instruction is extremely important (including tips and asides), and texts tend to be reminders of what has been learned in practice. Quantities of ingredients used in compounds and tonics tend to be imprecise because the person who is prescribing and/or mixing the remedy tailors it to the patient; however, great care is used in precisely making preparations, such as tinctures. For the modern herbalists with whom I studied, treatment is individualized to the patient, and the plant or ingredients used in treatment vary. That is why, even in modern herbals, several remedies are listed as being good for the same thing. There is no such concept, for example, that fennel (*Foeniculum* spp.) is the *only* plant to be used for bladder pain, or yarrow used solely for wounds. This way of proceeding explains what is, at first glance, a bewildering situation in the medieval texts, because nothing in them advocates one remedy over another for a given condition. Occasionally there will be an aside in a medieval manuscript to the effect that 'this remedy really works' or 'experienced physicians say this helps'. When reading these texts, the question is how medieval healers chose one remedy over another for a given condition, and why. Further, how did the reference works help in making that choice? How much tacit knowledge did the writer assume on the part of the reader?

With modern herbalists and *curanderos*, hands-on training, in some cases really an apprenticeship, is a major part of instruction. For the early Middle Ages, we know very little about how healers learned their diagnostic skills, knowledge of medicinal plants, and how to compound them into remedies. We can only infer this information from the texts that remain. Much more information is available about how medicine was taught and practised in the high Middle Ages.[37] However, these medical writings too are not fully comprehensible in, and of, themselves. If some type of apprenticeship is assumed in the medieval world for learning medicine and pharmacy, it helps to explain why the related texts are seemingly so abbreviated. An unwritten text, or the tacit knowledge possessed by that community, can be assumed to lie between each written line.

Modern herbalists do not always agree on a given plant as being best for any one condition, and each healer tends to have a small number of essential favourites. If those favourites are not available for some reason, or if the supply runs out, or the healer is in a locality far from home as was often the case with medieval monks and nuns, then the reference texts could be consulted for substitutes. Substitution of one plant for another was early recognized as a necessity, and a type of medical text known as *quid pro quo* arose.[38] I learned that knowing medicinal plants, how to make tinctures and infusions from them, how to compound medications, how to preserve the plants and so forth, was a basic part of the training for herbalists and *curanderos*. Perhaps this was also true in the Middle Ages.

Illustrations and tacit knowledge

Some of the early medieval herbals include plant illustrations that were copied from classical sources, and it must be kept in mind that considerable effort, if not expense, was required to include them.[39] The drawings do not appear lifelike to us, but it is presumptuous to think they had to be lifelike for a medieval person to find them useful (look at the lack of perspective in medieval art!). For example, see Figure 3.2. Such illustrations were copied again and again, and they must have had some value. If we assume medieval healers knew their plants in a fresh state, and possibly throughout the life cycle of the plants, the illustrations would have served perfectly well as aides-memoires. The leaves and blossoms as drawn may have been a kind of icon for the plant at that time. Such icons might have been copied over and over through the years because they came to symbolize a known plant, so anyone who knew the plant would recognize the icon.

Evaluating unfamiliar instructions in medieval medical texts

A number of medieval remedies specify that the ingredients be made in a certain kind of container, for example an iron or copper pot. Earlier scholars insisted that using a metal pot was for reasons of magic. But more critical minds have recently shown, on the contrary, that when the remedy was made in a metal pot, a chemical reaction occurred that made it more effective – or completely useless.[40] The directions to pick a plant on a given day, say Midsummer or St John's Day, have been attributed to

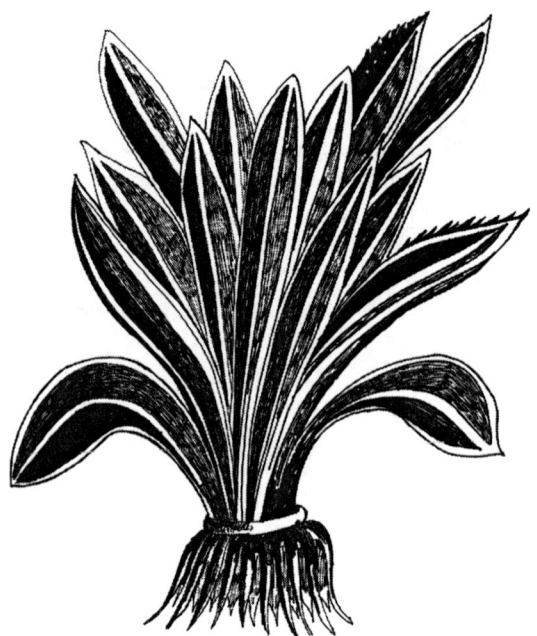

Figure 3.2 Original drawing of a plantain plant (*Plantago* spp.). Based on an illustration in the medieval manuscript British Museum Cotton Vitellius C III. It initially appeared in Anne Van Arsdall, *Medieval Herbal Remedies: The Old English Herbarium and Anglo-Saxon Medicine* (New York: Routledge, 2002) and is used with permission of the artist, Robby Poore, University of North Carolina at Chapel Hill. Note that this and certain other medieval plant drawings appear as though they may depict pressed plants.

superstition. Yet the time of year a plant is gathered depends on whether the flowers, leaves or roots will be used – each is collected at different times of the year. We use a calendar to specify days and months: the medieval texts tend to use saints' days or other familiar time markers. Herbalists or botanists, for example, who are familiar with gathering medicinal plants and roots at several times of the year and making them into medicines or remedies could help scholars interpret these seemingly non-rational parts of the old texts, using their specialized knowledge to help elucidate such material.

It must be admitted that the medieval medico-pharmaceutical writings certainly do contain other elements that set them apart from anything modern, such as charms and prayers, and they are nearly always branded as being non-rational. Yet, understood another way, they could make rational sense. The instruction, for example, to say three 'Our Father' prayers, while lying down after taking medicinal tea, or to sing a certain song while steeping an infusion can be seen, as earlier historians did, as superstition. Or it could also be translated into waiting a known period of time for medicine to take effect or for the ingredients to be properly infused – if one knew the duration of the prayer or the song. Directions to mark around a plant three times with the little finger and the thumb, then to pull the plant out and cut it into small pieces could be seen as a bit of medieval superstition – or as a way to loosen the soil so the roots of the plant would come out more easily. And the instruction found in medieval texts to talk to a plant while pulling it out and asking it to work well is not unusual: some practising herbalists today faithfully perform this ritual. In every instance, while working with the medieval writings, my choice was to assume a practical reason for the ingredient or instruction to be there, and then to seek what that reason might be. Generally, although certainly not always, a practical reason can be found for an ingredient or an instruction to be there, serving a useful purpose.[41]

Conclusion

Alternative ways have been suggested here to read, interpret and evaluate early medieval herbals and remedy books, in the belief that these texts have content that offers information of value. The value may be mainly cultural, partly medicinal and partly a new way to consider human needs. These writings are part of Western heritage and add to our understanding in a very real way as to how humans have coped with our health and well-being, our vanities, our illnesses. The roots of modern herbal medicine can certainly be traced to early medieval herbals and related medical texts, and it is important to make these texts and the related remedy books available in translation so that the whole tradition can be studied (the classical texts should obviously be included). Though many modern herbal practices and texts are much more science-based than those discussed here, there are still similarities between the old and the recent in the way health and healing are treated and medicines compounded. As stated earlier, it would be vanity to think we have nothing to learn from the healing traditions of the past and so-called alternative systems in the present. Finally, it is important not only to be able to understand the words of the medieval writings, the explicit knowledge they impart, but also to strive to understand them at a deeper level, closer to the way in which their intended users understood them. The history of medicine and pharmacy is preserved not only in its written texts, such as the herbals, but in the tacit knowledge behind them. That knowledge can, with creative effort and an open mind, to some extent be regained.

Deficiencies in textual scholars' understanding of herbalism can be corrected through collaboration between practising herbalists and scholars studying early medical texts from a number of eras. In turn, trained herbal practitioners and textual scholars could collaborate in translating the early texts, with the herbal practitioners using their technical, skilled knowledge to help interpret the ancient medico-pharmaceutical writings.

Recommended reading

Bierbaumer, Peter, and Helmut W. Klug, eds. *Old Names – New Growth: Proceedings of the Second Anglo Saxon Plant Name Society Conference, University of Graz, 6–10 June 2007*. Frankfurt: Peter Lang, 2009.

Mitchell, Piers D. *Medicine in the Crusades: Warfare, Wounds and the Medieval Surgeon.* Cambridge: Cambridge University Press, 2004.

Scarborough, John. *Pharmacy and Drug Lore in Antiquity: Greece, Rome, Byzantium.* Farnham: Ashgate, 2010.

Schleissner, Margaret R. *Manuscript Sources of Medieval Medicine: A Book of Essays.* New York: Garland, 1995.

Stock, Brian. *Listening for the Text: On the Uses of the Past.* Philadelphia: University of Pennsylvania Press, 1996.

Sweet, Victoria. *God's Hotel: A Doctor, a Hospital, and a Pilgrimage to the Heart of Medicine.* New York: Riverhead Books, 2012.

Wallis, Faith, ed. *Medieval Medicine: A Reader.* Toronto: University of Toronto Press, 2010.

Notes

1 Stephen J. Harris and Bryon L. Grigsby, eds., *Misconceptions About the Middle Ages* (New York: Routledge, 2008), 2. This collection of essays covers many aspects of the medieval period that suffer from modern misconceptions.

2 See specialized articles on the topic of remedy books and *Rezeptliteratur* in Ria Jansen-Sieben, ed., *Artes mechanicae en Europe medievale en middeleeuws Europa* (Brussels: Archives et bibliothèques de Belgique, 1989); Gundolf Keil and Paul Schnitzer, eds., *Das Lorscher Arzneibuch und die frühmittelalterliche Medizin* (Lorsch: Verlag Laurissa, 1991).

3 Anne Van Arsdall, *Medieval Herbal Remedies: The Old English Herbarium and Anglo-Saxon Medicine* (New York: Routledge, 2002), ch. 2 in particular concerning bias toward medieval medicine.

4 Pioneers in this approach include Loren MacKinney, John M. Riddle, Linda E. Voigts, M. A. D'Aronco and M. L. Cameron, some of whose works are cited here.

5 The school offered a three-year course of study leading to a degree in botanical medicine. It ceased to exist in 2004.

6 By traditional herbalist, I mean a person who knows how to grow and/or identify and gather medicinal herbs, knows how to use them in treatment, and uses a holistic approach toward diagnosis (mind/body and its systems), often in conjunction with modern diagnostic tests when needed. Today, professional herbal practitioners have training comparable to medical students: for example, the curriculum at Middlesex University in London leads to a Bachelor of Science (Hons) degree in Herbal Medicine.

7 Jerry Stannard, 'Medieval Herbals and Their Development', in *Herbs and Herbalism in the Middle Ages and Renaissance*, ed. Katherine E. Stannard and Richard Kay (Aldershot: Ashgate, 1999), chs 3 and 24. Collected papers retain their original pagination and are cited by chapter in this modern book.

8 See, for example, Andrew Chevallier, *The Encyclopedia of Medicinal Plants* (London: Dorling Kindersley, 1996); Penelope Ody, *Complete Guide to Medicinal Herbs* (New York: Dorling Kindersley, 1993); or the classic Maud Grieve, *A Modern Herbal: The Medicinal, Culinary, Cosmetic and Economic Properties, Cultivation and Folk-Lore of Herbs, Grasses, Fungi, Shrubs, and Trees with All Their Modern Scientific Uses*, ed. C. F. Leyel. Reprint of the 1931 ed., 2 vols (New York: Dover Publications, 1976).

9   Minta Collins, *Medieval Herbals: The Illustrative Traditions* (London: British Library, 2003), 13.
10 For a general history of medieval herbals, see Wilfrid Blunt and Sandra Raphael, *The Illustrated Herbal* (New York: Metropolitan Museum of Art, 1979). For a popular, non-scholarly view of herbals from medieval to early modern times, see Eleanour S. Rohde, *The Old English Herbals*, reprint of the 1922 ed. (New York: Dover Publications, 1971). For a well-known seventeenth-century herbal with roots in classical and medieval times, see David Potterton, ed., *Culpeper's Color Herbal* (New York: Sterling Publishing, 1983).
11 For a readable history of the period, see John M. Riddle, *A History of the Middle Ages, 300–1500* (Lanham, MD: Rowman and Littlefield, 2008). For medicine in particular, see Nancy G. Siraisi, *Medieval and Early Renaissance Medicine: An Introduction to Knowledge and Practice* (Chicago: University of Chicago Press, 1990).
12 Loren C. MacKinney, *Early Medieval Medicine: With Special Reference to France and Chartres*, 1937 ed. (New York: Arno Press, 1979), 5.
13 Augusto Beccaria, *I codici di medicina del periodo presalernitano (secoli IX, X, e XI)*, Storia e Letteratura (Rome: Edizioni di Storia e Letteratura, 1956). Beccaria lists the titles and location of hundreds of medical manuscripts for the period before 1100 CE across Western Europe.
14 One is a herbal, a translation of the Latin *Herbarius of Pseudo-Apuleius* (see Van Arsdall, *Medieval Herbal Remedies*). *Lacnunga* and the *Leechbook of Bald* are medical handbooks/herbals. For *Lacnunga*, see Edward Pettit, *Anglo-Saxon Remedies, Charms, and Prayers from British Library Ms Harley 585, the Lacnunga*, 2 vols (Lewiston, NY: Edwin Mellen Press, 2001). The difficult *Leechbook of Bald* is available in the antiquated version in vol. 2 of Thomas O. Cockayne, *Leechdoms, Wortcunning and Starcraft of Early England*, 3 vols (London: Kraus Reprint, 1965).
15 For the British Isles, see Maria A. D'Aronco, 'The Botanical Lexicon of the Old English Herbarium', *Anglo-Saxon England* 17 (1988): 15–33; Linda E. Voigts, 'Anglo-Saxon Plant Remedies and the Anglo-Saxons', *Isis* 70, no. 2 (1979): 250–68. For the continent, see Heimat- und Kulturverein Lorsch, *Das Lorscher Arzneibuch: Klostermedizin in der Karolingerzeit; ausgewählte Texte und Beiträge* (Lorsch, Germany: Laurissa, 2002).
16 In the US, herbalism is not a licensed practice and includes a variety of approaches, including folk healers (for example, in several US Hispanic, black and rural, mountainous white Appalachian communities). Schools for herbalists do exist, but few are accredited by federal or state governments.
17 S. W. F. Holloway, 'The Year 1000: Pharmacy at the Turn of the First Millennium', *Pharmaceutical Journal* 264, no. 7077 (2000): 32.
18 See Wilfrid Bonser, *The Medical Background of Anglo-Saxon England: A Study in History, Psychology, and Folklore* (London: Wellcome Historical Medical Library, 1963); Charles Singer, *From Magic to Science: Essays on the Scientific Twilight*, unabridged 1928 ed. (New York: Dover Publications, 1958).
19 Singer, *From Magic to Science*, 24. Singer liked to use the term 'leech' for a medieval physician, a terribly antiquated term derived from Old English for 'to treat', which adds even more of a pejorative aspect to Singer's remarks.
20 Van Arsdall, *Medieval Herbal Remedies*, 40–54; see 36–40 for an overview of medicine in the nineteenth century when a certain disdain for herbalism was emerging.

21 Peregrine Horden, 'What's Wrong with Early Medieval Medicine?', *Social History of Medicine* 24, no. 1 (2011): 5.
22 Horden, 'What's Wrong', 16.
23 See John M. Riddle, 'Research Procedures in Evaluating Medieval Medicine', in *The Medieval Hospital and Medical Practice*, ed. Barbara S. Bowers (Aldershot: Ashgate, 2007), 3–18; Bart K. Holland, ed., *Prospecting for Drugs in Ancient and Medieval European Texts: A Scientific Approach* (Amsterdam: Harwood Academic Publishers, 1996); and issues of journals, such as *Fitoterapia*, which are devoted to scientific laboratory evaluations of 'folk remedies'.
24 This work has been studied extensively. See Voigts, 'Anglo-Saxon Plant Remedies' and also Linda E. Voigts, 'A New Look at the Manuscript Containing the Old English Translation of the Herbarium Apulei', *Manuscripta* 20, no. 1 (1976): 40–59; D'Aronco, 'Botanical Lexicon'; Maria A. D'Aronco and M. L. Cameron, eds., *The Old English Illustrated Pharmacopoeia: British Library Cotton Vitellius C III* (Copenhagen: Rosenkilde and Bagger, 1998); M. L. Cameron, 'The Sources of Medical Knowledge in Anglo-Saxon England', *Anglo-Saxon England* 11(1982): 135–55; Van Arsdall, *Medieval Herbal Remedies*, which has a modern translation of the *Herbarium*. Several manuscripts containing this herbal have plant illustrations that are themselves the object of specialized study; see Collins, *Medieval Herbals*; Blunt and Raphael, *Illustrated Herbal*.
25 Van Arsdall, *Medieval Herbal Remedies*, 226–7.
26 Marcellus Empericus, *Marcellus über Heilmittel*, ed. Max Niedermann, 2 vols, Corpus Medicorum Latinorum, 5 (Berlin: Akademie-Verlag, 1968), ch. XXVI. The Niedermann edition has facing pages of the Latin original and a German translation. No English translation has been located.
27 This work has been studied extensively, though no modern translation yet exists, only Cockayne, *Leechdoms*, Book III, which Pollington has reissued with slight changes: Stephen Pollington, *Leechcraft: Early English Charms, Plant Lore, and Healing* (Cambridge: Anglo-Saxon Books, 2000). For studies of the work, see Marylin Deegan and D. G. Scragg, *Medicine in Early Medieval England* (Manchester: University of Manchester Centre for Anglo-Saxon Studies, 1989); Stephanie Hollis, 'The Social Milieu of Bald's Leechbook', *Avista Forum Journal* 14, no. 1 (2004): 11–16; Audrey L. Meaney, 'Variant Versions of Old English Medical Remedies and the Compilation of Bald's Leechbook', *Anglo-Saxon England* 13, December (1984): 235–68.
28 Book I, ch. XXXVIII, Cockayne, *Leechdoms*. Vol. 2, 91–2 (author's modernization).
29 It might be added that in medieval art, maps and jewellery, there is use of a language of symbols which we have had to learn to decipher but that the medieval person understood right away, i.e. they could could read or recognize the symbols.
30 For more on the topic of tacit knowledge in modern scientific communities, see Anne Van Arsdall, 'The Transmission of Knowledge in Early Medieval Medical Texts: An Exploration', in *Between Text and Patient: The Medical Enterprise in Medieval and Early Modern Europe*, ed. Florence L. Glaze and Brian K. Nance (Florence: SISMEL, 2011), 201–15.
31 For example in Harry M. Collins, *Changing Order: Replication and Induction in Scientific Practice* (Chicago: University of Chicago Press, 1992).
32 Michael Polani, cited in Collins, *Changing Order*, 1.
33 Dorothy Leonard and Sylvia Sensiper, 'The Role of Tacit Knowledge in Group Innovation', *California Management Review* 40, no. 3 (1998): 112.

34 Harry M. Collins, *Tacit and Explicit Knowledge* (Chicago: University of Chicago Press, 2010), 7.
35 Holloway, 'The Year 1000', 33.
36 For this not well-documented topic, see, for example, Elena Avila, *Woman Who Glows in the Dark: A Curandera Reveals Traditional Aztec Health Secrets of Physical and Spiritual Health* (New York: Putnam, 1998); Leonora S. M. Curtin, *Healing Herbs of the Upper Rio Grande* (Los Angeles: Southwest Museum, 1965); Michael Moore, *Los Remedios: Traditional Herbal Remedies of the Southwest* (Santa Fe: Red Crane Books, 1990); Eliseo Torres, *The Folk Healer: The Mexican-American Tradition of Curanderismo* (Albuquerque, NM: Nieves Press, n.d.).
37 See, for example, Michael R. McVaugh, *Medicine before the Plague: Practitioners and Their Patients in the Crown of Aragon 1285-1345* (Cambridge: Cambridge University Press, 1993); Florence E. Glaze, 'Prolegomena: Scholastic Openings to Gariopontus of Salerno's Passionarius', in Glaze and Nance, *Between Text and Patient*, 57-86; Florence E. Glaze, 'Speaking in Tongues: Medical Wisdom and Glossing Practices in and around Salerno, c. 1040-1200', in *Herbs and Healers from the Ancient Mediterranean through the Medieval West: Essays in Honor of John M. Riddle*, ed. Anne Van Arsdall and Timothy Graham (Farnham: Ashgate, 2012), 63-106; Nancy G. Siraisi, 'Theory, Experience, and Customary Practice in the Medical Writings of Francesco Sanches', in Glaze and Nance, *Between Text and Patient*, 441-63.
38 See, for example, Alain Touwaide, 'Quid Pro Quo: Revisiting the Practice of Substitution in Ancient Pharmacy', in Van Arsdall and Graham, *Herbs and Healers*, 19-61.
39 See Collins, *Medieval Herbals*; Blunt and Raphael, *Illustrated Herbal*; D'Aronco and Cameron, *Old English Illustrated Pharmacopoeia*.
40 For an example of such studies, see Cameron, 'Sources of Medical Knowledge'.
41 Because of space limitations, I omit here the vast but related topics of faith or meditation and ritual in healing. Certainly, prayers and ritual were an integral part of healing in the overwhelmingly Roman Catholic medieval period; Jewish medicine has its own rich history as well. For excellent papers on religion and medicine in the Middle Ages, see Peter Biller and Joseph Ziegler, eds., *Religion and Medicine in the Middle Ages* (Woodbridge: York Medieval Press in association with Boydell Press, 2001).

4

Early-modern Midwifery Manuals and Herbal Practice

Elaine Hobby

Introduction

Readers who think of literary criticism as a discipline focused solely on the beauties of works such as love poems, or the social dimensions of the great Victorian novels, might be surprised to learn that it can also help to establish a methodology for research into the history of Western herbal medicine. A brief outline of key concerns of literary criticism should, however, make the contribution clear. First, there is a founding assumption that close attention to the language of any text can reveal its implicit beliefs and sub-texts that might not be apparent on first reading. Second, literary criticism insists that books do not spring fully formed from their authors, but are the product of complex inter-relations between writers, the publishing industry and the reading public. Finally – and in part as a result of both these concerns – the discipline is inherently sceptical about the connections that might exist between what is said in a text and what happens (or happened) in reality. This chapter will draw its examples of herbal medicine from the relevant writings that I know best – midwifery manuals published in English between 1540 and 1670 – to show how a literary-critical perspective might contribute to the interdisciplinary project of writing a history of Western herbal medicine.

Early-modern midwifery manuals: Four waves

For the analysis that follows to make sense, it is necessary to start with a brief overview of the texts that are its concern. English-language midwifery manuals appeared in several waves. Before 1600 there was just one book, the German-based *The Birth of Mankind*, which first appeared in 1540 in a translation by a schoolmaster, Richard Jonas; revised and expanded in 1545 by the physician Thomas Raynalde, this best-seller passed through more than one dozen editions, and some of its remedies were taken, unacknowledged, into various later manuals.[1] Its 1634 edition appears to have prompted a rival publisher to bring out in 1637 a translation of a similar Swiss original by Jakob Ruf.[2] Ruf's *The Expert Midwife* had first appeared in German and Latin in 1554,[3] and its pharmacopoeia has significant overlaps with that of *The Birth of Mankind*, as might be expected given that both are essentially mid-sixteenth-century works, though reprinted later.

Where the German-speaking world is the first point of origin of British midwifery manuals, the second is France, with a translation of Jacques Guillemeau's training manual for French surgeons appearing as *Child-birth; or, the Happie Deliverie of Women* in 1612. This had its second edition in 1635, shortly after the appearance of a translation of the works of Guillemeau's teacher and colleague, Ambroise Paré, which included a volume on human reproduction.[4]

A third wave of publications was then initiated in the aftermath of the English Civil Wars by Nicholas Culpeper, as he set out to make medical knowledge cheaply available to the general public. His *Directory for Midwives*, drawing on his wide reading in Latin sources from various countries, appeared in 1651, intended as the first volume of a multi-part work on human health.[5] Subsequent editions, in 1652, 1653 and 1656, prompted the appearance of a competing publication, the anonymous, male-authored *The Compleat Midwifes Practice* in 1656.[6] This compilation drew extensively on *The Birth of Mankind*, Ruf, Guillemeau, and on Culpeper's *Directory for Midwives*, whilst scorning all of them, and further editions appeared in 1659, 1663, 1680 and several in the 1690s.[7]

Finally, again in explicit competition with Culpeper, in 1665 someone – perhaps a member of the Chamberlen family who were closely guarding their invention of midwifery forceps – published *Dr Chamberlain's Midwifes Practice*.[8] Based substantially on Culpeper, Guillemeau and *The Compleat Midwifes Practice*, but also adding new material, this book was the first of a flurry of publications in the next half-dozen years by James Wolveridge, William Sermon, Jane Sharp and Hugh Chamberlen. Wolveridge's *Speculum Matricis; or, the Expert Midwives Handmaid* (1671) was based largely on Ruf and Guillemeau.[9] That same year, Sermon's *The Ladies Companion* made extensive use of Guillemeau's manual while also promoting from its title-page sales of Sermon's 'most famous *Cathartique* and *Diuretique Pills*'.[10] The year 1671 also saw the appearance of Jane Sharp's *The Midwives Book*, which drew attention to its author's 30 years' experience as a midwife, but also borrowed materials from *The Compleat Midwifes Practice* and *Dr Chamberlain's Midwifes Practice*, as well as from Culpeper's *Directory for Midwives* and his translation of a work on female diseases by Daniel Sennert.[11] Then, in translating François Mauriceau's work under the title *The Diseases of Women* in 1672, Hugh Chamberlen claimed its superiority to the writings of Culpeper, Sharp, Wolveridge and Sermon, though its reliance on Paré and Guillemeau, as well as on the writings of the Hippocratic corpus and Galen, is clear.[12] Finally, the unpublished work-in-progress of a Derbyshire man-midwife, Percival Willughby, in the mid-1670s, records his reading of all of these and Ruf, as he set out to make his own contribution to the genre.[13] It is not possible, of course, to discuss all of these works in any detail in what follows; anyone seeking to make use of these materials should note, though, their complex inter-relationships and not assume that any remedy found in one of them is specific to the work in which it is first encountered.

Key characteristics of early-modern midwifery manuals

The key characteristics of these English-language midwifery manuals also need to be sketched if their uses and limits are to be understood. Most fundamental is the fact that, in common with medical thinking more generally in the period, they are based on ancient Greek and Roman understandings of the body and on humours theory; because those traditions also relied heavily on contributions from the medieval Islamic world, such elements are basic to the British scene, too. The names of Hippocrates (fifth century BCE), Galen (second century CE), and Avicenna (Ibn-Sina, c. 980–1037 CE), in particular, appear frequently, and anyone familiar with the writings of these authorities will recognize the presence of their thinking on dozens of additional occasions.

That is not to say that the manuals have no connections with developments in medical thinking in their own day. Of specific relevance to the history of herbal medicine is the interest of Raynalde, in particular, in sixteenth-century efforts to rediscover the pharmacopoeia of Dioscorides, which led him extensively to revise the remedies that had appeared in the first edition of his book in 1540.[14] A similar alertness to therapeutic practice is also indicated in the fact that both William Sermon, in 1671, and the author of *Dr Chamberlain's Midwifes Practice*, in 1665, included advertisements in their books for their own proprietary medicines, while Culpeper's *Directory for Midwives* in its later editions frequently cross-refers its reader to other Culpeper books.[15] Nonetheless, all of these examples of authorial engagement with current debates on practice appear in the context of an abiding respect for ancient texts and their recommendations.

Perhaps the most crucial characteristic of these English books, though, is a different aspect of the fact that their main immediate source was not British midwifery practice. Far from being original English compositions, these manuals were translations and recombinations of continental European sources. *The Birth of Mankind*, for instance, in print in English from 1540 to 1654, was based on a German midwifery textbook compiled by Eucharius Rösslin in 1513 from a range of medieval and ancient sources. That German book was designed for use in the training of midwives, as was Ruf's Swiss book of 1554, translated into English in 1637. Guillemeau's *Child-birth* and Mauriceau's *Diseases of Women*, similarly, were written by Frenchmen who could claim extensive experience of attending difficult births. Whereas their German, French and Swiss originals were mostly written by men charged by the state with responsibility for educating midwives and assessing their competence, the primary addressee of the English adaptations was a general reader interested in where babies came from and, perhaps, in self-medication.[16] The likelihood that the books' addressees are not those with medical training, but anyone who could read and afford a cheap text, needs to be borne in mind when seeking to use them as a source for the history of medical herbalism. That difference in reading audience was in part a result of the absence of any state training of midwives in Britain before the nineteenth century. Without a captive readership of aspiring midwives anxious to pass their examinations, British translator-authors and publishers had to spot a gap in the market and pitch their books accordingly. The fact that all these books include anatomical pictures – and a warning that these are not to be put to lewd purposes – is as much a response to

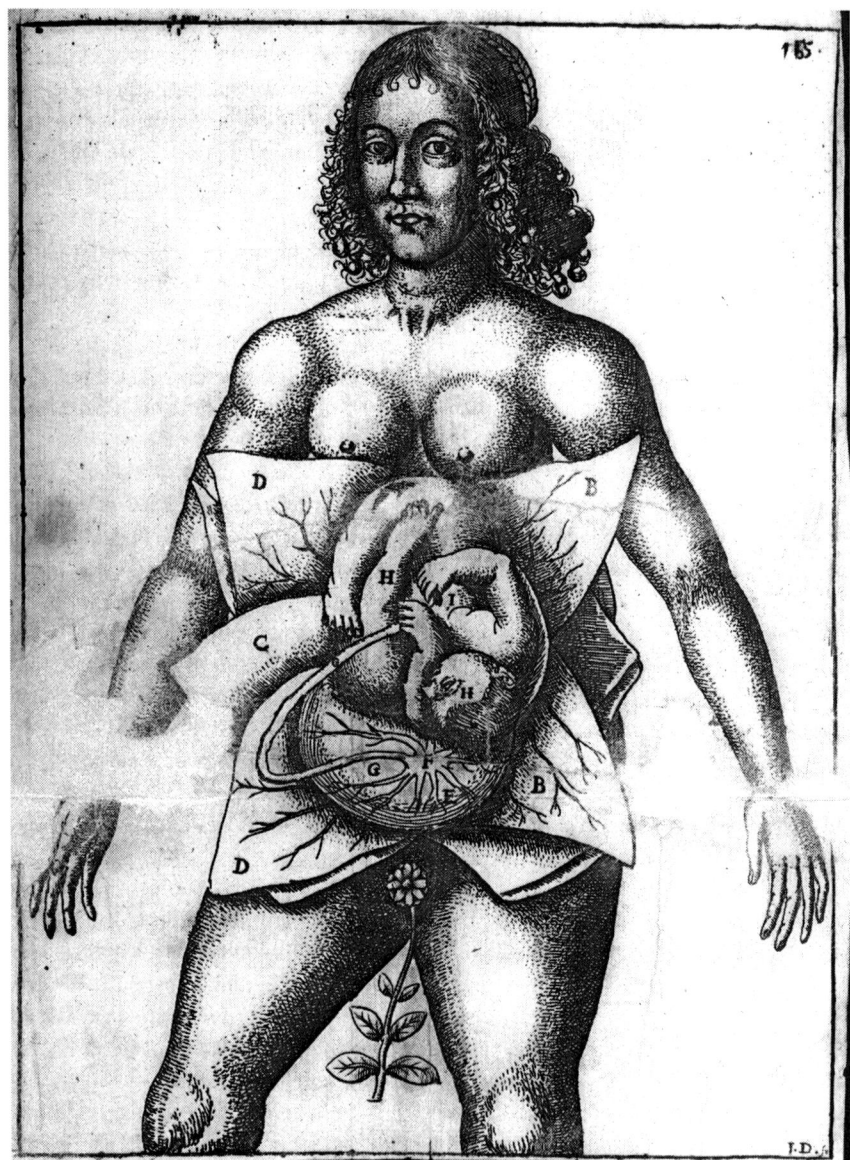

Figure 4.1 Illustration of a woman with foetus in utero: 'Dissection to expose child in the womb'. Illustration from Jane Sharp, *The Midwives Book. Or the Whole Art of Midwifery Discovered* (London: S. Miller, 1671), fold out plate between pages 154 and 155. Credit: Wellcome Library, London.

the interests of the general reader as it is an acknowledgement of the importance that midwives understand such matters. Indeed, it might even be the case that such pictures, rather than their therapeutic advice, were the books' main selling-point. Certainly, the fact that almost all surviving copies of the 1545 and 1552 editions of *The Birth of Mankind* lack these detailed drawings suggests that they were extracted by readers.[17] The anatomical illustration by John Dunstall for Sharp's *Midwives Book* is a particularly appealing example, showing the position of the foetus in the womb of a naked woman whose genitalia are covered – or emphasized – by the presence of a flower (see Figure 4.1).

Whatever their origins, however, all of these early-modern midwifery manuals contain remedies, ranging from advice about such matters as avoiding constipation in pregnancy, through guidance on help during the birthing process, to extensive discussion of such post-natal complications as 'flooding', fevers, and various disorders of the breasts and womb. All discuss how to treat infertility, and some (especially Guillemeau, Raynalde, Sharp) also include long sections on remedies for infants' diseases, which might indicate that their intended general readership wanted a single reference-source combining information about the health of pregnant women and babies. Though in some areas there are extensive disagreements between the manuals about what should be treated and how, they share some basic assumptions: both internal examination of the mother and the delivery itself should be facilitated through the use of lubricants (lily or almond oil, chicken- or duck-grease, egg-white); that the mother-to-be should be given a gentle enema at the onset of labour; and that a drying powder of such agents as bole Armeniac, sanguis draconis ('dragon's blood'), or myrrh, all of which could be obtained from an apothecary, should be applied to the stub of the umbilical cord. It is also the case that all of the manuals regularly refer to the use of pills and potions, vaginal pessaries and anal suppositories, and to external treatments such as ointments, plasters, baths and the fumigation of the sexual parts with therapeutic vapours. Although we cannot be certain whether this full range of treatment types was used in practice, the recommendation of such a variety of approaches to problems is ubiquitous, as is a routine recommendation of bleeding, cupping and scarification (scratching skin that has previously been cupped) as intrinsic therapeutic elements.

The relationship of texts to practice

The question of how far these books might be evidence of medical practice, and so useful in constructing a history of medical herbalism, is the final matter that needs to be considered before some examples of their remedies are discussed. The fact that they refer constantly to the authority of Hippocrates and Galen, for instance, might be thought either to indicate continuity in herbal medicine right back to the fifth century BCE, or, on the contrary, to suggest that such required deference to the ancients might mask a variable relation to practice in the early modern period. For example, much of what is said about the management of lochial bleeding in *Child-birth; or, the Happy Deliverie of Women* is drawn from discussions in the Hippocratic corpus.[18] In 1670,

James Wolveridge, basing that part of his book on Guillemeau, repeated those treatments again.[19] By contrast, in the following year, Jane Sharp, following Culpeper, recommended an entirely different set of remedies.[20] As a result, whereas Sharp in 1671 suggested the use of comfrey and knotgrass, or shepherd's purse and brambleleaves, to stem an excessive lochial flow, Wolveridge in 1670 was commending the plantain remedy that Guillemeau had attributed to Galen. Similarly, Wolveridge repeated Guillemeau's Hippocratic enema of marshmallow-roots and a dozen other ingredients for retained lochia, but Sharp, like Culpeper, suggested taking briony-water or gentian-roots in wine for the same disorder. Today's researcher has no certain way of knowing whether either author's recommendations came from contemporary practice, or from their repeating the advice in their own sources. It would be wise, however, to explore a variety of sources of this kind before deciding which ones to research further.

Some further complications in the puzzle of whether the repetition of remedies from one book to another indicates continuities in practice also appear when close comparisons between these texts are made, as literary criticism would recommend. For instance, as the modern edition of *The Birth of Mankind* makes clear, Raynalde was very interested in research that was going on in the 1540s to correct identifications of plants that had been used by the ancient Greeks (especially Dioscorides), and he systematically revised the remedies of the book's first version of 1540 in that light. He also added a chapter entitled 'Certain Expert Medicines', but very few of those that he proposed are repeated in later midwifery manuals, perhaps indicating a lack of confidence in them. By contrast, there is considerable continuity in remedies for infant diseases between *The Birth of Mankind* and other manuals, but the fact that most of these were taken from medieval Arabic medicine was somewhat downplayed in the anti-Islamic culture of early modern Britain. The chapter on illnesses that 'Chance to Children Lately Born' in *The Birth of Mankind*, for instance, opens by acknowledging that relevant materials can be found in Avicenna and Rhazes (Al-Razi, c. 865–925 CE), as well as in Hippocrates and Galen, but nowhere indicates that almost all of its remedies are copied from the Islamic sources.[21] Indeed, key Hippocratic texts on infant care, including *Dentition* and *Diseases of Women I*, were not used at all by Raynalde (or his source, Rösslin);[22] nor are Galen's works an identifiable point of origin. The careful adjustments that Raynalde made to many of the ingredients in 1545 suggests, though, that he expected his reader to make and use the remedies listed. That in turn indicates that a history of Western herbal medicine will need to be alert to its debts to Eastern sources, whether or not these are fully acknowledged in English-language texts. Meanwhile, of course, the possibility that connections exist between some of the remedies found in these books and those commended in the collections of medicinal recipes that circulated in manuscript throughout the Middle Ages needs to be explored in detail.[23] Only once the particular plants promoted in ancient, medieval Arabic and medieval European texts have been considered can an adequate assessment of Western herbal medicine's history be attempted.

The question of how far an analysis of the contents of texts might shed light on medical practice has a further dimension. As has already been outlined, early-modern midwifery manuals that were published in English are all heavily dependent on the continental European textbooks for trainee midwives (and sometimes surgeons) that they were translated from. If these books can serve as a reliable guide to therapeutic practice, therefore, they might do so more as a reflection of what went on in France, Germany or Switzerland, where the works of Guillemeau, Rösslin and Ruf were used in training, than as an indication of British herbal medicine. A particularly clear example of what is at issue here is found in the books' various observations on the importance of keeping a mother warm during and after delivery. Faithful to his continental sources (Guillemeau and Ruf), Wolveridge instructs, 'there is nothing worse to child-bearing women than the cold air', and that harm will follow if the birthing chamber is a 'cold, moist room'.[24] Believing that such advice is a trustworthy indicator of British norms, Adrian Wilson's much-cited description of common practices turns the mother's room into a 'physically and symbolically enclosed' space, with closely sealed windows and even a blocked key-hole.[25] Both Raynalde and Sharp, however, who often pause in their books to comment when continental practice differs from what they consider to be normal in England, recommend delivery in an airy, temperate room. Birth is 'hindered by overmuch cold or overmuch heat', Raynalde advises.[26] Echoing the guidance she had found in Culpeper, Sharp concurred: 'Keep her not too hot, for that weakens nature, and dissolves her strength, nor too cold'.[27] *Dr Chamberlain's Midwifes Practice*, again following Culpeper, is fully explicit:

> if it [the birth] be in winter, or cold weather, let the chamber wherein the labouring woman is, be warmed, but if it be in Summer, or hot weather, then let in the aire to refresh her, least her labour and the heat cause her to faint.[28]

These differences of view might suggest that the physician- and surgeon-led state midwifery systems of various continental countries might have produced hot, airless labours, and that British practice, being less regulated, was also more varied. The beautiful woodcut illustration from a Dutch version of Ruf's manual in 1616 (see Figure 4.2) might indicate a middle ground: whereas the border around the scene suggests close enclosure, the open door in the room's back wall might imply that the recovering mother has access to air. Whether or not there was variation in practice between different European countries, the literary critical practice of examining a range of texts and identifying their relation to one another certainly prompts greater care over what can be deduced.

There is similar evidence of possible British scepticism about continental prescriptions in some of the ways the English-language texts diverge from the models they translate. For instance, in place of Guillemeau's many pages of remedies that might be needed post-delivery, *The Compleat Midwife's Practice* 1663 edition reflects, departing completely from its source:

> There is great difference in the governing women in Child-bed: for she that thinks to order an ordinary labouring, or Countrey-woman, like a person of quality kills her; and she that thinks to govern a person of quality like an ordinary Countrey-woman, does the same to her. For the stomach and constitution of the one is tender and weak, and the constitution and stomach of the other is strong.[29]

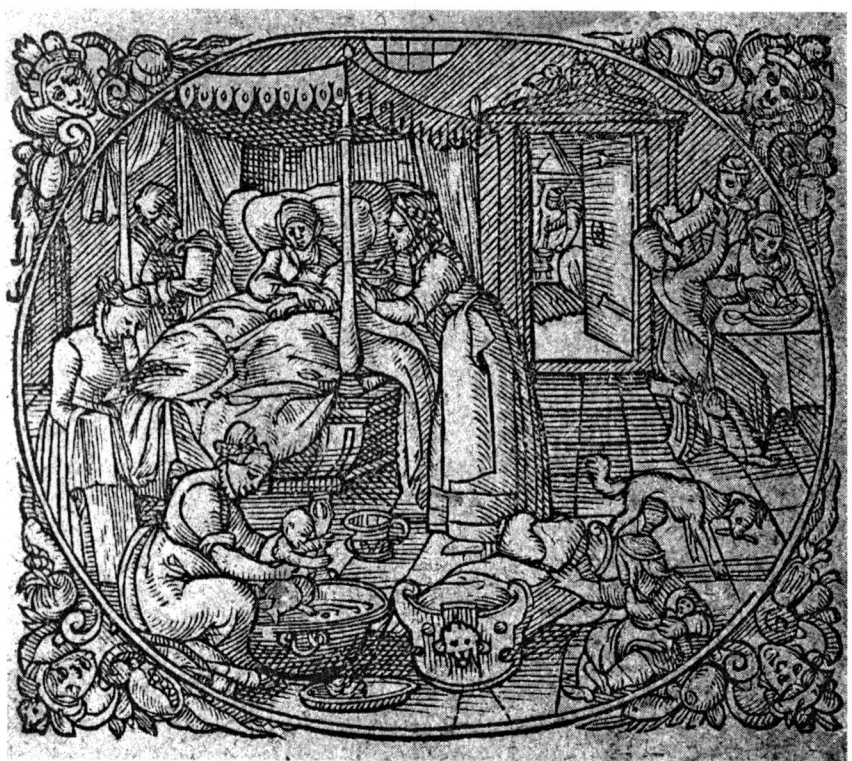

Figure 4.2 Lying-in room showing attendant, child being bathed and a midwife drinking her beer. Illustration from Jacobus Ruf (Rueff), *T'boeck vande vroet-wijfs. In't welcke men mach leeren alle heymelicheden vande vrouwen...* (Amsterdam: W. Jansz, 1616). Credit: Wellcome Library, London.

The remedies that follow in *The Compleat Midwife's Practice* are few and simple when compared with Guillemeau's text. It is notable, also, that the equivalent chapter in Sharp's book, which goes on to repeat Culpeper's remedies for child-bed women, opens by reiterating *The Compleat Midwifes Practice*'s warning that the treatments recommended for wealthy, delicate women will not be effective for 'hardy Country women', and vice versa.[30] Similarly, when revising *The Birth of Mankind* for its 1545 edition, Raynalde suggested a cheaper enema made from 'mallows, or hollyhock, with honey and sugar' that could be substituted for 'a pint of the broth of chicken, or other tender flesh' if the woman in labour needs treatment and is poor.[31] A modern reader alert to such continuities and changes between these texts might, therefore, be able to draw some tentative conclusions about medical practice.

Yet another indicator of the relation there might be between midwifery manuals' herbal medicines and the history of practice is the number of remedies the books contain, and the language that is used. Appearing before Culpeper had effected a revolution in British medical books by translating the apothecaries' pharmacopoeia into English, Guillemeau's numerous remedies are almost all in Latin. Appearing 60 years later, Mauriceau's preface to *The Diseases of Women* observes,

> I have not stuft it with a great number of long Receipts, which serve only to swell a Volumn, and confound their [i.e. readers'] Wits in the uncertainty of the choice of so many different Remedies, composed of Drugs which very often are unknown to them.[32]

It is worth remembering, therefore, that we cannot be certain that readers of these books would have used the recipes. Indeed, in some texts of the period, such as Sharp's source *Practical Physick* by Sennert, recipes are so very numerous that they could not possibly have had a direct relation to practice. There is ample evidence in the manuals, too, of an expectation that some remedies would have been purchased ready-made from an apothecary, rather than made from simples. The advertising in Sermon's *The Ladies Companion* and in *Dr Chamberlain's Midwifes Practice* of the authors' own proprietary medicines is a simple instance of such an expectation. Richard Jonas's advice to his readers in the first edition of *The Birth of Mankind* that ingredients with unfamiliar names 'are such for the most part which are to be had only at the apothecaries', being of them right well known' is another indicator of anticipated practice, as is Percival Willughby's assumption that 'oile of charity' and 'emplaster de smegmate' can be acquired ready-made.[33] Also worth pondering for significance is the fact that whereas Sharp's source, Sennert, refers to the apothecary's product 'sealed earth', she instead calls it by its Latin name, 'terra sigillata'.[34] Given Sharp's more general insistence on writing in plain English because 'It is not hard words that perform the work',[35] it might be that her usage here indicates that the Latin name had become accepted as the normal term by the time that she was writing in 1671, and that any reader would have asked the apothecary for 'terra sigillata'.

Readers and publishers of early-modern midwifery manuals

The uncharacteristic appearance of a Latin term in Sharp's book also connects to another aspect of both *The Midwives Book* and *The Birth of Mankind*. These works declare a commitment to making medical information available to a general reader (for Sharp, especially a woman reader) in straightforward language. This mission connects them to Nicholas Culpeper's allied aim – an ambition that results in Culpeper's work routinely being attacked by all his competitors – and differentiates them from Wolveridge's bookish *Speculum matricis*, and its inheritance of Guillemeau's Latin remedies. This explicit agenda also, though, suggests a need for caution when seeking to use them as sources: these books do not purport to be scientifically objective, but are instead written with a social mission in mind. Of particular relevance here might be Richard Jonas's repeated modification, in his (the first) edition of *The Birth of Mankind*, of Rösslin's advice to a reader to consult a 'wise learned doctor' when seeking to treat any complicated or difficult condition, '[i]f you may have such a one', as Jonas observed (and such observations were left intact in all future versions of the book, despite the other revisions made by physician Thomas

Raynalde).[36] According to *The Birth of Mankind*, a reader armed with this book can seek to cure many worrying illnesses; perhaps that is indeed evidence of a greater reliance on self-medication amongst the English than amongst Germans; perhaps, on the other hand, it indicates that Jonas, a humanist schoolmaster, wished to see a world in which physicians had less control over the prescribing of remedies.

An additional aspect of these early modern texts that literary criticism would urge us to be mindful of is one that has been alluded to by implication several times already. It was not only the books' authors, but also their publishers, who had an agenda. In the era when these books appeared, copyright belonged not to authors but to publishers (usually, the individuals named as the booksellers).[37] Even more than is the case in later centuries, therefore, decisions about what is printed and when, and whether any subsequent editions are updated, were market-led. This had various results, including, for instance, that no further changes were made to *The Birth of Mankind*'s remedies between its second edition in 1545 and its final appearance in 1654, despite substantial developments in medical theory and practice. Publishers' opportunistic attempts to market their own rival title once a book sold by someone else was successful might also explain the flurry of titles in the 1650s and in the period 1665–72. On the one hand, this could have had the result that recommendations from old French, German and Swiss sources continued to appear in English into the late seventeenth century, making it necessary to question the validity of these texts for a history of Western herbal medicine. (Sermon and Wolveridge's reuse of Guillemeau and Ruf are obvious examples.)[38] On the other hand, the fact that the booksellers, whose very survival depended on their ability to judge the marketplace, perceived a flowering of interest in medical matters at particular moments could guide our research. For instance, the best-selling midwifery manual of the seventeenth century, Culpeper's *Directory for Midwives*, contains rather few remedies. Maybe it was because readers wanted these books to include such information that from 1671 onwards, the *Directory for Midwives* was normally published with a 'Second Part', Culpeper's translation of Sennert's *Practical Physick*.[39] Sennert's book was far from new, its Silesian-born author having died in Germany in 1637.[40] It was, though, packed with (old-fashioned) remedies, and perhaps thereby helped the continuing sales of Culpeper's book.

Humours theory and therapeutic principles

Whereas many of the matters outlined thus far might seem to suggest that literary criticism provides troubling complications for anyone seeking to use printed texts as a source for the history of medical herbalism, there is a respect in which the approach can remove a confusion. Literary critics are expected to identify the conventions of culture and genre that lie behind a text, and thereby understand not only how matters are addressed but also the implicit assumptions that have led to such questions being discussed at all. In the case of early-modern midwifery manuals (and, indeed, of medical texts in that period more generally), the fundamental assumptions are those of humoral theory: health is achieved and maintained by paying attention to an individual's balance of the qualities hot and cold, wet and dry, and all plants have a natural capacity to help adjust those relations. In this model, however, it is not only materials ingested or applied externally that have an effect. Instead, treatment must always take account of six factors known (strangely, to a modern ear) as the 'non-naturals'. Guillemeau explains, for instance:

> [So t]hat a woman with child may enjoy her perfect health, she must diligently observe that which consisteth in the use of the sixe things not naturall, which are the Aire, Meate and Drinke, Exercise and Rest, Sleeping and Waking, Fulnesse and Emptinesse, and the Passions of the Minde.[41]

It is because of this framework that all the manuals discuss diet, exercise, and the significance of a pregnant woman's state of mind, and include recommendations also on sleeping patterns and even on where best to live, so as to ensure good air.[42] Indeed, all these books have explanations akin to Sharp's warning that 'change of weather may cause miscarriage, saith *Hippocrates*, when the winter is hot and moist, and the Spring cold and dry that follows it, the women that conceive in that Spring will easily abort'.[43] Once this paradigm and its associated conventions are grasped, it is no longer puzzling that Raynalde should have added to *The Birth of Mankind* remedies for freckles or smelly armpits, or that Sermon should have promoted his diuretic pills as a fertility drug. Raynalde's 'Bellifying Receptes' (beautifying remedies) are offered as cures for humoral imbalances that result not in illness but in 'such things as commonly chance to men and women without any imperishment of their health'.[44] Sermon, believing, in common with his contemporaries, that women are naturally inclined to be cold and moist, but that an excess of those qualities can result in infertility, advises use of his '*Cathartique* and *Diuretique Pills*; for they most certainly expell all superfluous Humidity or Moistness from the womb, etc and not only so, but strengthen the parts, and so causeth Conception'.[45]

Treatment for post-partum abdominal swelling: Literary-critical analysis

With the aim of demonstrating how these various literary-critical concerns can guide the use of early-modern midwifery manuals, some representative remedies will now be discussed. The first example comes from the section of *The Birth of Mankind* that suggests treatments for a newly delivered mother who is suffering from fever and a swollen abdomen. The chapter opens:

> It is also to be understood that many times after the deliverance, happeneth to women other [either] the fever or ague, or swelling or inflation of the body, other tumbling in the belly, or else commotion or settling out of order of the mother [uterus] or matrix. Cause of the which things is sometimes lack of due and sufficient purgation and cleansing of the flowers [menstrual blood] after the birth, or else contrariwise, overmuch flowing of the same, which sore doth weaken the woman. Also, the great labour and stirring of the matrix in the birth.

Then as oft as it cometh for lack of due purgation of the flowers, there must be ministered such things the which may provoke the same; whether it be by medicines taken at the mouth, or by lotion and washing of the feet, or by fumes, or odour, or emplastration, or by decoction of herbs serving to that purpose, or else by ointments and such other things, according as the person or the peril doth require. Of the which things, few or no women be ignorant. And ye must take diligent heed that she be exactly and utterly purged. To this be agreeable all such simples the which provoke urine and open the veins, making free way for the blood to pass, and send the humours and matter downward, as motherwort, asarum, savine, pennyroyal, parsley, chervil, aniseed, fennel-seed, juniper berries, rue, bayberries, germander, valerian, thyme, cinnamon, spikenard, and such other. All those things, as they do provoke and cause urine, so do they also provoke and cause the flowers to depart. Howbeit, as near as ye can, use none of these things without the counsel of an expert physician, lest whilst ye help one place, ye hurt another. Also, to sneeze helpeth much to this matter, and to hold in the breath enclosing the nose and the mouth. Also, fumigation made of the eyes of salt fishes, or of the hoof of a horse underneath, provoketh the flowers. If ye profit not by this means, then being able to bear it, let her blood in the vein called saphena, under the ankles of the feet; for this provoketh flowers chiefly of all other things.[46]

These instructions are present in all editions of *The Birth of Mankind* between its first edition in 1540 and its final appearance in 1654, Thomas Raynalde, the physician who revised many of its remedies in 1545, having changed only one word: the technical term 'simples' is substituted for Richard Jonas's vaguer 'things' of the first edition. It might therefore be speculated that although Raynalde assumed that the word 'simples' would be meaningful to a general reader, it was not a term that sprang to mind for schoolmaster Jonas when he was making his translation from Rösslin's *Rosegarden*.[47] That aside, these two writers share the fundamental assumptions that lochial flow ('flowers') is a variant of menstruation, and that its purpose is purgation and cleansing. Because in humours theory both menstruation and urination serve to remove excess fluid from the body, the very same herbs that have a diuretic effect will stimulate the lochia: 'All those things, as they do provoke and cause urine, so do they also provoke and cause the flowers to depart'. The writers also take it for granted that appropriate remedies might be 'taken at the mouth', or consist of plasters, fumigations or ointments. In a manner consistent with medical principles that date right back to the Hippocratic corpus, they also believe that muscular contractions of the uterus can be stimulated by causing a woman to sneeze while blocking her nose and mouth, and that bleeding her from her ankles can increase blood-flow downwards, including from the womb. That closing sequence of treatments, including its fumigation made from fish-eyes and horse-hoof, is probably taken direct from Avicenna's *Canon of Medicine* 3.12.2.35–6, which lists precisely these treatments in this order.[48] This Islamic heritage is not acknowledged in the text, and the advice passes seamlessly into Western tradition.

On first acquaintance with this passage, a modern reader might be most struck either by the strangeness of some of the assumptions that are clearly taken for granted by both a sixteenth-century schoolmaster and by a physician of the period, or by the fact that several of the herbs listed as stimulants to lochial bleeding are today thought to have an abortifacient action. It might indeed be that these are the most important aspects of passages of this kind. All the midwifery manuals of the period include similar advice, though with a wide range of different herbs listed, and investigating those plants might be a good step in establishing medical herbalism's history.[49] All except for thyme appear in John Goodyer's 1655 translation of Dioscorides' *De materia medica*, making possible an evaluation of their accepted properties at that time.[50] A literary critic, however, trained in close analysis of texts, might compare these instructions directly with their appearance in Rösslin's *Rosegarden*, and thereby be struck by additional thoughts. First, a literary critic would notice that in place of Rösslin's firm injunction that 'one should use these things [i.e. herbs] under the advice of a wise learned doctor',[51] *The Birth of Mankind* is less insistent about the need for such an authority. The 'counsel' of 'an expert physician' should be sought 'as near as ye can', Jonas wrote.[52] A comparable downplaying of the role of physicians occurs repeatedly in the English book, with the cumulative effect that the English reader is assumed to have more control over their own treatment than the German midwife is allowed. Close attention to textual detail, in other words, stimulates further thinking about what relation there might be between what Jonas and Raynalde say and how herbal medicine was understood or practised in their era.

Such a discrepancy comes to seem all the more telling when it is noticed, secondly, that whereas *The Birth of Mankind* indicates that 'few or no women be ignorant' of the remedies that can be used to stimulate bleeding from the uterus, the German source limits such knowledge to 'many honourable women'.[53] This suggests either that women in England were generally more knowledgeable than those in Germany about such herbs, or that the English translators were more positive about female expertise than the German midwife-trainer had been. Either way, there is an implicit assumption in Jonas's choice of words that his women readers know how to stimulate menstrual bleeding: this is general female knowledge, not the preserve of specialist practitioners in his view.[54]

Treatment for difficulties in breast-feeding: Literary-critical analysis

With a view in part to drawing attention to quite how wide a range of remedies is found in midwifery manuals, the second example of what a literary critic might note is taken from Jane Sharp's discussion of problems that can arise when breastfeeding. Her advice opens:

> The immediate causes of great Breasts is partly natural by birth, the passages being loose and large; and sleep and idleness furthers it, and much handling of them heats and draws the blood thither: their causes are not many. It is best to prevent their growing too big at first, for it is not easily done afterward: Cooling Diet, and drying and astringent repercussive Topical means are the best, Binding

things help loose breasts, and make them hard; all cold Narcotick stupefying Medicaments are forbidden, they will bind the Vessels, but they abate Natural heat, and will let no milk breed.

When children are weaned, Discussers and Driers will do well to consume the Moisture that is superfluous. Take the Meal of Beans and Orobus, of each two ounces and a half; Powder of Comfrey roots half an ounce, Mints three drams; Wormwood, Cammomile Flowers, Roses, of each two drams; when they are boiled with two ounces of oil of Mastick, make a Cataplasme [plaster]: or take red Roses, Myrtle leaves, Horstail, Mints, Plantain, a handful of each; Flowers of sowr Pomegranates two Pugils, boil all in Vinegar and red wine, and with a spunge lay it warm to the breasts, and let it dry on.

If Milk be too much in the breasts after the child is born, and the child be not able to suck it all, the breasts will very frequently inflame, or Imposthumes breed in them; they swell and grow red, and are painful, being overstretched, whence hard tumours grow: too much blood is the cause of it, or the child is too weak, and cannot draw it forth. Sometimes it goeth away without any remedies, but if you need help then hinder the breeding of more milk, and try to consume that which is bred; if the child cannot draw it forth, Glasses are made to suck it forth. The woman must eat and drink in moderation, and use a drying diet: if she nurse not the child her self, or if the child be weaned, to dry up the milk, take a good quantity of Rozin, mingle it with Cream, and being lukewarm lay it all over the breasts; or make a plaister to dry up the Milk, with Bean meal, red Vinegar, and oil of Roses, lay it on warm.[55]

This passage appears in a part of *The Midwives Book* where Sharp is drawing extensively on Sennert's *Practical Physick*, and is typical of what she does, trimming and reshaping the German text to fit her own needs. The result is much shorter than Sennert's version, with several alternative remedies being omitted entirely.[56] Other instructions are summarized, so that Sennert's warning that 'Hemlock, Henbane, and other Narcoticks are forbidden' becomes Sharp's brusquer 'all cold Narcotick stupefying Medicaments are forbidden', perhaps indicating that Sharp believes that her reader knows what 'stupefying Medicaments' are. Both writers share, though, an assumption that the 'non-naturals' have a fundamental impact on any physical condition: 'sleep and idleness' can cause breasts to become large ('idleness, [and] much sleep' in Sennert's version). Similarly, since the presence of milk in the breasts relates to the body's overall level of moistness, remedies that 'consume the Moisture that is superfluous' are the ones that will be effective. Finally, there is sufficient detail in the recipes given to allow a knowledgeable reader to make her own remedies; perhaps Sharp's systematic reduction in the number of remedies that Sennert had included indeed indicates a desire on her part that the range not be baffling.

Comparing Sharp's passage with its source in Sennert, as a literary critic would routinely do, also makes evident another difference between these writings as a source for a history of medical herbalism. In forming her advice that congestion in breasts can be eased either by having a child suckle, or by using a special glass sucking-instrument, Sharp had passed silently over a third suggestion in Sennert that also appears in the work of some other continental authors: 'in women that give suck, the Child will draw them, or a Puppy'.[57] Putting a puppy to a woman's breasts was a remedy that she chose not to repeat.

Literary criticism's contribution to a history of herbal medicine

What, then, might literary criticism contribute to the project of writing a history of Western medical herbalism? Fundamentally, literary critics believe that in order to make an adequate interpretation of a text, we need to know what kind of book it is, how it came to be as it is, and whom it is addressed to. Having established such an understanding of our sources, we can avoid coming too rapidly to conclusions about what they might indicate about practices in the past, and start to establish what they show us, between the lines. As a result of their sheer number, and their attempt to address a general readership, early-modern midwifery manuals are a rich potential source. They need, though, to be used with care.

Recommended reading

Goodyer, John. *The Greek Herbal of Dioscorides*. Edited by Robert T. Gunther. Oxford: Oxford University Press, 1934.
Green, Monica H., ed. *The Trotula: A Medieval Compendium of Women's Medicine*. Philadelphia: University of Pennsylvania Press, 2001.
Raynalde, Thomas. *The Birth of Mankind: Otherwise Named the Woman's Book*. Edited by Elaine Hobby. Farnham: Ashgate, 2009.
Sharp, Jane. *The Midwives Book, or, the Whole Art of Midwifry Discovered*. Edited by Elaine Hobby. New York: Oxford University Press, 1999.

Notes

1   Thomas Raynalde, *The Birth of Mankind: Otherwise Named the Woman's Book*, ed. Elaine Hobby (Farnham: Ashgate, 2009). Its advice (or that of its own source, the Soranus-based Latin translation by Muscio) on the management of malpresentation is also reproduced in later manuals. The earlier version was Eucharius Rösslin, *The Byrth of Mankynde Newly Translated out of Laten into Englysshe*, trans. Richard Jonas (London: T[homas] R[aynald], 1540). Readers interested in midwifery are also directed to ch. 7 of this volume, where Nicky Wesson discusses the difficulties of finding sources for plants used in childbirth in early modern times.

2   Jakob Ruf (or Rueff), *The Expert Midwife, or an Excellent and Most Necessary Treatise of the Generation and Birth of Man* (London: Printed by E. Griffin for S. Burton, 1637). The title-page includes the phrase 'the birth of Man', and the dedicatory epistle copies Raynalde, *Birth of Mankind* in opening with the unusual word 'Albeit'. These details suggest direct competition with the 1634 *Birth of*

Mankind. Perhaps the appearance in this year of a petition from midwives resisting Peter Chamberlen's attempt to control their licensing was also a factor in the appearance of these books at that time. See Helen King, 'Chamberlen, Peter (1601–1683)', *Oxford Dictionary of National Biography* (Oxford: Oxford University Press, 2004); online ed., May 2012, http://www.oxforddnb.com/view/article/5067 (accessed 27 June 2013).

3   See Hildegard E. Keller and Hubert Steinke, 'Jakob Ruf's *Trostbüchlein* and *De Conceptu* (Zürich, 1554): A Textbook for Midwives and Physicians', in *Scholarly Knowledge: Textbooks in Early Modern Europe*, ed. Emidio Campi et al. (Geneva: Librairie Droz, 2008), 307–32.

4   Ambroise Paré, *The Workes*, trans. Thomas Johnson (London: Printed by Thomas Cotes and R. Young, 1634); Jacques Guillemeau, *Child-birth, or, the Happie Deliverie of Women* (London: A. Hatfield, 1612), 2nd ed., *Child-birth; or, the Happy Delivery of Women* (London: Anne Griffin, for Ioyce Norton, and Richard Whitaker, 1635).

5   Nicholas Culpeper, *A Directory for Midwives or, a Guide for Women, in Their Conception, Bearing, and Suckling Their Children* (London: Printed by Peter Cole, 1651); subsequent editions appeared in 1652, 1653, 1656, 1660, 1662, 1668, 1671, 1675, 1676, 1681, 1684, 1693 and 1700, and many more thereafter. His plan that this be the first of many works on health is declared in his dedicatory epistle to the first edition. For more on Culpeper, see also ch. 5 in this book.

6   *The Compleat Midwifes Practice... By T.C. I.D. M.S. T.B. Practitioners* (London: Printed for Nathaniel Brooke at the Angell in Cornhill, 1656); subsequent editions in 1659, 1663 and 1680. Quotations in this chapter are from the 1663 edition entitled *The Compleat Midwife's Practice* (book title with an apostrophe). There is no reason to believe that this compilation is by midwives, despite wishful thinking in Doreen Evenden, *The Midwives of Seventeenth-Century London* (Cambridge: Cambridge University Press, 2000), 8–11. Perhaps a member of the Chamberlen family was involved; see below.

7   It also included a selection from case studies originally published in French by midwife Louise Bourgeois in *Observations diuerses, sur la sterilité, perte de fruict, foecondité, accouchements, et Maladies des femmes* (Paris: A. Sougrain, 1609); and from 1663 some remedies attributed to the king's physician-in-ordinary, Theodore de Mayerne.

8   *Dr. Chamberlain's Midwifes Practice* (London: Printed for Thomas Rooks, 1665). For possible candidates as author, see Helen King, 'Chamberlen family (per. c. 1600–c. 1730)', in *Oxford Dictionary of National Biography* (Oxford: Oxford University Press, 2004); http://www.oxforddnb.com/view/article/58754 (accessed 27 June 2013).

9   James Wolveridge, *Speculum matricis; or, the Expert Midwives Handmaid* (London: Printed by E. Okes, sold by Rowland Reynolds, 1671). This had first appeared the previous year as *Speculum matricis hybernicum; or, the Irish Midwives Handmaid*, but reference to Ireland was removed from the title page, perhaps because that association with Wolveridge's place of residence was thought to be hampering its sales.

10 William Sermon, *The Ladies Companion or the English Midwife* (London: Edward Thomas, 1671).

11 Jane Sharp, *The Midwives Book, or, the Whole Art of Midwifry Discovered*, ed. Elaine Hobby (New York: Oxford University Press, 1999). Daniel Sennert's *Practical Physick* first appeared in English as Daniel Sennert, *Practical Physick*, trans. Nicholas

Culpeper (London: Printed by Peter Cole and Edward Cole, 1661). Other editions followed, especially with Sennert's book presented as 'The Second Part' of Culpeper, *Directory for Midwives* from 1668. References in this chapter are to the 1668 edition. Some of Sharp's borrowings from Sennert and other manuals are indicated in the footnotes to the modern edition.

12 François Mauriceau, *The Diseases of Women with Child*, trans. Hugh Chamberlen (London: Printed by John Darby, sold by R. Clavel, W. Cooper, Benjamin Billingsley and W. Cadman, 1672); reissued the following year under the title *The Accomplisht Midwife* (London: J. Darby for B. Billingsley, 1673).

13 Willughby's unfinished manuscript drafts of two books were finally published as Percival Willughby, *Observations in Midwifery: As Also the Country Midwifes Opusculum or Vade Mecum*, ed. Henry Blenkinsop (Warwick: H. T. Cooke, 1863).

14 See the modern edition of *Birth of Mankind* for specific revisions made by Raynalde in the light of these changes. New understandings of human anatomy are discussed in all of the manuals after 1545.

15 Sermon's pills are not only referred to on the title page of his book, but also recommended at key moments of his book as certain cures for amenorrhoea and related conditions (A4ᵛ, 15, 17, 34, 56, 84, 137, 203). The advertisements section that precedes *Dr. Chamberlain's Midwifes Practice* indicates that 'An excellent powder, to procure the easie delivery in Childe-bearing women, being a secret of the Authors' can be bought at the same shop of Thomas Rooke where the manual itself can be purchased (A4).

16 Willughby's decision, when working on his *Observations in Midwifery*, to focus on 'handy operation' and not 'meddle with diseases, or medicines' might have depressed his sales had his book ever been completed.

17 The only perfect copy of the 1545 edition of *Birth of Mankind* is in the Wellcome Library. The text refers in detail to the pictures, making it most unlikely that the book was intended to appear without them. See 'Introduction', in Raynalde, *Birth of Mankind*, xxvii–xxx.

18 Guillemeau, *Child-birth* (1612), 222–32.
19 Wolveridge, *Speculum matricis*, 117–20.
20 Sharp, *Midwives Book*, 179–80; compare Culpeper, *Directory for Midwives*, 149–51.
21 Raynalde, *Birth of Mankind*, 161–84.
22 Hippocrates, 'Dentition', in *Hippocrate. Vol. 13 Des lieux dans l'homme [and other works]*, trans. Robert Joly (Paris: Belles Lettres, 1978); Hippocrates, 'Diseases of Women I', in Emile Littré, ed., *Oeuvres complètes d'Hippocrate*. Vol. 8 (Paris: J. B. Baillière, 1839[–1861]).
23 An excellent starting-point for research into medieval manuscript sources is Monica H. Green, ed., *The Trotula: A Medieval Compendium of Women's Medicine* (Philadelphia: University of Pennsylvania Press, 2001).
24 Wolveridge, *Speculum matricis*, 31 and 116; see also Paré, *Works*, 612–13.
25 Adrian Wilson, *The Making of Man-Midwifery: Childbirth in England, 1660–1770* (Cambridge, MA: Harvard University Press, 1995), 26.
26 Raynalde, *Birth of Mankind*, 101.
27 Sharp, *Midwives Book*, 176.
28 *Dr. Chamberlain's Midwifes Practice*, 120.
29 Guillemeau, *Child-birth* (1612), 189–209; *Compleat Midwife's Practice* (1663), 114.
30 Sharp, *Midwives Book*, 175.
31 Raynalde, *Birth of Mankind*, 104.

32 Mauriceau, *Diseases of Women*, sig. A7ᵛ.
33 Raynalde, *Birth of Mankind*, 208; see also 122, 130; Willughby, *Observations in Midwifery*, 39.
34 Sennert, *Practical Physick*, 208; Sharp, *Midwives Book*, 251.
35 Sharp, *Midwives Book*, 12.
36 See 'Introduction', in Raynalde, *Birth of Mankind*, xxxi–xxxii.
37 See John Barnard, D. F. McKenzie and Maureen Bell, eds., *The Cambridge History of the Book in Britain. Vol. 4, 1557–1695* (Cambridge: Cambridge University Press, 2002).
38 For instance, the first 25 pages of Wolveridge's book, *Speculum matricis*, provide a synopsis of Ruf, *Expert Midwife*, 1–80; most of Sermon's remedies are copied from Guillemeau, *Child-birth* (1612).
39 See, for instance, the editions of Culpeper, *Directory for Midwives*, in 1671, 1675, 1681 and 1695.
40 See the Worth Library, 'Daniel Sennert at the University of Wittenberg', http://www.alchemyandchemistry.edwardworthlibrary.ie/Chymistry-at-the-Universities/Wittenberg (accessed 13 May 2013).
41 Guillemeau, *Child-birth* (1612), 18. See also Vivian Nutton, 'Humoralism', in *Companion Encyclopedia of the History of Medicine*, ed. W. F. Bynum and Roy Porter (London: Routledge, 1993), 281–91.
42 See, for instance, Ruf, *Expert Midwife*, 67–9; repeated Wolveridge, *Speculum matricis*, 110; Sermon, *Ladies Companion*, 36. Related disquisitions also appear in Sharp, *Midwives Book*, 153, and in *Dr. Chamberlain's Midwifes Practice*, 107–8.
43 Citing Hippocrates, *Aphorisms* 5.12, Sharp, *Midwives Book*, 171.
44 Raynalde, *Birth of Mankind*, 197–202.
45 Sermon, *Ladies Companion*, 15.
46 Raynalde, *Birth of Mankind*, 124–5.
47 Jonas translated Rösslin's *De partu hominis* to create *The Birth of Mankind*. That Latin version of Rösslin's work was itself a translation, Rösslin's book having been published in German in 1513. For full details of these relationships, see 'Introduction', in Raynalde, *Birth of Mankind*.
48 Avicenna, *Liber tertius naturalium. De generatione et corruptione*, trans. S. van Riet and introduction by Gérard Verbeke (Leiden: Brill, 1987).
49 See also remedies to stimulate the lochia in Ruf, *Expert Midwife*, 92–5; Wolveridge, *Speculum matricis*, 117 (taken direct from Guillemeau, *Child-birth* (1612), 231, as is Sermon, *Ladies Companion*, 156); Mauriceau, *Diseases of Women*, 330.
50 John Goodyer, *The Greek Herbal of Dioscorides*, ed. Robert T. Gunther (Oxford: Oxford University Press, 1934). See Raynalde, *Birth of Mankind*, 'Medical Glossary', for a key locating these simples in Goodyer's translation.
51 Rösslin's *Rosegarden* was translated into English in 1994 by Wendy Arons as *When Midwifery Became the Male Physician's Province: The Sixteenth Century Handbook: The Rose Garden for Pregnant Women and Midwives* (London: McFarland, 1994), and that edition is the source of all quotations from the German book. It should be noted, when comparing it with Raynalde, *Birth of Mankind*, that Jonas's source was not the German work but a Latin translation. My edition of Raynalde, *Birth of Mankind*, draws attention to significant discrepancies between the German and Latin versions. This passage in Arons, *When Midwifery Became*, 72.
52 Raynalde, *Birth of Mankind*, 125.
53 Arons, *When Midwifery Became*, 72.

54 Midwifery manuals often warn their readers not to use uterine stimulants to cause miscarriage. See, for instance, Raynalde's 'Prologue to the Women Readers' that he added in 1545 to Raynalde, *Birth of Mankind*, 18; Sharp, *Midwives Book*, 221; Culpeper, *Directory for Midwives*, 78; Louise Bourgeois in *Compleat Midwife's Practice* (1663), 24–5; Ruf, *Expert Midwife*, 59–61. Jonas is unusual in stating his belief that women have such knowledge in any case.
55 Sharp, *Midwives Book*, 249–50.
56 See Sennert, *Practical Physick*, 204–8.
57 Sennert, *Practical Physick*, 206. See similar advice in Guillemeau, *Child-birth* (1612), 18; Pare, *Workes*, 613.

5

An Anatomy of *The English Physitian*

Graeme Tobyn

Introduction

In 1652, Nicholas Culpeper (1616–54) released his most famous work, *The English Physitian: Or, an Astrologo-Physical Discourse of the Vulgar Herbs of This Nation: Being a Compleat Method of Physick.*[1] It has been described as 'one of the most popular and enduring books in publishing history, perhaps the non-religious book in English to remain longest in continuous print'.[2]

In this chapter I aim to provide a detailed dissection or 'anatomy' of the structure and contents of the *English Physitian* with a particular emphasis on the origins and relationships between elements of the text. First, I will outline the approach that Culpeper used in producing texts for publication, and the various editions of the *English Physitian* made available. Second, I consider how historical writers have portrayed Culpeper. Third, I examine the Culpeper texts compared with those of John Parkinson (c. 1567–1650) and discuss similarities and differences and argue that past scholarship has mistakenly portrayed Culpeper's text as an original work. A detailed examination of the astrological provenance of the *English Physitian* lies outside the focus of this chapter, although some brief comments are warranted; rather, I will explore here some of the herbal content that offers an understanding of the overall construction of the work. My central contention is that, contrary to current scholarship which views the *English Physitian* as original and drawing on a range of earlier authorities, the majority of the herbal entries are directly obtained from the work of the apothecary and Royal Herbalist to Charles I, John Parkinson.[3] These findings are based on a comparative study of a sample of the entries in the *English Physitian* (1652) and its swiftly released, expanded second edition the *English Physitian Enlarged* (1653) with those same herbs in John Parkinson's *Theatrum botanicum: The Theater of Plants* (1640)[4] and, to a lesser extent, his *Paradisi in sole paradisus terrestris* (1629).[5] This borrowing from the works of Parkinson was recognized in the seventeenth century by at least one reader who wrote, 'This booke was collected out of Parkinson's herball' on the title page of a pirated edition of the *English Physitian*.[6]

Culpeper's texts and his approach to publications

Culpeper's identification of a single source from which to fashion a useful text in English was his usual way of working, in an age when copyright did not exist and publishers obtained works through a variety of means to maximize their profits from sales. The *Pharmacopoeia Londinensis* of the College of Physicians was one such source which was translated by Culpeper from Latin into English with explanations, controversially acerbic comments and his own additions to form *A Physical Directory* (1649), his first entry into print which had an immediate impact, enjoyed large sales and brought him immediate fame.[7] Further works followed and his translation of Galen's *Ars medica* appeared as *Galen's Art of Physick* (1652), and works of the astrologers Abraham ibn Ezra (c. 1089–1164) and Noel Duret (1590–1650) were rendered into English, commented on and expanded in *Semeiotica Uranica* (1651).[8] Culpeper's enemies proposed that his *A Directory for Midwives* (1651) was founded upon the work of Papius and others[9] although he had not acknowledged this. In the *English Physitian*, Parkinson appears on a list of sources entitled 'authors made use of in this treatise',[10] although, as we will see, this list, a roll call of the standard medical authorities, actually reflected the names excised in Culpeper's editing of Parkinson's herbal entries. Parkinson's *Theatrum botanicum*, like *The Herbal, or Generall Historie of Plantes* (1597)[11] of John Gerard (c. 1545–1612), barber-surgeon, one time curator of the Chelsea Physic Garden and 'herbarist' to James I, was an expensive, large and copiously illustrated folio. It contained more than 1,700 pages describing over 3,800 plants known to European writers. Parkinson's friend, the botanist and translator of Dioscorides, John Goodyer (c. 1592–1664), had purchased a copy on 24 August 1640 for 36 shillings plus three shillings for the binding.[12] Praise for Parkinson's magnum opus is revealed in Culpeper's foreword in *A Physical Directory*:

> It is a base dishonourable unworthy part of the Colledg of Physitians of London to train up the people in such ignorance that they should not be able to know what the Herbs in their Garden are good for; both Gerrhard's *Herbal*, and Parkinson's which is an hundred times better, being of such a price, that a poor man is not able to buy them.[13]

This praise was set alongside Culpeper's claimed purpose in reproducing knowledge from the best English herbals in a cheap and thus accessible form.

Editions of the *English Physitian*

Culpeper's *English Physitian* was a small folio of 158 numbered pages without pictures, sold for 3d, the price of a pound of sweet almonds[14] and about 150 times cheaper than *Theatrum botanicum*. The version of Culpeper's herbal that continued to be reprinted after his early death, and for centuries to come, originated with the second, expanded octavo edition of the work *The English Physitian Enlarged: with Three Hundred and Sixty Nine Medicines, Made of English Herbs*, which appeared within a year of the first edition. This enlarged edition included 46 new herbs (and the removal of one, apples)[15] which brought the total number of entries to 328. Since at least 10 per cent of the entries in both editions discuss two or occasionally three native species under one name, the total number of herbal medicines described in the text could without difficulty be made to attain the 369 medicines stated in the sub-title of the work. Editions of 'Culpeper's herbal' were still being issued into the twenty-first century.[16] A census of the surviving copies of the works of Culpeper, including his herbal, their provenance and analysis of changes to the text over the past three centuries of editions has still to be undertaken.[17] For instance, a section in the *English Physitian* on 'Directions' for gathering simples and making medicines is also reproduced in modern editions but in an abbreviated form, lacking a horoscope example in the last chapter. I have not found this astrological judgement, which Culpeper called 'the Key of the Work',[18] in editions of Culpeper's herbal issued after 1665, the year of the death of Culpeper's main publisher, Peter Cole, who shared his radical political and religious views.[19]

Culpeper in the eyes of historians

Culpeper's reputation among historians of medicine in the past has not been high. As an apprenticed apothecary who abandoned his training on the eve of the English Civil War to set himself up as a physician, practising illegally in London, he attracted strong condemnation from supporters of the College for his unsolicited translation of the *Pharmacopoeia Londinensis* and has long since been dubbed a quack.[20]

Even when the *English Physitian* came under scrutiny by writers in the twentieth century who were interested in, or sympathetic to, the use of herbal medicine, the work did not find a place alongside other notable English herbals of the sixteenth and seventeenth centuries. Agnes Arber (1879-1960) in her *Herbals, Their Origin and Evolution: A Chapter in the History of Botany 1470-1670*,[21] still the standard work in English on the history of herbals, approached the materials from the botanical point of view and left untouched the medical aspect of the herbals which she consulted, due to her lack of expertise in the area.[22] She felt able, however, to contrast 'the works of the genuine herbalists of the sixteenth and seventeenth centuries', principally the works of William Turner (c. 1508-68), *A New Herball*, Gerard's *Herball* and John Parkinson, with contemporary books that dealt with what she regarded as pseudo-scientific themes of the doctrine of signatures and botanical astrology.[23] It is here that we find Culpeper, the 'most notorious exponent' of this astrological botany, with which 'England became badly infected' in the seventeenth century, alongside William Coles (1626-62), 'a keen and enthusiastic collector of herbs' who carried the doctrine of signatures to its extreme in his writings.[24] Culpeper's most recent biographer, Benjamin Woolley, has suggested that Arber thought the *English Physitian* a mystical work on account of its astrological content. In comparison, Coles, who was critical himself of Culpeper's insistence on the necessity of astrology to physicians, must have seemed to Arber as more grounded among the plants he discussed. Indeed Coles expressed his own view of Culpeper:

for ought I can gather, either by his Books, or learne from the report of others, he was a man very ignorant in the forme of simples. Many Books indeed he hath tumbled over, and transcribed as much out of them, as he thought would serve his turne, (though many times he were therein mistaken) but added very little of his own.[25]

Another well-known study of English herbals is by Eleanour Sinclair Rohde (1881–1950), *The Old English Herbals* (1922). This author styled Parkinson as 'the last of the great English herbalists' and, by comparison, Culpeper was an 'old rogue' who 'wrote a number of medical works which do not concern us here, but his name will always be associated with his herbal'.[26] Through this work, Culpeper became 'the most notable exponent of this debased lore', prevalent in the later seventeenth century in England, of the influence on herbs of the heavenly bodies, 'a travesty rather than a reflection of the ancient astrological lore'.[27] Rohde's study, however, does not make clear what this ancient astrological lore might have been debased by, or how Culpeper's version differed from the venerable 'ancient' sources.

Culpeper's rehabilitation as an important medical figure commenced in 1962 with an article by F. N. L. Poynter. His own studies of Culpeper led him to assert that the general opinion of him as a 'vituperative quack' who well reflected the turbulence of the English Civil War period and as 'the founder of a modern herbalist cult which flourishes at the expense of orthodox medicine' was so false as to be able to be characterized as 'anti-historical'.[28] Culpeper's provision for English doctors of 'a comprehensive body of medical literature in their own tongue' through his translations of the leading European medical writers of his age showed Poynter that:

> If our concern is with the history of medicine as it was professed and practised, then Culpeper is a figure of outstanding importance, for he had a far greater influence on medical practice in England between 1650 and 1750 than either Harvey or Sydenham.[29]

Increasing awareness of Culpeper's significance has led to the appearance of three biographies and a television documentary in the last 20 years. The first biography, which employed fictional scenes to amplify the few details that exist concerning Culpeper's life, sought 'to highlight his influence in medicine and to clean his memory from the simplistic epithet of being a nonsensical quacksalver'.[30] This required removing 'the shell of mystical astrology from Culpeper's personality and work', and was achieved by a simplistic discussion of medical astrology in what is considered a substandard work.[31] My own work *Culpeper's Medicine: A Practice of Western Holistic Medicine* (1997) considered the practical medical and astrological aspects. This was followed by Benjamin Woolley's *The Herbalist: Nicholas Culpeper and the Fight for Medical Freedom* (2004), an enthusiastic account of Culpeper's political struggle to return medicine to the people, on which a television documentary was based.[32]

The contents of the *English Physitian*

The title-page of the *English Physitian* provided an outline of what the reader could expect to find within its pages, principally a 'compleat method of physick', not with 'outlandish' foreign herbs whose provenance, authenticity and suitability for English temperaments were unknown, but through the use of English herbs 'being most fit for English bodies', those which divine providence had planted close by and to which Puritan writers were drawing attention as God-given efficacious medicines.

The introductory material includes a list of 'authors made use of in this treatise', from Aegineta to Tragus, and 'a catalogue of the herbs and plants &c in the treatise, appropriated to their several planets', from Saturn to the Moon.[33] This ordering of the *materia medica*, which facilitated the selection of herbs on astrological indications, reverted to alphabetical ordering by plant name in the enlarged edition of 1653, perhaps as a result of feedback from readers or owing to Culpeper's ill health and inability to monitor the changes his publisher made to it.[34] Both lists were preceded by the 'Epistle To the Reader' in which Culpeper commenced by citing historical examples of the prizing of knowledge on the uses of medicinal herbs, among whom 'the worthies of our own nation, Gerard, Johnson and Parkinson are not to be forgotten'.[35] He then objected that neither these nor any other authors had explained how herbs cured or why different herbs were used for treating different parts of the body. Instead of reasons, Culpeper said, they quoted old authors in parrot fashion, as if they were true. 'And if all that they say be true,' he asked, 'why do they contradict one another?'.[36] Culpeper then claimed that he pursued his own study of simples, 'most of which I knew by sight before', to discover the reason of their operation.[37]

Culpeper argued that every thing in the world was a composition of contrary elements harmoniously blended according to God's design within a unity of the creation.[38] Man, wrote Culpeper, was an epitome or microcosm of creation. His sicknesses were caused naturally by the various operations of the microcosm, but the microcosmic, elemental world could be influenced by the wider macrocosm, by God and by the natural powers inherent in the planets and stars he set in motion.[39] It was in astrological signs that Culpeper found his answer:

> therefore he that would know the reason of the operation of herbs must look up as high as the stars: I always found the disease vary according to the various motions of the stars; and this is enough one would think to teach a man by the effect where the cause lay.[40]

Here, Culpeper emphasized the importance of reason and experience, claiming that he had consulted with his brothers, 'Dr. Reason and Dr. Experience', in order to publish the results.

Culpeper justified writing his own herbal by arguing that famous and learned authors who had already written much in English on herbs did not share his intentions. First, they did not provide an explanatory account of the operation of herbs: how a herb might have a special healing affinity for a part of the body through a macrocosmic astrological correspondence. Second, a reader of Gerard or Parkinson would come across expensive exotic plants ('outlandish' herbs)[41] not obtainable in England, or at least not outside London, whereas Culpeper's native plants were remedies to be found in the reader's garden, fields and hedgerows. Among the translations which Culpeper made in those years was a work by the virtually unknown Simeon Partliz (1590–1640) on a comparison of Galenic and Paracelsian medicine, *A New Method of Physick*, only published after Culpeper's death.[42] That Culpeper should have prepared such a text for publication is illustrative of the increasing currency in England in the 1650s of Paracelsian ideas. A key tenet of Paracelsus (1493–1541) was that every land has its own diseases and its own cures:[43] 'There is no disease but hath his own proper and peculiar medicine and remedy: and every place furnisheth you with simples enough for its cure'.[44]

Thus the focus of the *English Physitian* on 'sympathetic' treatment using like-for-like correspondences between the microcosmic plant and human body and the macrocosmic stars goes beyond the approach of Galenic pharmacology.[45] A Galenic approach dominated the catalogue of simples which Culpeper inserted into his translation of the *Pharmacopoeia Londinensis* of the College of Physicians in 1649, from which knowledge of a plant's primary qualities of heat, cold, dryness or moisture derived its use in opposing the qualities of a disease (*contraria contrariis curentur*). The 'instructions for the right use of the Book',[46] at the end of the epistle, were consequently astrological rules for the use of herbs by sympathy or antipathy according to the part affected and the significations of disease in horoscopes cast at the onset of illness or at the time of consultation.[47] An example was given in this section for the blessed thistle (*Cnicus benedictus*), and interested readers were referred to a prolonged discourse under wormwood (*Artemisia absinthium*) in the herbal.[48]

Following Cole's advertisement for his titles penned by Culpeper and other authors is the herbal itself, consisting of 283 entries on native herbal simples, from adder's tongue (*Ophioglossum vulgatum*) to yarrow (*Achillea millefolium*). Each entry includes common names of the herb, and then subdivisions similar to those found, for instance, in Gerard's and Parkinson's herbals: a physical description of the plant, the places where it may be found, the time in the year of its flowering and seeding and then its medicinal 'vertues and use'. Culpeper omitted only discussion of the Latin and Greek names for the plants, and the classical authorities of Dioscorides (c. 40–c. 90 CE), Pliny (c. 24–79 CE) and Galen (c. 130–c. 200 CE). Descriptions were omitted in 85 of the 283 entries in the *English Physitian*, (and 103 of the 328 entries in the *English Physitian Enlarged*), where Culpeper thought the plants were so well known as not to need describing. For example, angelica (*Angelica archangelica*), bay (*Laurus nobilis*), saffron (*Crocus sativus*) and blessed thistle required no description.[49] Among those plants needing to be described were mustard (*Brassica nigra*), jack-by-the-hedge or garlic mustard (*Alliaria petiolata*), English tobacco (*Nicotiana* spp.), dandelion (*Taraxacum officinale*) and foxglove (*Digitalis purpurea*).[50] In seven cases, the entries concerned two or three species, but descriptions of the less common ones were omitted.

After the herbal comes the section on 'Directions' for gathering and preserving the medicinal parts of herbs, including leaf, flower, root, bark or seed, and juices, and the best times for collecting them. These instructions included considerations of optimal phases in a herb's growth cycle that yielded the most potent medicine and of the propitious astrological time to infuse the natural power of its corresponding planet. Observe these astrological rules, Culpeper asserted, and 'you may happen to do wonders'.[51]

Thanks to his apothecary training, Culpeper was well versed in the standard preparations of his day which he described in a further section: this section included distilled waters, syrups and juleps, decoctions, oils, electuaries and lohochs, conserves and preserves, ointments, plasters and poultices, troches and pills. The book closes with an index of the medicinal indications of the herbs described followed by another advertisement from the publisher.

How original is the *English Physitian?*

The brevity of the *English Physitian* contrasts sharply with the folio editions of Gerard and Parkinson, in which are descriptions of all the forms of each plant known to them, native and foreign. This difference has perhaps encouraged a superficial assessment of Culpeper's work as entirely original. For instance, Mary McCarl, author of a study into Culpeper's published works, thought the *English Physitian* his only original work; Thulesius was of the opinion that 'it was really his own work and not a mere translation'; while Woolley judged that 'it combined Nicholas's own, obviously extensive experience of herbs with information drawn from more than forty authorities', including Parkinson and Gerard.[52]

Bilberries

However, an examination of many of the entries in the *English Physitian* reveals that they are skeletons of those in Parkinson's works. In order to show the way that Culpeper drew heavily from Parkinson's work, to form this first group of entries, I will use the example of bilberries (*Vaccinium* spp.) as depicted by both authors. Parkinson provided considerable detail. Under 'Whortle berries', Parkinson identified nine different kinds of bilberries, including Spanish, French and Cretan varieties. He distinguished native bushes with black or red berries, the former growing in heaths, woods and barren hills including 'Hampsteede Heath, Fincheley, and Saint Johns wood, not farre from London'; the latter on northern hills in Lancashire and Yorkshire.[53] Culpeper provided some of this detail: he listed locations for black bilberries as forests, heaths and barren places – with no mention of Parkinson's London locations – and Lancashire and Yorkshire for the red berries.[54] Times of flowering and fruiting were the same in both texts. A comparison of the two native species bears closer examination. Parkinson's detailed descriptions of the two native species, black and red bilberries, includes:

> Vaccinia nigra vulgaria, Blacke whorts or Bill berries. This small bush creepeth along upon the ground, scarce rising halfe a yard high; with divers small darke greene leaves set on the greene branches, which it spreadeth abroad on both sides, but not always one against another, somewhat like unto the smaller Myrtle leaves, but not so hard, and a little dented about the edges: at the foot of the leaves come

forth small hollow pale blush coloured flowers, the brimmes ending in five points, with a reddish thred in the middle, which passe into small round berries of the bigness and colour of Juniper berries but of a purple sweetish sharp or sowre juice; which doth give a sad purplish colour to their hands and lips that eate and handle them, especially if they break them; containing within them divers small seed: the roote groweth aslope under ground, shooting forth in sundry places as it creepeth: this looseth the leaves in winter.[55]

Culpeper, in his entry, preferred the name 'Bilberries' and described only two kinds, the black and the red in the same order as Parkinson.

Bilberries, called also (by som) Whorts and Whortleberries Of these I shal only speak of two sorts, which are commonly known in England viz. the Black and the Red bilberries. And first of the Black.

This small bush creepeth along the ground scarce rising half a yard with divers small dark green leaves set on the green branches, not always one against the other, and a little dented about the edges; at the foot of the leaves com forth small, hollow pale, blush coloured flowers, the brims ending in five points, with a reddish threed in the middle which pass into small round berries of the bigness and colour of juniper berries but of a purple sweetish sharp taste; the juice of them giveth a purplish colour to their hands and lips that eat and handle them, especially if they break them. The root growth asloop underground, shooting forth in sundry places as it creepeth; this loseth its leaves in winter.[56]

Leaving aside the matter of spelling and punctuation and the differences in presenting two rather than nine examples, the descriptions are almost identical. On the black bilberry, Culpeper left out mention of 'divers small seed' and may have felt that it was obvious that the plant 'spreadeth abroad on both sides'. He needed to keep his herbal as brief as possible, if it was to be sold very cheaply, and so found it unnecessary to describe the taste of the black berries as both sharp and sour, or of the red as acid and astringent rather than sharp. Among the entries I have studied, this example of the use of Parkinson's descriptions is typical, unlike Culpeper's original descriptions which can be found in entries for beets and blites, and buckshorn from the enlarged edition.[57]

Turning next to the 'vertues' of bilberries, Parkinson wrote at length:

The Bill berries doe coole in the second degree, and doe a little binde and dry withal: they are therefore good in hot agues, and to coole the heat of the stomacke and liver, and doe somewhat binde the belly, and stay castings, and loathings, but if that they be eaten by those that have a weake or a cold stomacke, they will much offend and trouble it saith Camerarius, and therefore the juice of the berries being made into a syrupe, or the pulpe of them made into a conserve with sugar, will be more familiar to such, and helpe those paines, the cold fruite procured; and is good for all the purposes aforesaid, as also for those that are troubled with an old cough, or with an ulcer in the lungs or other disease thereof: with the juice of the berries painters to colour paper or cards, doe make a kinde of purple blew colour, putting thereto some allome and Galles, whereby they can make it lighter or sadder as they please. And some poor folks as Tragus sheweth, doe take a potfull of the juice strained, whereunto an ounce of allome, foure spoonfuls of good wine vinegar, and a quarter of an ounce of the waste of the copper forgings, being put together, and boyled all together, into this liquor while it is reasonable, but not too hot, they put their cloth, wooll, thred or yarne therein, letting it lye for a good while, which being taken out and hung up to dry, and afterwards washed with cold water will have the like turkie blew colour, and if they would have it sadder, they will put thereto in the boiling an ounce of broken gaules: Gerard saith, that hee hath made of the juice of the red berries, an excellent crimson colour, by putting a little allome thereto: the red Whorts are taken to be more binding to the belly, womens courses, spitting of blood, and any other fluxe of blood or humours, to be used as well outwardly, as inwardly.[58]

In comparison, Culpeper's shortened 'vertue and use' of bilberries stated:

The black bilberries are good in hot agues and to cool the heat of the liver and stomach; they do somewhat bind the belly, and stay vomitings and loathings; the juice of the berries made into a syrup, or the pulpe made into a conserve with sugar, is good for the purposes aforesaid as also for an old cough or an ulcer in the lungs, or other diseases therein. The red whorts are more binding and stop womens courses and spitting of blood or any other flux of blood or humours, being used as wel outwardly as inwardly.[59]

While Culpeper's entry was so much shorter as to appear quite different, he extracted from Parkinson's entry all of the medical indications and uses, and in the same order in which Parkinson wrote them. These were abbreviated in the margin of the page, to facilitate easy identity of indication or part affected, as 'agues, stomach, liver, vomiting, apetit lost, cough, phtisick [consumption], fluxes'.[60] Culpeper chose not to inform his readers that bilberries are, according to Galenic pharmacology, cold in the second degree. He omitted the observation of the German physician and botanist Joachim Camerarius (1534–98) cited by Parkinson and, in so doing, strengthened the impression that a syrup or conserve of bilberries was the required medicinal form. Camerarius' name was credited in the list of authors made use of at the beginning of the *English Physitian*.

Another characteristic of the abbreviation of Parkinson's text was the omission of all non-medical uses. Thus Culpeper ignored the example from Tragus, that is, Hieronymus Bock (1498–1554) the German physician, botanist and herbal-writer, of fixing the juice of the black berries with astringent alum or oak galls for colouring paper and card or prepared as a dye for cloth and wool, such as the crimson colour Gerard had claimed to have obtained. Tragus and Gerard were also included in Culpeper's list of authors.

Asparagus

In another example of this first group of entries, that of asparagus (*Asparagus officinalis*), Culpeper had to draw from Parkinson's *Paradisi in sole* for the physical description, which he then reproduced almost exactly.[61] Both Culpeper and Parkinson mentioned that asparagus grew wild in Appleton meadow in Gloucestershire, which the poor gathered to sell more cheaply than garden asparagus sold in London.[62]

On the 'vertues and use' of asparagus, Culpeper's order of actions and conditions once again followed Parkinson's exactly. He ignored Parkinson's questioning of some beliefs concerning asparagus and its cultivation and in this case also excised some of the medical detail. Strangury was not defined, pain of 'the reins' was a sufficient term to cover kidney and back pains, and the bites of poisonous spiders and 'other serpents' were omitted. Through this excision, the indications for jaundice, frenzy and epilepsy and use for pains in the breast and stomach were lost. For the sake of brevity, Culpeper may have omitted completely the uses and risks of asparagus cited by Parkinson from the physicians Chrysippus of Cnidos of the fourth century BCE and Avicenna (980–1037 CE).[63] Culpeper had recorded in *A Physical Directory* that the root was temperate in quality and advocated its decoction in cooling white wine, which was the recommended medicinal form of a seemingly safe herb in the *English Physitian*.[64]

Hemlock and fluellin

A second group of entries are also drawn from Parkinson, although they have significant additions made by Culpeper. Telling statements in two examples are useful. Under hemlock (*Conium maculatum*), Culpeper copied exactly the description (omitting only that the stem is hollow), the location and time of flowering of 'cicuta vulgaris major, the common greater hemlock', one of seven species described by Parkinson.[65] He left out the latter's comments on the execution of Socrates (b. 469 BCE) by hemlock and the amusing story from Pietro Andrea Matthioli (1501–77) concerning asses drugged by the narcotic herb, but retained the references to Pliny's and Tragus' examples of curing those who ate hemlock root by mistake, thinking them parsley or parsnip roots. Parkinson advised that hemlock could safely be applied topically to inflammations, tumours and swellings, but not, as some advocated, to the male genitalia in cases of venereal disease, nor to women's breasts to curtail their swelling and repress their milk, 'by reason the places are so tender and full of vitall spirits, it often proveth that the remedy is more dangerous then the disease'.[66] Culpeper repeated this safe external use, adding 'save the privy parts [genitalia]', which appeared in parentheses. In this example, Culpeper commenced his entry with a query regarding 'my authors [Parkinson's] judgment':

> I wonder why it may not be applied to the privities in a priapismus, or continual standing of the yard, it being very beneficial for that disease; I suppose my authors judgment was first upon the opposite disposition of Saturn to Venus in those faculties and therefore he forbid the applying of it to those parts that it might not cause barrenness, or spoil the spirit procreative, which if it do, yet applied to the privities it stops lustful thoughts.[67]

Culpeper here identified a single source (Parkinson) whose entry on hemlock he specifically qualified with his viewpoint based on astrological theory. Parkinson's concern for the danger to procreative vital spirits was reinterpreted as the threat of affliction to Venus by a poisonous Saturnine plant, and augmented by an observation on how to diminish the excesses of Venus and avoid the danger of contracting venereal disease.

In the other example, that of fluellin or lluellin (*Kickxia elatine*), Culpeper took an oblique line from Parkinson as the basis to mount another attack on the College of Physicians. Once again the descriptions of two sorts of fluellin (Parkinson's third, which only differed in the colour of the flowers, was omitted), their locations and their time of flowering was the same in both herbals, even as far as Culpeper repeating the exact locations of Southfleet in Kent and three places in Huntingdonshire cited in Parkinson. The virtues of the herbs in each entry were also the same actions and uses, and in the same order. Parkinson added a story, as a witness to the efficacy of the herb and lay knowledge, of a man whose nose was being eaten away by a canker. His doctors appointed a surgeon to cut off the remnant of his nose in order to preserve the rest of the body, but a simple barber, overhearing the order, asked if he could be given a little time to try to save the nose by a use of fluellin which his master had taught him. The juice and decoction of the herb was taken internally and the herb applied externally and the nose saved and the body returned to health. Parkinson commented that:

> This occasion doth make me thinke, that not onely in this herbe, but in many other simple herbes, our forefathers found helpe of many diseases, and therefore used fewer compounds: and were we in these times as industrious, to search into the secrets of the nature of herbes, as the former ages were, and to make tryall of them, we should no doubt finde the force of simples, many times no lesse effectuall than of compounds: but of this enough, yet not too much, for as I might provoke some learned to bee more industrious, and not like droanes onely to sucke the honey from others hives.[68]

Culpeper had alighted on an opinion close to his heart, that of the benefits of native simples versus the compounds prescribed by physicians. Only at the end of his entry in the *English Physitian* did he refer to the cure of this patient, and to its use for virulent sores and 'ulcers of the French pox' (syphilis). Culpeper took up Parkinson's simile of drones to make his point about the ignorance of physicians in regard to herbs:

> Bees are industrious and go abroad to gather honey from each plant and flower, but drones lie at home and eat up what the bees have taken pains for; just so do the Colledg of Physitians lie at home, and domineer, and suck out the sweetness of other men's labours and studies, them selves being as ignorant in the knowledge of herbs as a child of four years old, as I can make appear to any rational man by their last Dispensatory, now then to hide their ignorance, there is no readier way in the world, than to hide knowledg from their countrymen, that so no body might be able so much as to smel out their ignorance, when simples were more in use, mens bodies were better in health by far than now they are, or shall be if the Colledg can help it.[69]

The examples of hemlock and fluellin represent a second grouping, where the material taken from Parkinson was amplified by additional observations from Culpeper's own knowledge and experience, contained in as little as a single sentence or as much as a whole paragraph. Into this grouping fall 28 out of the 105 entries considered, evident in examples from the *English Physitian* such as butcher's broom (*Ruscus aculeatus*), where Culpeper appended 'the common way of using it',[70] and clary (*Salvia sclarea*), a remedy for the back but not therefore a treatment for 'the running of the reins' (urinary incontinence) or 'the whites in women' (leucorrhoea)[71] as Parkinson suggested.[72]

Some extra material included by Culpeper concerned gathering of the plant parts according to season (ash tree, *Fraxinus excelsior*), or the use of cleavers (*Galium aparine*), watercress (*Nasturtium officinale*) and dandelion (*Taraxacum officinale*) as spring cleansers for the body. Alchemical preparations such as distilled waters (water betony, *Scrophularia auriculata*), a salt of chamomile (*Matricaria recutita*) and the production of an alchemical panacea from greater celandine (*Chelidonium majus*) went beyond Parkinson's record of their medicinal forms and highlight Culpeper's interest in, and growing knowledge of, the new medicine of Paracelsus and Van Helmont (1579–1644), very much in vogue in the 1650s.[73]

Heartsease and stinking arrach

A third grouping of items in the *English Physitian* including those entries which are quite unlike those of Parkinson, in terms of their construction and the order of actions and indications, total seven out of the 105 items I have studied in the *English Physitian*, but 15 out of the 22 items from the enlarged edition. One such example, from the enlarged edition, is heartsease (*Viola tricolor*). Parkinson wrote of its temperament, its viscous juice and its usefulness in hot diseases of the lungs, agues, the falling sickness (i.e. epilepsy), itchy skin conditions and wounds.[74] Culpeper's focus was on the 'antivenerean' effect of this saturnine plant, made by decoction into a syrup, or distilled in an alembic as a remedy for the 'French pox' (syphilis). More briefly he added that 'the spirit of it is excellent good for the convulsions in children, as also for the falling-sickness, and a gallant remedy for inflammations of the lungs and breast, pleurisie, scabs, itch &c'.[75] These other uses of heartsease do seem similar to those in Parkinson, but appear to have been added almost as an afterthought, incomplete ('&c'), written in a different order and to be effected by a different preparation of the plant than that noted by Parkinson.[76]

A second example is 'wild and stinking arrach' (*Atriplex foetida*).[77] Parkinson recorded its use in one line: to help women pained and strangled by the mother by smelling the stinking plant.[78] Culpeper borrowed his description of *Atriplex sylvestris olida vel foetida*, 'stinking wilde arrache', then filled most of a column in the *English Physitian* with its virtues, seemingly derived from its favoured location and the resulting astrological signature, as a universal remedy for the womb.[79] Digressions into the 'sympathetical' use of a herb, by virtue of the astrological or, much less often, the visual signature of the plant – the doctrine of signatures – could dominate, as in the case of arrach, taking the entry far beyond Parkinson's scope. Usually, however, the medicinal uses of a plant constituted the bulk of the information.

Sampling the texts

These examples are based on 127 entries drawn from the first half of Culpeper's expanded herbal, equalling 39 per cent of the total of 328 of the version, and ad hoc sampling from the remainder of the text which, as a work in progress, I have compared with their equivalents in Parkinson's *Theatrum botanicum*. Of these, 105, or 37 per cent of the content of the *English Physitian*, also appeared in the *English Physitian Enlarged*, while 22 constitute 48 per cent of the material of the enlargement of the latter. Thus my selection contains slightly more of the material of the enlargement and very slightly less of the original entries than would be the case if I had started with the last entry in the herbal and worked backwards. Out of the 105 entries examined in the earlier work, 70, or two-thirds, follow the first group pattern in the examples of bilberries and asparagus above, where Culpeper's physical description and list of a herb's actions and indications is replicated from, and in the same sequence as in Parkinson's entries. Interestingly, however, of the 22 entries found only in Culpeper's enlarged edition, only six share this similarity. This suggests that Culpeper drew more from his own knowledge in preparing material for the enlargement, perhaps for reasons of time or his own ill health which had become grave in 1653.

Conclusion

In the process of anatomizing Nicholas Culpeper's *English Physitian*, I have shown that the major source for the larger part of plant descriptions examined was that of the most recent and best herbal in the English language, John Parkinson's *Theatrum botanicum*. Culpeper methodically excised Parkinson's references to classical authorities for entries in the *English Physitian*, and took plant descriptions from Parkinson's other work *Paradisi in sole*, when the native simple had been depicted there instead. Culpeper thus made more accessible the knowledge of native plants that God had provided as cures, and sought to free his English readers from the monopoly of medically learned men in pursuit of his stated aim, the 'liberty of the subject'.[80]

In the *English Physitian*, Culpeper's additional purpose was to embellish knowledge of simples with the practice of astrological medicine. He represented this in his own original way and thus where Culpeper's entries differ from Parkinson's, especially in the new entries contained in the *English Physitian Enlarged*, these are regularly constituted along astrological lines and draw clearly on Culpeper's own interest in correspondences between the macrocosm and microcosm. However, the key astrological component has itself long since been excised.

Apart from the astrological additions, Culpeper's herbal, the *English Physitian*, is substantially indebted to the work of John Parkinson in a way largely unrecognized by researchers. Thus, Parkinson's descriptions of native English herbs contained in the expensive *Theatrum botanicum*, that was never reprinted, have been read and appreciated down the centuries only thanks to Culpeper. The contribution of Culpeper continues to offer fertile ground for historical research.

Recommended reading

Arber, Agnes. *Herbals, Their Origin and Evolution: A Chapter in the History of Botany, 1470–1670*. 3rd ed. Cambridge: Cambridge University Press, 1986.
Curry, Patrick. *Prophecy and Power: Astrology in Early Modern England*. Cambridge: Polity, 1989.
Furdell, Elizabeth L. *Publishing and Medicine in Early Modern England*. Rochester, NY: Rochester University Press, 2002.
Tobyn, Graeme. *Culpeper's Medicine: A Practice of Western Holistic Medicine*. New ed. London: Singing Dragon, 2013.
Tobyn, Graeme, Alison Denham, and Margaret Whitelegg. *The Western Herbal Tradition: 2000 Years of Medicinal Plant Knowledge*. Edinburgh: Churchill Livingstone/Elsevier, 2011.
Woolley, Benjamin. *The Herbalist: Nicholas Culpeper and the Fight for Medical Freedom*. London: HarperCollins, 2004.

Notes

1 Nicholas Culpeper, *The English Physitian: Or, an Astrologo-Physical Discourse of the Vulgar Herbs of This Nation* (London: Printed by Peter Cole, 1652). Henceforth, all references are to this edition and referred to as the *English Physitian*. Mary McCarl has shown that pirated editions of this text can be distinguished by their spelling of the title as '*English Physician*'. Mary R. McCarl, 'Publishing the Works of Nicholas Culpeper, Astrological Herbalist and Translator of Latin Medical Works in Seventeenth-Century London', *Canadian Bulletin of Medical History* 13, no. 2 (1996): 226, n. 2.

2 Benjamin Woolley, *The Herbalist: Nicholas Culpeper and the Fight for Medical Freedom* (London: HarperCollins, 2004), 316.

3 Anna Parkinson, *Nature's Alchemist: John Parkinson, Herbalist to Charles I* (London: Frances Lincoln, 2007). See also ch. 12 by Jill Francis in this book.

4 Nicholas Culpeper, *The English Physitian Enlarged* (London: Printed by Peter Cole, 1653); John Parkinson, *Theatrum botanicum: The Theater of Plants, or, an Herball of a Large Extent* (London: Tho. Cotes, 1640).

5 John Parkinson, *Paradisi in sole paradisus terrestris* (London: H. Lownes and R. Young, 1629).

6 Nicholas Culpeper, *The English Physician* (London: W. Bentley, 1652), frontispiece. This example is also cited by Jonathan Sanderson who recognized that Culpeper derived the main text of the *English Physitian* from Parkinson's *Theatrum botanicum* although without analysis of the differences. Jonathan Sanderson, 'Nicholas Culpeper and the Book Trade: Print and the Promotion of Vernacular Medical Knowledge 1649–65' (unpublished PhD thesis, University of Leeds, 1999), 115, 159–61.

7 Nicholas Culpeper, *A Physical Directory or a Translation of the London Dispensatory, Made by the College of Physicians in London* (London: Peter Cole, 1649); Graeme Tobyn, *Culpeper's Medicine: A Practice of Western Holistic Medicine* (Shaftesbury: Element, 1997), 14–17. Woolley, *Nicholas Culpeper*, 288–97.

8 Nicholas Culpeper, *Galen's Art of Physick* (London: Printed by Peter Cole, 1652);

	Nicholas Culpeper, *Semeiotica Uranica, or, an Astrological Judgment of Diseases from the Decumbiture of the Sick* (London: Printed for Nathaniell Brookes, 1651).
9	Nicholas Culpeper, *A Directory for Midwives or, a Guide for Women, in Their Conception, Bearing, and Suckling Their Children* (London: Printed by Peter Cole, 1651); McCarl, 'Publishing the Works', 236.
10	*English Physitian*, B2^v.
11	A second edition was issued in 1633. It is this version that was reprinted in its entirety by Dover Publications in 1975 and is still available today.
12	See D. E. Allen, 'Goodyer, John (c. 1592-1664)', in *Oxford Dictionary of National Biography* (Oxford: Oxford University Press, 2004); http://www.oxforddnb.com/view/article/57486 (accessed 27 June 2013); Parkinson, *Nature's Alchemist*, 271.
13	Nicholas Culpeper, *A Physical Directory, or, a Translation of the Dispensatory Made by the Colledge of Physitians of London* (London: Printed by Peter Cole, 1650), B2^r.
14	Woolley, *Nicholas Culpeper*, 319.
15	*English Physitian*, 5; Sanderson, 'Nicholas Culpeper', 151, n. 73, mistakenly calculates 47 additions.
16	I have analyzed the herb entries also in a hardback edition printed several times in the twentieth century. It includes 110 additional entries and some contractions of the original entries, which otherwise are identical with those in the *English Physitian Enlarged*. See Nicholas Culpeper, *Culpeper's Complete Herbal* (London: W. Foulsham and Co., n.d.). A more recent paperback edition benefits from the inclusion of a translation of the *Pharmacopoeia Londinensis* and is *Culpeper's Complete Herbal: A Book of Natural Remedies for Ancient Ills* (Ware: Wordsworth Editions, 1995).
17	McCarl, 'Publishing the Works', 254. McCarl has appended to her article a complete list of Culpeper's works published up to the end of the seventeenth century.
18	*English Physitian*, 242 (i.e. 252, the pagination being erroneous).
19	Elizabeth L. Furdell, *Publishing and Medicine in Early Modern England* (Rochester, NY: Rochester University Press, 2002), 41-5.
20	For instance, Burton Chance, 'Seventeenth Century Ophthalmology as Gleaned from Works of Nicholas Culpeper Physician-Astrologer (1616-1653)', *Journal of the History of Medicine and Allied Sciences* 8, no. 2 (1953): 197-209.
21	Agnes Arber, *Herbals, Their Origin and Evolution: A Chapter in the History of Botany, 1470-1670*, 3rd ed. (Cambridge: Cambridge University Press, 1986). Arber's work was reprinted in 1938 and again in 1986 in the Cambridge Science Classics series.
22	Ibid., xi. Andrew Wear, *Knowledge and Practice in English Medicine, 1550-1680* (Cambridge: Cambridge University Press, 2000), 67, n. 54.
23	Arber, *Herbals*, ch. 8, 247. For more on Turner and Parkinson, see chs 11 and 12 respectively. For other references to Gerard, see also chs 10, 11 and 12.
24	Ibid., 252-4, 261.
25	Woolley, *Nicholas Culpeper*, 317; William Coles, *The Art of Simpling. An Introduction to the Knowledge and Gathering of Plants* (London: Printed by J. G. for Nathaniel Brook, 1656), 77. Under pressure from Elias Ashmole (1617-92), the publisher cancelled the page containing this quote from the second edition of *The Art of Simpling* in 1657; Sanderson, 'Nicholas Culpeper', 152-3.
26	Eleanour S. Rohde, *The Old English Herbals*, reprint of the 1922 ed. (New York: Dover Publications, 1971), 163-7.
27	Ibid. See also Joan Thirsk, 'Rohde, Eleanour Sophy Sinclair (1881-1950)', in *Oxford Dictionary of National Biography* (Oxford: Oxford University Press, 200); http://www.oxforddnb.com/view/article/38541 (accessed 28 June 2013).

28 F. N. L. Poynter, 'Nicholas Culpeper and His Books', *Journal of the History of Medicine and Allied Sciences* XVII, no. 1 (1962): 152–3.
29 Ibid., 152–3; Tobyn, *Culpeper's Medicine*, xiii; Woolley, *Nicholas Culpeper*, 349–52.
30 Olav Thulesius, *Nicholas Culpeper, English Physician and Astrologer* (New York: St Martin's Press, 1992), 186.
31 Ibid., 187; Martha Baldwin, 'Review of *Nicholas Culpeper: English Physician and Astrologer*, by Olav Thulesius', *Journal of the History of Medicine and Allied Sciences* 49, no. 1 (1994): 120–2; Furdell, *Publishing and Medicine*, 42, n. 60.
32 Woolley's biography was serialized as a 'book of the week' on BBC Radio 4 and turned into a documentary for BBC 4, *Rebel Physician*, narrated by the author and broadcast on 17 November 2006.
33 *English Physitian*, C6^r and C1^r–C5^v.
34 Culpeper had some dialogue with his readers. The new herb entry in the *English Physitian Enlarged*, 68, on 'cives' (chives, *Allium schoenoprasum*), finds him writing, 'I confess I had not added these had it not been for a letter I received of a Country Gentleman who certified me that amongst other herbs I had left these out'.
35 *English Physitian*, A1^r–A2^r. This section was omitted in the *English Physitian Enlarged* to make way for the publisher's instructions on how to identify the new bona fide edition from the pirated copies of the *English Physitian* which prompted the revision.
36 *English Physitian*, B1^r.
37 Ibid., A2^r.
38 This unity embraced both visible and invisible components: the mortal body and the immortal soul, or the Aristotelian manifest qualities of herbs that explained their heating or cooling actions on the body and Galen's proposal of occult qualities or hidden properties pertaining to the whole substance of a herb whose operation could not be attributed to its manifest qualities. For a discussion of the complex ideas involved in manifest and hidden qualities, see Brian P. Copenhaver, 'Natural Magic, Hermetism and Occultism', in *Reappraisals of the Scientific Revolution*, ed. David C. Lindberg and Robert S. Westman (Cambridge: Cambridge University Press, 1990), 261–302, especially 270–5.
39 Culpeper had summarized the hermetic theory of the three worlds, the elemental, celestial and intellectual, which was a key construct of Renaissance occult philosophy that influenced Paracelsus and his followers, in the premonitory epistle to the reader in Nicholas Culpeper, *Pharmacopoeia Londinensis; or, the London Dispensatory* (London: Printed for Peter Cole, 1653), C1^r–C1^v.
40 *English Physitian*, A2^v.
41 Ibid., A2^v.
42 Simeon Partliz, *A New Method of Physick, or, a Short View of Paracelsus and Galen's Physic*, trans. Nicholas Culpeper (London: Peter Cole, 1654).
43 Further background on Paracelsian medicine can be found in Allen Debus, *The English Paracelsians* (London: Oldbourne, 1965); Charles Webster, 'Alchemical and Paracelsian Medicine', in *Health, Medicine and Mortality in the Sixteenth Century*, ed. Charles Webster (Cambridge: Cambridge University Press, 1979), 301–4. On astrology, see Patrick Curry, *Prophecy and Power: Astrology in Early Modern England* (Cambridge: Polity Press, 1989).
44 Partliz, *New Method of Physick*, 539.
45 *English Physitian*, B1^r–B2^r. Tobyn, *Culpeper's Medicine*, 162–8. John R. R. Christie, 'The Paracelsian Body', in *Paracelsus: The Man and His Reputation, His Ideas and*

Their Transformations, ed. Ole P. Grell (Leiden: Brill, 1998), 279, uses the term 'similarity' in relation to the selection of remedies. Readers interested in Galen are directed to ch. 9 in this book.

46 *English Physitian*, C5^r–C5^v.
47 Ibid., B1^r–B2^r.
48 Ibid., B1^v–B2^r, 238–41.
49 Ibid., B1^v, 4, 11, 212.
50 Ibid., 42, 56, 87, 88, 224.
51 Ibid., 5.
52 McCarl, 'Publishing the Works', 237; Thulesius, *Nicholas Culpeper*, 103; Woolley, *Nicholas Culpeper*, 319.
53 Parkinson, *Theatrum botanicum*, 1455–9. In these examples I have kept the spelling and punctuation but omitted italicizations and irregular use of capital letters.
54 *English Physitian*, 15–16.
55 Parkinson, *Theatrum botanicum*, 1455.
56 *English Physitian*, 16.
57 Ibid., 13, 18; *English Physitian Enlarged*, 45.
58 Parkinson, *Theatrum botanicum*, 1459.
59 *English Physitian*, 15.
60 Ibid., 15.
61 Parkinson, *Paradisi in sole*, 503.
62 Parkinson, *Theatrum botanicum*, 454–6.
63 Culpeper seemed more open to the views of Chrysippus (died c. 312 CE) that basil (*Ocimum basilicum*) could be poisonous, *English Physitian*, 11; Graeme Tobyn, Alison Denham and Margaret Whitelegg, *The Western Herbal Tradition: 2000 Years of Medicinal Plant Knowledge* (Edinburgh: Churchill Livingstone/Elsevier, 2011), 221–3. Chryssipus does not appear in Culpeper's list of authors.
64 Culpeper, *Physical Directory*, 4, in both 1649 and 1650 editions.
65 Parkinson, *Theatrum botanicum*, 934.
66 Ibid.
67 *English Physitian*, 63.
68 Parkinson, *Theatrum botanicum*, 554.
69 *English Physitian*, 56.
70 Ibid., 21.
71 Ibid., 35.
72 Parkinson, *Theatrum botanicum*, 60.
73 Woolley, *Nicholas Culpeper*, 372, n. 32.
74 Parkinson, *Theatrum botanicum*, 757.
75 *English Physitian Enlarged*, 119.
76 Parkinson, *Theatrum botanicum*, 757.
77 *English Physitian*, 6.
78 Parkinson, *Theatrum botanicum*, 747–50.
79 *English Physitian*, 6.
80 Culpeper, *Physical Directory*, 1649, A1^r.

Part Two

Using Archival Sources: Extending the Evidence Available

Introduction

Susan Francia and Anne Stobart

Since the late twentieth century, with the growth of social history as a valid academic field, social historians have been using new methodologies and asking new questions.[1] Medical history has also sought new ways to look at the history of health, using a variety of social perspectives such as the patient's point of view, and the use of aggregate data to investigate the field of public health. And, like social history, medical history has started to use new types of sources. As Roy Porter put it:

> There is more to medicine than the written record… [there are] customary beliefs about illness and the body, the self and society… [and] medical beliefs and practices before and beyond the literate tradition.[2]

In a similar way, research in the history of herbal medicine also needs to look beyond the traditional medical literary sources relating to practice and to investigate beliefs about illness and about plants used as medicines, utilizing as wide a range of sources as possible.

Medieval diaries allow us a glimpse into a world where many of the uses of plant-based medicaments were common knowledge, for example, as attested in the twelfth-century writings of Alexander Neckham (1157–1217 CE), a young English scholar in Paris:

> The apothecaries sold aromatic spices, which were required in every kitchen except the humblest. People who were troubled with nervous stomachs, which needed warming, would carry around with them various spices which they ate like our modern candy.[3]

Manorial records have been used by social historians to research families and village communities in medieval times, and writers such as Barbara Hanawalt have used these and other records such as coroners' records to investigate the intimate details of family life, some of which pertain to sickness and cause of death.[4] By approaching these documents from a different angle, such records could also be explored by researchers interested in investigating knowledge of plant medicines. Legal records can also offer a view into people's personal lives, including their health. Popular texts, folk carols, ballads, poems, plays and sayings may all be considered for attitudes to health and sickness.

Printed and household recipe collections are further potential sources in the early modern period which can be found in county record offices. Here again, personal items such as diaries and letters can reveal the intimate healing methods of a private household, and their access to, and knowledge of, plant-based remedies. They may also show conflicts with a medical professional regarding the use of herbal remedies. For example, in seventeenth-century letters to her husband, Bridget Fortescue wrote of her fear of using the physician's favourite remedy, Jesuit's bark (*Cinchona* spp.). The doctors conceded that she might be right in her differing view of the right remedy to take, possibly because of her status as a wealthy patient. Bridget wrote of her preferred remedy, 'snakeroot', claiming that she had herself 'cured many Agues' with it and triumphantly noting that her remedy worked 'with out the helpe of the nasty Barke'.[5] Detailed studies such as these can provide further depth and understanding of daily life and household health care.[6]

Many other archives in the UK may provide sources for research in the history of herbal medicine, including the John Lindley (1799–1865) library managed by the Royal Horticultural Society, and the library of the Royal College of Physicians.[7] In the USA, in addition to numerous substantial manuscript archives, the Cincinatti-based Lloyd Library and Museum, with extensive holdings in the history of pharmacy, medicine, botany and related sciences, deserves further exploration.[8]

Herbariums (annotated collections of plant samples) are another carefully archived source, for example the Royal Botanic Gardens at Kew and the Natural History Museum in London.[9] Medicine chests and apothecary cabinets are widely found in local museums and in stately homes, and some of these organizations are enthusiastic participants in living history events, appreciating interest in accurate recreation of past practices.

The Internet offers further support for access to new sources. For example, interpretation of handwritten recipes is much assisted by having visual access to the original manuscript pages, as in the online Wellcome Library collection of digitized sixteenth- to nineteenth-century recipe books.[10] In addition to information sites, the Internet can host tools for further acquiring and developing knowledge, such as the Portal for the Medieval Plant Survey.[11]

In this section of the book we have brought together scholarly examples which extend the range of sources in use for the study of herbal history. Richard Aspin makes the pertinent remark that, historically, herbal knowledge and expertise was so integral to everyday life that it had little need to be documented, and we therefore need to search out ways of obtaining the details. His chapter uses legal documents and draws on the vast numbers of testamentary records to examine their potential contribution to understanding herbal history, discussing some of the challenges faced in finding, understanding and interpreting such sources.

Susan Francia draws out the significant role of cumin in the later medieval period, effectively as a currency for payment of a range of items, thus highlighting its importance in the medieval world. As well as trade accounts, a variety of documents have been largely ignored, and the interpretation of the importance of cumin has not hitherto been attempted. Trade accounts offer the potential researcher a rich source of historical evidence for the use of plants as foods and medicines, and there are many other plants and spices which could be investigated in this way.

There are some other areas for which location of the sources is less readily achieved, and Nicky Wesson explores this particular problem with reference to childbirth in the early modern period. Her chapter on the uses of herbal medicines in childbirth provides an overview of the limitations that might affect availability of sources. She also investigates information found in other sources, including recipe collections.

Notes

1. See, for example, John Tosh with Seán Lang, *The Pursuit of History: Aims, Methods and New Directions in the Study of Modern History* (Harlow: Pearson Longman, 2006).
2. Roy Porter, *The Greatest Benefit to Mankind: A Medical History of Humanity from Antiquity to the Present* (London: Fontana Press, 1999), 30.
3. Urban T. Holmes, *Daily Living in the Twelfth Century Based on the Observations of Alexander Neckam in London and Paris* (Madison: University of Wisconsin Press, 1952), 135–6.
4. Barbara A. Hanawalt, *The Ties That Bound: Peasant Families in Medieval England* (New York: Oxford University Press, 1986).
5. Anne Stobart, '"Lett Her Refrain from All Hott Spices": Medicinal Recipes and Advice in the Treatment of the King's Evil in Seventeenth-Century South-West England', in *Reading and Writing Recipe Books, 1550–1800*, ed. Michelle DiMeo and Sara Pennell (Manchester: Manchester University Press, 2013), 216. Bridget's remedy of snakeroot has not been definitively identified.
6. For example, Judith M. Spicksley, ed., *The Business and Household Accounts of Joyce Jeffreys Spinster of Hereford 1638–1648* (Oxford: Oxford University Press for the British Academy, 2012); Jane Whittle and Elizabeth Griffiths, *Consumption and Gender in the Early Seventeenth-Century Household: The World of Alice Le Strange* (Oxford: Oxford University Press, 2012). Both texts contain sections which consider health practices, including services and remedies purchased.
7. Royal Horticultural Society (RHS), 'Lindley Libraries: the nation's gardening collections', http://www.rhs.org.uk/About-Us/RHS-Lindley-Library (accessed 16 June 2013); Royal College of Physicians Library, http://www.rcplondon.ac.uk/resources/library (accessed 16 June 2013).
8. Lloyd Library Museum, http://www.lloydlibrary.org/ (accessed 15 June 2013).
9. For example, 'Volumes 1–7. Plant specimens from Sloane's Voyage to Jamaica (1687-1689)', http://www.nhm.ac.uk/research-curation/research/projects/sloane-herbarium/ (accessed 15 June 2013); see also http://www.kew.org/collections/herbcol.html (accessed 15 June 2013).
10. The Wellcome Library Recipe Project can be found at http://wellcomelibrary.org/about-us/about-the-collections/archives-and-manuscripts/digitised-recipe-books-project/ (accessed 15 June 2013).
11. Helmet W. Klug and Roman Weinberger, 'Modding Medievalists: Designing a Web-Based Portal for the Medieval Plant Survey/ Portal der Pflanzen Des Mittelalters', in *Herbs and Healers from the Ancient Mediterranean through the Medieval West: Essays in Honor of John M. Riddle*, ed. Anne Van Arsdall and Timothy Graham (Farnham: Ashgate, 2012), 329–57. See also the website at http://medieval-plants.org/ (accessed 17 June 2013).

6

The Use of Trade Accounts to Uncover the Importance of Cumin as a Medicinal Plant in Medieval England

Susan Francia

Introduction and methodology

The history of medicinal plants, like the history of medicine in general until recent times, has traditionally been written using textual sources, most of which were written or compiled by people belonging to the wealthier classes. As a result, we have only a fragmentary understanding of how plants were viewed, or how they were used, by the population at large, and very little understanding of who exactly had access to them or to knowledge of their use. As any glance at the work of social historians over the past 40 years will show, it is necessary to use a wide variety of sources in order to access the historical lives of ordinary people. This is particularly true in trying to understand the history of medicinal plant use, and it is something which has not yet been done to any extent.

Social historians use sources such as wills, probate accounts, household accounts, diaries and letters to reconstruct the lives of ordinary people in the past.[1] Legal records are another invaluable source.[2] All these sources can also yield an insight into how, historically, people viewed and used plants as medicines. Other sources include records and accounts from hospitals, hospices and apothecaries. Records of almshouses and workhouses and parish records also yield information on payments for medical treatment, often specifying the medicaments purchased. The use of plant medicines in history may also be accessed through studying in detail the trade in, and use of, one particular plant, and this is the method used in this chapter. Records of where such a plant was traded, in what quantities, and for what purposes, can give us an insight into a world very different to that of today, where ideas about the health of the body and about medicine are unfamiliar to us. Anne Van Arsdall's chapter in this book gives a detailed study on this concept of our unfamiliarity with historical thinking about medicine and health, and the need to place ourselves, as far as possible, inside the minds of those who lived in the past in order to understand their lives.

This chapter is based on a number of different types of sources, in order to gain an insight into the medieval circulation and use of one particular type of medicinal plant: cumin, also spelt cummin (*Cuminum cyminum*). It has been chosen because of the high incidence of its use in rent payments in medieval England. Records of rent payments in cumin, trade accounts, port tax documents, monastic and household accounts, and records from medieval gardens are married with textual records of both the medicinal and culinary uses of cumin, to provide a picture of a world in which cumin was not only extremely popular, but was circulating in large quantities, and being used for medicinal as well as culinary purposes.

Rents and tithes

In medieval England, rents for agricultural land or for rural or urban property were often paid in items other than money. Spices were used to pay rents, and pepper (*Piper nigrum*) and cumin were used far more often than any other spice. It is not the purpose of this chapter to explain the tangled history of rent payments in medieval England, but a few words may usefully be said. All land was legally owned by the Crown, and therefore all landowners actually held land from the Crown as tenants or subtenants of some kind, not as what we would nowadays call freeholders. In order for land to be bought or sold, it usually had to be encumbered by some sort of annual rent payment, to make it clear that it was leasehold. Medieval documents detail a perplexing tangle of tenures, revealing how customs were changing over time, with a general trend towards the replacement of rents in kind or in service by cash, which was already beginning to be evident by the time the Hundred Rolls were written in 1279 CE. Some documents also detail a monetary equivalent for a cumin rental payment, showing us at least how it was valued in that particular place and time, although this also shows wide variation. Land changed hands a great deal in medieval England, and rents were often passed on as encumbrances to the next owner, or even added to, at the time of exchange.

This chapter uses the example of medieval Oxfordshire, starting by focusing on the year 1279, when the Hundred Rolls were produced (see Figure 6.1). In 1279, Robert, son of Robert of Romney, a free tenant in Steeple Aston in Wootton Hundred in north Oxfordshire, paid the yearly rent for his holding of 3½ yardlands with 1 lb of cumin plus 2d to the lord of the demesne.[3] He was by no means the only landholder to pay for his holding in cumin. In Oxfordshire alone, in the same year, in the Hundred of Bampton in the south-west of the county, seven landholders paid their rents in cumin, in amounts of either ½ or 1 lb.[4] Also in the same year, in the south-east of the county, Sir Geoffrey de Lewknor was continuing to pay in cumin for a portion of his estate, ½ a hide which had been subject to a payment of 1 lb of cumin plus 24s to Lewknor Church for least a hundred years, since Master Nicholas de Lewknor paid 1 lb of cumin to the almoner of Abingdon Abbey at some point in the late 1100s.[5] Again in 1279 in Cowley, now part of the city of Oxford, William Burgan held ½ a hide of land for 1 lb of pepper and of cumin.[6] And in the north-east of the county, at Souldern, the year 1279 also saw Thomas de Lewknor paying his annual rent for the manor of 1 lb

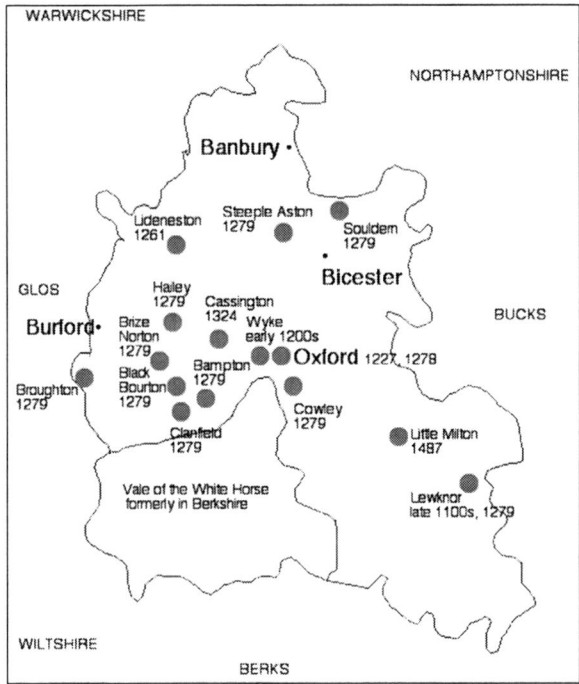

Figure 6.1 The use of cumin (*Cuminum cyminum*) to pay rents in medieval Oxfordshire. Illustration drawn by S. Francia.

cumin to the mesne lord, while in 1285 the same mesne lord, Thomas de Arderne, paid his own annual rent of 1 lb of cumin to John de Lovetot.[7]

In 1227 the citizens of Oxford bought a house for the use of the Grey Friars, and bound themselves to pay its former owner a yearly rental of 1 lb of cumin, and by 1278 the same friars had been granted another house at an annual rental of 1 lb of cumin.[8] Also in the early 1200s, Ralph Russel granted land in Wyke, near Oxford, to John, son of Alexander, which was encumbered by a rent of 1 lb of cumin on the Feast of St Michael, payable to William de Wyke.[9] And on 12 July 1261, a court of inquisition investigating the estate of the deceased Maeumus, son of Richard de Eytrop, detailed one hide of land let to tenants in Lideneston (Lidstone) in north-west Oxfordshire, which was held from Robert de Broc for a yearly rent of 1 lb of cumin plus 1d.[10] Later centuries also saw the use of cumin to pay rents. In 1324 the manor of Cassington, west of Oxford, brought in money rents of 37s, together with 1 lb of pepper and ½ lb of cumin.[11] And in 1487 various messuages and lands in Little Milton, in the south-east of the county, were held of Great Milton manor by a yearly payment of 1 lb of cumin.[12]

We have, then, evidence of cumin in use for rental payments in Oxfordshire over a period of 300 years, from the late twelfth to the late fifteenth century. Further research would certainly turn up more documents. And Oxfordshire was by no means unique in having landholdings which levied rentals in cumin. Cumin was widely used to pay rents in medieval England, in both rural and urban areas. A large number and a wide variety of sources cite rents of cumin, in amounts from 1 oz to 5 lbs, sometimes together with other spices and/or a monetary payment. The use of cumin for rental payment is widely evidenced in a range of documents, including the Hundred Rolls, the Calendars of the Patent Rolls, Close Rolls and Charter Rolls, the Pipe Rolls of bishoprics, cartularies and records of cathedrals and monasteries, city records, baronial records and calendars of Inquisitions Post Mortem.

It is clear that cumin was often used in that class of rents which consisted of very small amounts of either money or a spice or product, and which were sometimes in the nature of quit-rents, a small fixed amount of rent, payment of which released the tenant from manorial services or freed the occupier of the land from the intrusion of others' rights in it, for example access for hunting. This is evidenced, for example, by a quitclaim of the north Oxfordshire manors of Broughton and Northnewenton, two miles south-west of Banbury (and 11 miles from Robert in Steeple Aston), which involved, among other items, the advowson of Broughton Church in Oxfordshire and a rent of 1 lb of cumin for a property in Buckinghamshire.[13] But nominal rents were so very widespread that it seems probable that they were also used as a legal device, in a period when the conveyance of land was technically impossible, in order to grant land and the concomitant services of any tenants to another, to be held on behalf of the grantor at a token rent.[14] The most common spices demanded as such a rent payment appear to have been pepper and cumin, and in some areas cumin proved more popular than pepper.[15] It may be that token rents, like those paid with cumin, were often paid by freeholders. Robert of Steeple Aston was clearly a freeholder. Christopher Dyer also identifies free tenants as paying nominal rents, sometimes in spices.[16] But it is frequently difficult to identify the free tenant from the unfree, since such distinctions gradually broke down; for example, the Hundred Rolls of Bampton in Oxfordshire identifies seven freeholders who pay rent in cumin (from ½ lb to 1 lb), and the one person who is listed under the heading 'cotters' as paying rent with cumin is also listed separately as a freeholder himself, and as someone to whom others owe rent.[17]

Monastic accounts are another good source for medieval medicine, and monasteries not only took cumin as rental payments, but also tithed it to the poor. Monasteries designated some of their rental income to their obedientiaries, so that we find in 1288 the abbot and convent of Tavistock Abbey 'demise and let to farm all their land of La Doune' – that is, Downhouse, near Tavistock – 'which Richard Cola formerly held of them in villeinage', to Peter de Doneslond for 23 years, at an annual rent of 12s payable on St Rumon's Day, with 1 lb of pepper and 1 lb of cumin to the salsarius.[18] A salsarius was a monk responsible for buying salted meats and fish for the monastery. The high value which medieval people set on cumin is also evidenced by the fact that cumin was among the items given by monks to the poor. As early as the year 867 CE, the Abbey of St Bertin, in northern France, made a survey of its possessions and listed items for dispensing to the poor, which included cumin, gallnut, cinnamon (*Cinnamomum* spp.) and cloves (*Syzygium aromaticum*).[19] And cumin also shows up in England in tithes donated to the poor or sick, as at the *leprosarium* at Brook Street in Essex, which was granted a tithe (tenth) of all the fodder, flax, cumin, geese, meat, cabbage, leeks, pears and onions from certain properties of William Doo, in order to remit his sins and those of his family.[20] Cumin was clearly very widely available, and easily obtained. It was also very much in demand. Such, indeed, was the quantity of cumin which seems to have been in circulation in medieval England that it is difficult for the twenty-first-century mind to appreciate how very popular it was among medieval people, and to understand the many and varied uses to which it was put.

Cultivation of cumin

How did medieval people obtain so much cumin? Was it grown in England? *Cuminum cyminum* Linn. (Apiaceae) is native from the eastern Mediterranean to India (see Figure 6.2). The word cumin is derived from the Arabic *kamun*, either via the Spanish *comino* and the French *cumin*, or via the Latin *ciminum/cuminum* via Greek.[21] It is uncertain to what extent cumin was cultivated in medieval Europe, or whether it was ever cultivated to any extent in England. The early ninth-century decree by Charlemagne (742–814 CE) on gardens gives a list of plants to be grown in every imperial garden, which includes cumin.[22] And the monastery of St Gall in modern-day Switzerland had a garden in 820 CE where cumin was grown.[23]

The warmer climate of early medieval England certainly afforded the possibility for cultivation. It was definitely grown in eastern England in the mid-twelfth century, when the lepers of St John's Hospital, Brook Street, in Essex, were given a tithe of cumin, as detailed earlier. And it was clearly still possible to grow it in the England of 1597, since Gerard's Herbal states that:

> cumin is husbanded and sowne in Italy and Spaine, and is very common in other hot countries.... I have proved the seeds in my garden, where they have brought forth ripe seed much fairer and greater than any that comes from beyond the seas. It is to be sown in the middle of spring; a showre of rain presently following much hindreth the growth thereof... myself did sow it in the midst of May, which sprung up in six daies after: and the seed was ripe in the end of July.[24]

But the evidence that cumin was not cultivated to any extent in medieval England is more convincing, and much more extensive. A fourteenth-century list of plants grown in the Infirmarer's Garden of Westminster Abbey, and various other abbeys throughout England, shows that a very wide variety of medicinal plants were in cultivation, but cumin does not appear in any of these gardens.[25] It may be that it could only flourish in the drier areas of eastern England, on light sandy soils, more comparable to its native conditions. It is evident that many European monasteries were purchasing, rather than growing, cumin in medieval times,[26] and cartularies of English monasteries indicate an interest in obtaining supplies of cumin.[27] The accounts of Selby Abbey and the cellarer's accounts of Battle and Durham show that cumin was being imported from the Mediterranean, while Bolton Abbey bought cumin from St Botolph's Fair at Boston.[28] And the Order of St Lazarus of Jerusalem in England (c. 1150–1544) were keen to obtain supplies of cumin, as detailed in their charters.[29]

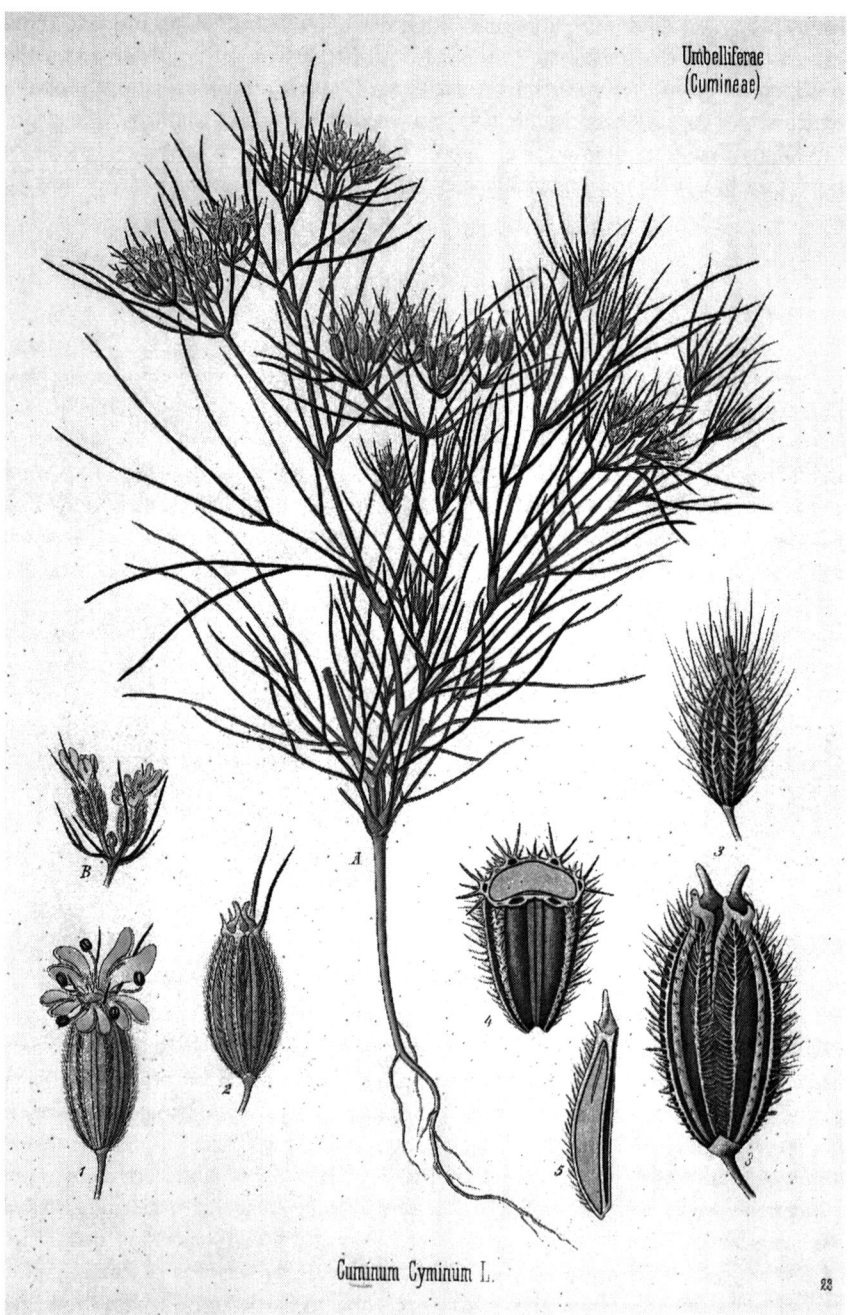

Figure 6.2 Cumin (*Cuminum cyminum*). Illustration from Gustav Pabst, ed., *Köhler's Medizinal-Pflanzen in naturgetreuen Abbildungen mit kurz erläuterndem Texte*, illustrations by Walther Müller and C. F. Schmidt (Germany; Gera-Untermhaus, 1887), 198. Courtesy of Missouri Botanic Garden, USA.

Trade in cumin

International trade

Clearly the medieval population of England was able to source cumin easily, and it was imported rather than grown. So where did it come from? As early as the twelfth century, English merchants established trade links with Spain, exporting woollen cloth and importing spices. Trade accounts give ample evidence that cumin was imported from Spain and Portugal into medieval England on a large scale, and was transported around in large quantities. Cumin was introduced into cultivation in Islamic Spain in the tenth or eleventh century,[30] so it is likely that the cumin imported into England from Spanish ports was grown there. It was certainly used a great deal in Spanish cookery, as the number of recipes containing cumin in the thirteenth-century 'Anonymous Andalusian Cookbook' attests: there are 65 recipes which incorporate cumin in some way.[31] Documents of 1283 and 1289 detail merchants bringing cumin from Spain and Portugal.[32] And on 5 June 1352, five Spanish merchants came before the Mayor of London in order to prove that 12 bales of cumin belonged to them.[33]

An embargo on trade from the Netherlands to England in 1371 produced records listing the consignments held up at the port of Sluis, which included the phenomenal amount of 16,400 lbs of cumin, 6,600 lbs of pepper and 6,600 lbs of ginger (*Zingiber officinale*). The cumin was valued at £1 7s 10d per bale, and the pepper at £8 12s 11d per bale.[34] While in 1388, a Genoese ship coming from Spain, en route for Middelburg in the Netherlands, ran aground on the dunes off Sandwich and offloaded half of its cargo, which included cumin, to sell.[35] Documentary evidence shows that the port of Sandwich imported spices, including cumin, from at least 1298: cumin arrived regularly in ships' cargoes and was manifestly the main spice imported.[36] Italian merchants also brought spices to London, to be distributed by the pepperers (later grocers) of London.[37]

Cumin was imported in quite large quantities. The laws of Edward the Confessor (c. 1003–66), written after 1115, specified that any foreign merchant entering the City of London with pepper or cumin should not sell less than 15 lbs at a time.[38] Port trade accounts from the mid-fifteenth century show amounts of 3 cwt being regularly imported. From 1290, tolls payable at the market in Ludlow show that local goods being sold included meat, grain, flour, pulses, onions and garlic, butter and honey, but that wine, cumin, fish and salt came from farther away, and tolls were levied on cumin by the horse-load.[39]

Internal trade distribution

In English towns, spices were distributed by agents, fairs and markets, or sold through apothecaries' shops, while in the countryside mendicant friars and travelling merchants acted as distributors. The geographical range over which merchants distributed their goods is evidenced in toll disputes, which show that, for example, in 1312 the sheriff of London distrained a merchant of Andover for payment on six bales of cumin.[40] Spices imported into English ports found their way into all parts of the country. Edinburgh was charging tolls on cumin in the fifteenth century.[41]

The brokerage books of Southampton for 1435–6 and 1443–4 show that carts travelled throughout the year from Banbury, in Oxfordshire, (a market town ten miles away from Robert of Steeple Aston) to Southampton, taking down wool, cloth and corn, and bringing back wines and spices such as cumin, which had been brought into the port on Venetian and Genoese galleys.[42] So Robert could have obtained his 1 lb of cumin from Banbury market. But he need not have gone to market to buy cumin. Travelling salesmen known as chapmen traversed the countryside, bringing spices into rural areas. The 1446 probate inventory of Thomas Gryssop, a chapman of York, lists a large stock of spices, giving a view of the variety of spices sold by travelling salesmen.[43] A thirteenth-century play known as *Le Dit de l'Herberie*, by the satirist Rutebeuf (c. 1230–85), also mentions preachers as selling spices, and gives a vivid image of the quantities of cumin traded:

> Good people, I am not one of these impoverished preachers or poor traders in simples who pitch up in front of churches with their tattered old cloaks, carrying boxes and bags, and who spread out a carpet: why, they have more bags than dealers in pepper and cumin![44]

And an old song criticizing the mendicant friars also indicates that they were selling spices: 'Many a dyvers spyse in bagges about they bear'.[45]

There were complaints about the greed and power of men who captured the market in *materia medica*. In 1385 the botanist Henry Daniel criticized the ignorance of apothecaries, who were to be found in every town in order to supply the growing demand for spices, perfumes and compound medicines. In the early fourteenth century in Norwich there were 34 apothecaries, as well as a *forum unguentorum* or *apothecaria* where their goods were sold.[46] If Robert travelled from Steeple Aston to Oxford, he could have bought his cumin in the specialist market there, as in thirteenth-century Oxford a district near St Mary's was known as the Apothecaria, where merchants sold herbs and spices in booths.[47]

However, Robert of Steeple Aston may not have needed to travel even to Banbury to buy his cumin, or to wait for a chapman or friar to come to his village with a pack on his back. Small tenant farmers in rural areas also sometimes had trades to provide an extra income, and among the different trades which have been identified is that of the 'espicer',[48] which indicates that some people living in country areas could have been buying and selling spices. The term 'grocer' was not widely used until the late fourteenth century, or the fifteenth century in rural areas, and before this they were known by names such as 'John le Espicer'. Spice was at that time a general term for all kinds of aromatic culinary and medicinal items.[49]

Householders' and monastic accounts

Householders' accounts also tell us something of the consumption pattern for cumin. One of the earliest surviving English household accounts, for a household in the late twelfth century, lists the occasional expenses for spices purchased, which were salt, pepper, cumin, saffron (*Crocus sativus*) and sugar.[50] Another late-twelfth-century household, which may have been the London household of the Abbot of Bury St Edmunds, bought 1 lb of cumin for 1d.[51] Householders might make special journeys to towns in order to purchase spices: the Le Strange household of Hunstanton travelled to Lynn several times a year during the 1340s to buy various spices, including cumin.[52] Wealthy households might buy cumin in very large amounts: in the thirteenth century the household of Henry III (1207–72) bought cumin in quantities of 20 lbs.[53] Peasants also used spices for special celebrations: in Norfolk in the fifteenth century a parish gild organized a feast for 100 people, buying pepper, cloves, mace (*Myristica* spp.), conniseed, sugar and dates, paying the cook 16d in wages; it is not unreasonable to assume that such groups also used cumin on occasion.[54] Throughout England, parish gilds often organized feasts as a way of raising funds for their church and community.[55]

Cumin was also acknowledged to be an essential commodity for monks: in 1230 the Prior of Tutbury made an agreement with the (maximum of 15) monks pertaining to the monks' kitchen, in which he was liable to provide 3 lbs of cumin per year.[56] And the master of William le Gros's hospital at Hedon was criticized in 1334 because he had not distributed the inmates' entitlement of pepper, cumin, salt, wax, oil, cheese and butter.[57] Monastic household accounts record cumin purchased during the period from the thirteenth to the sixteenth century at Creake Abbey in Norfolk, Holy Trinity Priory in Dublin, Selby Abbey in east Yorkshire, Whalley Abbey in Lancashire, and by both the Bursar and the Cellarer at Durham Cathedral Priory. The Bursar bought 10 lbs of cumin from Boston Fair in 1314–15, at a cost of 20d.[58] In Oxfordshire the accounts of Bicester Priory for 1327 list cumin among the spices kept.[59]

Medicinal uses

It is clear that cumin was imported in large quantities and was freely available to buy in all parts of England. The question then arises as to what medieval people actually wanted it for. The answer to this lies in its medicinal and culinary value. This chapter does not address the question of whether remedies containing cumin actually 'worked', but takes as its premise the view that, as Joan Thirsk has said, the life that people lived in the past was different from ours, and we are obliged to see history on their terms.[60]

In medieval England the idea of separating diet and medication was completely alien. Concepts of health, current since ancient times in both Europe and the Islamic world, were based on the need to keep a balance in the body. While many of the ways in which medieval ideas about this were expressed seem foreign to us, the emphasis placed on fresh air, exercise and a balanced diet appears very sensible to a modern readership. Various preparations were therefore popularly used both by the sick and the healthy, for example electuaries: paste-like preparations containing sugar or honey and a number of herbs and spices, were taken regularly in wine after dinner, as *digestifs*, to settle the stomach (in the same way that modern liqueurs, such as Benedictine, based on herbs, are still used today). Cumin acts as a carminative, and would therefore have had the desired beneficial effect.[61] Electuaries could also be eaten, rather like sweets, and were popular ways of taking herbs and spices, so Robert's father and landlord is likely to have used them on a regular basis. The electuary made of cumin was known as diacyminum, and was so popular that recipes were unnecessary.[62] Electuaries were also used as treatments for the sick, and appear in various medical compendia circulating in medieval England. That they were highly prized is shown by accounts of Robert Montpellier, apothecary to the king, who supplied 6½ lbs of diacyminum on 4 February 1265, followed by a further 10 lbs on 22 February 1265, at 10d per lb. The king, Henry III, was ill at that time.[63] Both cumin and its compound, diacyminum, are found in recommendations for many different kinds of problems. The *Compendium of Medicine*, produced by Gilbertus Anglicus (c. 1180–c. 1250) sometime before 1250, was translated from Latin into English in the early fifteenth century, and circulated widely. The text has at least five references to diacyminum and more than 25 references to cumin; uses include digestive ailments, loss of appetite, liver problems, coughs, toothache, earache, eye complaints and palsy. For stomach ache, it refers to both the simple herb and the compound medicine, diacyminum, in the same section:

> Ache of þe stomake
> ... and let him vse diacinimum... and let him vse a poudir y-made of comyn, and canel, and coliandre seed.
> [Stomach ache
> ... and let him use diacyminum... and let him use a powder made of cumin, and cinnamon, and coriander (*Coriandrum sativum*) seed.][64]

The 1398 translation into English by John de Trevisa (c. 1342–c. 1402) of Bartholomeus Anglicus' *De proprietatibus rerum* of c. 1240, one of the most influential of the medieval encyclopaedias, also includes cumin for treating skin blemishes and bruises:

> Wormode wiþ poudre of comyn and hony doþ awey moles and splekkes and ache þat comeþ of smytynge. [Wormwood (*Artemisia* spp.) with cumin powder and honey does away moles and skin blemishes and ache that comes from beating.][65]

Cumin was also used in the Middle Ages for various kinds of infections, including the common cold, as shown in the fifteenth-century text known simply as *A Leechbook*, which contains, altogether, 37 recipes using cumin:

> ffor rewm þt comyth of cold... tak comyn lorere bayes and stamp hem togedł hete hem in a vessell ouł þe fire and put hem in a bagge and lay to þe sike hede.
> [for a cold, take cumin and laurel (*Laurus* spp.) berries, and crush them together, and heat in a vessel over the fire, and place in a bag and lay it to the sick head.][66]

We also have evidence that monastic infirmarers kept cumin among their medicaments. The Infirmarer of St Mary's Abbey, York, was required to keep cumin along with other 'spices and unguents necessary for the sick'.[67] And, in 1285–6, among the ready-made electuaries purchased by the Infirmarer of St Benet Holme was one containing cumin.[68] The Westminster Abbey Infirmarer's Rolls indicate that there was an exceptionally high consumption of electuaries during the months of the plague, in 1349–50. They also give an unusually detailed itemization of pharmaceutical products bought in the year 1350–1, including diacyminum for a monk called J. Walyngford.[69]

Cumin was also used in veterinary medicine, especially as a treatment for colic.[70] And, rather more surprisingly, cumin was used to preserve human body parts. The ancient Egyptians had used it in mummification, and archaeological work at Wymondham Abbey in Norfolk uncovered a medieval sealed lead case containing human remains packed in cumin and coriander.[71]

Cumin clearly retained its popularity as a medicine, for in the late 1500s the Elizabethan schoolmaster John Conybeare recorded the following recipe for the medicinal use of cumin:

> Take a handfull of flowers of camomil, and half a handfull of cummin, and mingle them together, and make two bagges of the breadth of your eares, and lay them thereunto. A medicine for the megrime truelie proved.[72]

So Robert's landlord could have used his rent payment of cumin to doctor his horses, or to provide himself with electuaries mixed into wine after dinner, or to stock his household medicine cupboard. But was knowledge of the medicinal uses of cumin readily available to all levels of the population? During the fourteenth and fifteenth centuries, there was a large increase in the number of medical manuscripts in circulation, and vernacular writings were in use in homes to a considerable extent.[73] And legal records show that medical knowledge comparable to that found in books such as the Middle English translation of Gilbertus Anglicus was by no means confined to practitioners or to medical texts: in the courts, lay people often gave legal judgements on medical matters. Medical knowledge did not belong only to specialists: knowledge of the practice, recipes and vocabulary found in the medical texts was found on many levels in medieval English society.[74]

Culinary uses

Having established that cumin was very widely available, and was used for its medicinal properties, let us turn to the question of how medieval people used it in cooking, always remembering that they saw no separation between food and medicine. It has often been assumed that the copious use of spices in medieval food was to disguise the taste of tainted meat, but there are many everyday recipes using only vegetable produce which include quantities of spices. In fact, in the past people ate a wide variety of foods which have fallen out of fashion, and which we sometimes no longer identify as foodstuffs. Food in the past was not monotonous or lacking in nutrition; rather, as Joan Thirsk says, 'the variety that people enjoyed in the past was different from ours, but that obliges us to see it on their terms'.[75] There was a fashion in medieval England for highly spiced food, comparable to Middle Eastern food of today. Cumin was certainly used in monastery kitchens: the late twelfth/early thirteenth century collection of poems attributed to Walter Mapes (1140–c. 1208) includes a monastic cook who grinds cumin along with other spices: 'Crocum, garophyllum, piper et cyminum, cocus terit, conficit, onerat catinum [Cook pulverizes saffron, cloves, pepper and cumin, makes the dish and fills the bowl]'.[76]

It is also probable that medieval people knew more about the dietary uses of herbs and spices than most people do today.[77] Cumin was valued as a stimulant to the appetite in medieval times,[78] as well as a *digestif* to settle the stomach after a meal.

In medieval England, culinary tastes, as in every other era, went through changes of fashion. In the eleventh century, a pan-European style of cookery, which included a new selection of foreign spices, became popular, under the influence of the Anglo-Norman aristocracy, which belonged to a European society with a shared culture and had extensive contacts in the eastern and southern Mediterranean. This fashion was widespread among those of high status, but it also influenced society as a whole.[79] The cuisine of the gentry and the aristocracy was a striking mixture of Arab, French and Italian styles and ingredients, altered by local taste, which created many dishes unique to England.[80] The lord of Steeple Aston in Oxfordshire would probably have wished to mark his social and economic status through the copious use of spices in everyday fare.

The European character of culinary taste can be seen in the similarities of cookery manuals popular in France and England. A popular fourteenth-century French cookery manual called the *Le Viandier de Taillevent* features recipes which use cumin for everyday food such as soups, not food for special occasions. It contains two sections on potages and broths, which were distinctive items of late medieval French cookery, including potages containing cumin, which were known as *comminée*. Thus, for example, there is a *comminée de poisson*, and a *comminée d'almandes* using chicken.[81] And in about 1390 in England, a cookery book was written by the master cooks of Richard II (1367–c. 1400), and was known as *The Forme of Cury*, containing recipes such as chicken with cumin, poached eggs in cumin sauce, comyn (*comminée*) and blank de sur (see below).[82] This was followed by the *Liber cure cocorum* (including recipes using cumin with chicken, whelks with 'goode comyne', and *comminée* made of veal, mutton and pork),[83] the *Noble Boke off Cookry* (cumin with chicken, whelks, etc.) and others.[84]

A typical item of this type of cuisine which contained cumin, and was only to be found in England, was the 'blandissorye', similar to but not the same as the French *blanc manger*. The spelling indicates that it probably came from Syria (i.e. white food from Syria).[85] One recipe used eggs, milk, cumin, saffron, rice flour or white bread, and cheese, and was suitable for use in Lent; in the *Forme of Cury* it was called 'Blank de Sur' and instructions were:

For to make Blank de Sur
Tak the zolkys of Eggs sodyn and temper it wyth mylk of a kow and do ther'to Comyn and Safroun and flowr' of ris or wastel bred mycd and grynd in a morter and temper it up wyth the milk and mak it boyle and do ther'to wit of Egg' corvyn

smale and tak fat chese and kerf ther'to wan the licour is boylyd and serve it forth.[86]

Cumin was also used in confectionery. Spices, like candied cumin seeds, were used among wealthy people as a final course, along with fruits, wafers and hippocras, which was itself a highly spiced wine. We also have an example from literature, as Sir Thopas, a character depicted by Chaucer (c. 1343–1400), eats candied cumin seeds, along with liquorice (*Glycyrrhiza glabra*) and 'gingerbread', which in fourteenth- and fifteenth-century manuscripts is a kind of toffee-like sweet, made of honey and ginger: [87]

> They fette hym... spicerye Of gyngebred... And lycorys and eek comyn With sugre.
> [They made him... spices of ginger toffee... and liquorice and also candied cumin seeds.][88]

We may question whether the cookery manuals portray a realistic view of food in the Middle Ages, since they were for the most part written by royal chefs or for people of standing; but there is evidence from contemporary writers such as the poor schoolmaster Alexander of Neckham (1157–1217), who describes his lodgings in Paris in the twelfth century, where chicken is flavoured with cumin for his meal. He also describes the apothecaries, who sold aromatic spices which were used in every kitchen apart from the very poorest; and he gives a vivid image of ordinary people who suffered from 'nervous stomachs', and carried around various spices to eat by the handful, much like our modern day sweets.[89] But the key to understanding the very great popularity of cumin lies in the fact that it was widely used to flavour breads, cheeses, and probably also to flavour beer, the three staples of everyday life for most of the population. It is believed that the Gauls used cumin to flavour beer.[90] An early fourteenth-century farming handbook, known as the *Liber commodorum ruralium*, described a cheesemaking process in which ground cumin was added at the curdling stage.[91] Various types of cheeses flavoured with cumin seeds can still be bought in England, the Netherlands and several other countries.

Affordability

Cumin was, therefore, very popular, and widely available, even in rural areas. But was it only the relatively wealthy who could afford to use it? The question of prices and wages in the medieval era is a notoriously difficult one, for many reasons. Prices fluctuated wildly, and both prices and wages varied across geographical regions. But a very general idea can be gained by using statistical information from the Global Price and Income History Group, which gives data for certain spices. Although cumin is not one of them, data exists for pepper and ginger (both used in rent payments) and also for sugar. Between the years 1209 and 1500, the daily wage of an English farm worker would have purchased 2 to 6 oz of pepper, 1 to 4 oz of ginger, or 1 to 5 oz of sugar.[92]

In some documents, rent payments of cumin or pepper are described with a cash value. Again, these vary enormously, but cumin is generally, though not always, assessed at a lower price than pepper. It would therefore seem reasonable to assume that a farm worker could have purchased cumin in amounts slightly higher than pepper for his daily wage. Although he could not have used it every day, he could have afforded to buy small amounts as medicine at need, or for use in cooking on special occasions. Craft workers, who earned up to twice the wage of the farm worker, would have been able to use cumin more often. And, as we have already seen, spices were purchased for parish feasts.

Conclusion

Cumin was very highly prized in medieval England, and was circulating in large quantities. The international character of Anglo-Norman culture and cuisine, with its strong Arab influence, created a society in which both the aristocracy and the gentry were concerned to emulate a Middle Eastern style of diet, with its emphasis on highly spiced foods, and this influence spread throughout society. Cumin was used as a flavouring and in confectionery. Landholders demanded rents in cumin more than any other spice except pepper. Those who had to pay their rents in cumin could buy it from travelling chapmen, mendicant friars, fairs, market stalls, shops or special emporia in towns. There were even people living and trading as 'espicers' in rural villages. It would not have been difficult to get hold of cumin in medieval times. And poorer people could have used it occasionally. Indeed, cumin was dispensed to the poor and to the sick as a work of charity. Cumin was also considered to be a valuable medicinal product for various ailments, both human and veterinary, and was used on an everyday basis by healthy people in the form of electuaries for *digestif* drinks, or as a flavouring for such staple foods as bread, cheese and beer.

So, Robert of Steeple Aston in north Oxfordshire would not even have had to leave home to buy his cumin. It could have come up to Banbury and Oxford from Southampton on carriers' carts, imported on Genoese ships out of Spain, where it had been introduced by the Muslims. A landlord could choose to sell his cumin for cash, or to cook with it or to use it medicinally. He might save it for one of the great feasts, such as at Christmas, or use it in everyday fare such as potages and soups. If he was wealthy enough he might take it in wine after dinner to settle the stomach. He would certainly have aspired to use spices as often as possible as a marker of his social status.

Or, if the rent-payer had a monastic landlord, the cumin might go into the infirmarer's or cellarer's stores at the abbey or monastery. But the rent-payer himself (or herself) might also use cumin. Those who paid rents in cumin were often relatively well-off freeholders or villeins themselves, and may have been able to afford to use it in everyday food. Robert, son of the Lord Robert of Romney, was probably such a person. But even a poor rural peasant could have used it on special occasions. In a culture in which the use of spices was highly valued, people of all social levels seem to have used them to the extent that their income allowed: and cumin appears to have been as highly valued as pepper in medieval England.

Recommended reading

Carlin, Martha, and Joel T. Rosenthal, eds. *Food and Eating in Medieval Europe*. London: Hambledon, 1998.
Dyer, Christopher. *Making a Living in the Middle Ages: The People of Britain, 850–1520*. New Haven, CT: Yale University Press, 2002.
Getz, Faye M., ed. *Healing and Society in Medieval England: A Middle English Translation of the Pharmaceutical Writings of Gilbertus Anglicus*. Madison, Wisconsin: University of Wisconsin Press, 1991.
Rawcliffe, Carole. "'On the Threshold of Eternity": Care for the Sick in East Anglian Monasteries'. In *East Anglia's History: Studies in Honour of Norman Scarfe*, edited by Christopher Harper-Bill, Carole Rawcliffe and Richard G. Wilson. Woodbridge: Boydell Press, 2002, 41–72.
Thirsk, Joan. *Food in Early Modern England: Phases, Fads, Fashions, 1500–1760*. London: Hambledon Continuum, 2007.

Notes

1. A detailed account of the many types of records available to the social historian can be found in Kate Tiller, *English Local History: An Introduction*, 2nd ed. (Stroud: Sutton, 2002).
2. For a comprehensive study of the use of coroners' records to reconstruct the everyday lives of medieval people, see Barbara A. Hanawalt, *The Ties That Bound: Peasant Families in Medieval England* (New York: Oxford University Press, 1986).
3. Record Commissioners, *Rotuli Hundredorum: Temp. Hen. III. and Edw. I. In Turr' Lond' Et in Curia Receptæ Scaccarij Westm. Asservati*. Vol. 2 (London: George Eyre and Andrew Strahan, 1818), ii, 861–3. I am indebted to Deborah Hayter for bringing this reference to my attention, and for her translation.
4. Eric Stone, ed., *Oxfordshire Hundred Rolls of 1279* (Oxford: Oxfordshire Record Society, 1968), 28, 35, 42, 51, 71.
5. Record Commissioners, *Rotuli Hundredorum*, ii, 782.
6. Ibid., 713.
7. Ibid., 823; Herbert E. Salter, ed., *The Feet of Fines for Oxfordshire, 1195–1291*. Vol. 12 (Oxford: Oxford Record Society, 1930), 222.
8. Andrew G. Little, *The Grey Friars in Oxford* (Oxford: Printed for the Oxford Historical Society at the Clarendon Press, 1892), 13, 295.
9. Gift: [Charter of Ralph Russel]. Deeds for parishes in South-east Oxfordshire. P400/D/1, Oxfordshire Record Office, Oxford. I am grateful to Dr Elizabeth Gemmell for bringing this reference to my attention, and for her transcription.
10. J. E. E. S. Sharp, ed., *Calendar of Inquisitions Post Mortem and Other Analogous Documents Preserved in the Public Record Office. Vol. I. Henry III* (London: HMSO, 1904), 137–43.
11. Alan Crossley, ed., *A History of the County of Oxford*. Vol. 12. *Woolton Hundred (South), Including Woodstock*, The Victoria History of the Counties of England (Oxford: Published for the Institute of Historical Research by Oxford University Press, 1990), 44–8.
12. Mary D. Lobel, ed., *A History of the County of Oxford*. Vol. 7. *Dorchester and Thame*

Hundreds (London: Oxford University Press for the Institute of Historical Research, 1962), 117–46.
13   *Calendar of the Close Rolls... Vol. 3. Richard II. A.D. 1385–1389* (London: HMSO, 1921), 78.
14   R. W. Eyton makes this point in the case of a 'conveyance' of demesne land in Shropshire in 1255: R. W. Eyton, *Antiquities of Shropshire*. Vol. 6 (London: John Russell Smith, 1858), 255.
15   See, for example, Charles W. Foster, ed., *Final Concords of the County of Lincoln from the Feet of Fines Preserved in the Public Record Office*. Vol. II (Lincoln: Lincoln Record Society, 1920), where the subject index under 'rents' lists 29 entries for cumin but only 15 for pepper; Gerald A. J. Hodgett, ed., *The Cartulary of Holy Trinity, Aldgate* (Leicester: London Record Society, 1971) has 26 entries for cumin but only 12 for pepper.
16   Christopher Dyer, *Standards of Living in the Later Middle Ages: Social Change in England, c. 1200–1500* (Cambridge: Cambridge University Press, 1989), 11.
17   Stone, *Oxfordshire Hundred Rolls*, 27–8, 35, 41–2, 51, 71.
18   Herbert P. R. Finberg, *Tavistock Abbey: A Study in the Social and Economic History of Devon* (Cambridge: Cambridge University Press, 1951), 249.
19   Roy C. Cave and Herbert Henry Coulson, *A Source Book for Medieval Economic History* (New York: Biblo and Tannen, 1965), 315.
20   Carole Rawcliffe, *Leprosy in Medieval England* (Woodbridge: Boydell and Brewer, 2006), 324.
21   'cumin | cummin, n'., OED Online, Oxford University Press; http://www.oed.com/view/Entry/45801?redirectedFrom=cumin (accessed 27 June 2013); Wikipedia, 'Cumin', http://en.wikipedia.org/wiki/Cumin (accessed 16 June 2013).
22   Reinhard Schneider, ed., *Kapitularien*, Historische Texte Mittelalter 5 (Göttingen: Vandenhoeck and Ruprecht, 1968). See also Karolus Magnus (747–814), 'Capitulare de villis', available at http://www.hs-augsburg.de/~harsch/Chronologia/Lspost08/CarolusMagnus/kar_vill.html (accessed 16 June 2013).
23   Phyllis P. Bober, *Art, Culture and Cuisine: Ancient and Medieval Gastronomy* (Chicago: University of Chicago, 1999), 210.
24   Marcus Woodward, *Leaves from Gerard's Herball* (New York: Dover Publications, 1969), 170.
25   John Harvey, 'Westminster Abbey: The Infirmarer's Garden', *Garden History* 20, no. 2 (1992): 97–115.
26   Peter Spufford, *Money and Its Use in Medieval Europe* (Cambridge: Cambridge University Press, 1989), 39.
27   David Marcombe, *Leper Knights: The Order of St Lazarus of Jerusalem in England, c. 1150–1544* (Woodbridge: Boydell Press, 2004), 145.
28   Graham Keevill, Mick Aston and Teresa Hall, eds., *Monastic Archaeology: Papers on the Study of Medieval Monasteries* (Oxford: Oxbow Books, 2001), 70–2.
29   Marcombe, *Leper Knights*, 145.
30   John Harvey, 'Garden Plants of Moorish Spain: A Fresh Look', *Garden History* 20, no. 1 (1992): 73.
31   See 'An Anonymous Andalusian Cookbook of the 13th Century: Translated by Charles Perry', available online at http://www.daviddfriedman.com/Medieval/Cookbooks/Andalusian/andalusian_contents.htm (accessed 16 June 2013).
32   Reginald R. Sharpe, ed., *Calendar of Letter-Books in the City of London* (London: J. E. Francis, 1899), A1275–98, f. 110.

33 Arthur H. Thomas, ed., *Calendar of the Plea and Memoranda Rolls Preserved among the Archives of the Corporation of the City of London at the Guildhall*. Vol. 1 (Cambridge: Cambridge University Press, 1926), Roll A4 1337–43, membr. 3.
34 Brian Moffat, ed., *SHARP Practice 6. The Sixth Report on Researches into the Medieval Hospital at Soutra, Scottish Borders/Lothian, Scotland* (Fala, UK: SHARP, 1998), 28.
35 *Calendar of the Close Rolls. Vol. 3*, 275–6.
36 Joan Thirsk, *Food in Early Modern England: Phases, Fads, Fashions, 1500–1760* (London: Hambledon Continuum, 2007), 315.
37 Christopher Dyer, *Making a Living in the Middle Ages: The People of Britain, 850–1520* (New Haven, CT: Yale University Press, 2002), 206–8.
38 Cave and Coulson, *Source Book*, 200.
39 G. C. Baugh, ed., *A History of Shropshire*. Vol. 4. *Agriculture*, The Victoria History of the Counties of England (Oxford: Oxford University Press for the Institute of Historical Research, 1989), 26–71.
40 James Masschaele, *Peasants, Merchants and Markets: Inland Trade in Medieval England, 1150–1350* (New York: St Martin's Press, 1997), 113.
41 James D. Marwick, ed., *Extracts from the Records of the Burgh of Edinburgh. A.D. 1403–1528* (Edinburgh: Printed for the Scottish Burgh Records Society, 1869), Appendix: Table of tolls and customs.
42 Brian Foster, ed., *The Local Port Book of Southampton for 1435–36*. Vol. 7, Southampton Record Series (Southampton: Southampton University, 1963); Olive Coleman, ed., *The Brokerage Book of Southampton, 1443–1444*, vol. 1 (Southampton: Southampton University, 1960).
43 Thirsk, *Food in Early Modern England*, 317.
44 Michel Zink, ed., *Oeuvres Complètes. [Rutebeuf]*, 2 vols (Paris: Bordas, 1990). Vol. 2, 247.
45 Charles W. E. Bardsley, *English Surnames: Their Sources and Significations*, 2nd ed. (London: Chatto and Windus, 1875), 370.
46 Rawcliffe, *Leprosy*, 216–17.
47 Eleanour S. Rohde, *Herbs and Herb Gardening* (London: Medici Society, 1936), 4.
48 Henry S. Bennett, *Life on the English Manor: A Study of Peasant Conditions 1150–1400* (Cambridge: Cambridge University Press, 1960), 67.
49 Bardsley, *English Surnames*, 370.
50 Martha Carlin and Joel T. Rosenthal, eds., *Food and Eating in Medieval Europe* (London: Hambledon, 1998), 34, n. 28.
51 Christopher M. Woolgar, ed., *Household Accounts from Medieval England, Part 1, Introduction, Glossary, Diet Accounts (I)* (Oxford: Oxford University Press for the British Academy, 1992), 108.
52 Christopher Woolgar, 'Diet and Consumption in Gentry and Noble Households: A Case Study from around the Wash', in *Rulers and Ruled in Late Medieval England: Essays Presented to Gerald Harriss*, ed. Rowena E. Archer and Simon Walker (London: Hambledon, 1995), 29.
53 *[Calendar of the] Close Rolls Preserved in the Public Record Office... Henry III, A.D. 1227–[1272]* (London: HMSO, 1902–38), 164.
54 Catherine B. Firth, 'Village Gilds of Norfolk in the Fifteenth Century', *Norfolk Archaeology* 18 (1914): 185.
55 Many vivid examples are detailed in Eamon Duffy, *The Voices of Morebath: Reformation and Rebellion in an English Village* (New Haven, CT: Yale University Press, 2003).

56 Michael W. Greenslade, *The Victoria History of the Counties of England*. Vol. 3. *A History of the County of Stafford* (London: Oxford University Press for the Institute of Historical Research, 1970), 331–40.
57 Rawcliffe, *Leprosy*, 324.
58 Brian Moffat, ed., *SHARP Practice 3: The Third Report on Researches into the Medieval Hospital at Soutra, Lothian/Borders Region, Scotland* (Edinburgh: SHARP, 1989), 79–82.
59 William Page, *The Victoria History of the Counties of England. Vol. 2. A History of the County of Oxford* (London: Constable, 1907), 165–213.
60 Thirsk, *Food in Early Modern England*, xi.
61 Tolou Allahghadri et al., 'Antimicrobial Property, Antioxidant Capacity and Cytotoxicity of Essential Oil from Cumin Produced in Iran', *Journal of Food Science* 75, no. 2 (2010): H54–61; Maud Grieve, *A Modern Herbal: The Medicinal, Culinary, Cosmetic and Economic Properties, Cultivation and Folklore of Herbs, Grasses, Fungi, Shrubs and Trees with All Their Modern Scientific Uses*, ed. C. F. Leyel, repr. of 1931 ed. (London: Peregrine Books, 1976), 243.
62 Rawcliffe, *Leprosy*, 214.
63 Geoffrey Trease, 'The Spicers and Apothecaries of the Royal Household in the Reigns of Henry III, Edward I and Edward II', *Nottingham Medieval Studies* 3 (1959): 19–52.
64 Faye M. Getz, ed., *Healing and Society in Medieval England: A Middle English Translation of the Pharmaceutical Writings of Gilbertus Anglicus* (Madison: University of Wisconsin Press, 1991). This book has a glossary for all the recipes containing cumin and diacyminum.
65 Barthollomew Glanvill, *De proprietatibus rerum*, in 19 books; translated into English by John de Trevisa, Western Manuscripts Add. 27944, 215 a/b, British Library, London.
66 Warren R. Dawson, ed., *A Leechbook or Collection of Medical Recipes of the Fifteenth Century: The Text of Ms No. 136 of the Medical Society of London, Together with a Transcript into Modern Spelling* (London: Macmillan, 1934), 240.
67 Herbert H. E. Craster and Mary E. Thornton, eds., *The Chronicle of St. Mary's Abbey, York, from Bodley Ms. 39*, vol. CXLVIII (Durham: Surtees Society, 1934), 98.
68 Carole Rawcliffe, '"On the Threshold of Eternity": Care for the Sick in East Anglian Monasteries', in *East Anglia's History: Studies in Honour of Norman Scarfe*, ed. Christopher Harper-Bill, Carole Rawcliffe and Richard G. Wilson (Woodbridge: Boydell Press, 2002), 62.
69 E. A. Hammond, 'The Westminster Abbey Infirmarer's Rolls as a Source of Medical History', *Bulletin of the History of Medicine* 39 (1965): 270.
70 David M. R. Culbreth, *A Manual of Materia Medica and Pharmacology* (Philadelphia: Lea Brothers and Co., 1906), 448.
71 Christopher M. Gerrard, *Medieval Archaeology: Understanding Traditions and Contemporary Approaches* (London: Routledge, 2003), 48.
72 Frederick C. Conybeare, ed., *Letters and Exercises of the Elizabethan Schoolmaster John Conybeare: Schoolmaster at Molton, Devon, 1580 and at Swimbridge, 1594* (London: Henry Frowde, 1905), 73.
73 R. Robbins, 'Science and Information in English Writings of the Fifteenth Century', *Modern Language Review* 39 (1944): 3; Linda E. Voigts, 'Multitudes of Middle English Medical Manuscripts', in *Manuscript Sources of Medieval Medicine: A Book of Essays*, ed. Margaret R. Schleissner (New York: Garland, 1995), 192.

74 Getz, *Healing and Society*, Introduction.
75 Thirsk, *Food in Early Modern England*, xi. See the introduction to this book for a clearly written deconstruction of the myth that food in the past was lacking in variety and nutritional value.
76 Thomas Wright, ed., *The Latin Poems Commonly Attributed to Walter Mapes* (London: Printed for the Camden Society, by John Bowyer Nichols and Son, 1841), 248.
77 Reay Tannahill, *Food in History*, revised ed. (Harmondsworth: Penguin, 1988), 167.
78 Terence Scully, ed., *The Viandier of Taillevent: An Edition of All Extant Manuscripts by Taillevent* (Ottawa: University of Ottowa Press, 1988), 54.
79 Christopher M. Woolgar, Dale Serjeantson and Tony Waldron, eds., *Food in Medieval England: Diet and Nutrition* (Oxford: Oxford University Press, 2006), 269.
80 Constance B. Hieatt, 'Medieval Britain', in *Regional Cuisines of Medieval Europe: A Book of Essays*, ed. Melitta W. Adamson (New York: Routledge, 2002), 23.
81 Scully, *Viandier of Taillevent*, 54, 288.
82 Samuel Pegge, *The Forme of Cury: A Roll of Ancient English Cookery Compiled, About A.D. 1390* (London: J. Nichols, 1780).
83 Richard Morris, ed., *Liber cure cocorum* (Berlin: Published for the Philological Society by A. Asher and Co., 1862).
84 Robina Napier, ed., *A Noble Boke Off Cookry Ffor a Prynce Houssolde or Eny Other Estately Houssholde Reprinted Verbatim from a Rare Ms. In the Holkham Collection* (London: Elliot Stock, 1882).
85 Constance B. Hieatt and Sharon Butler, eds., *Curye on Inglysch: English Culinary Manuscripts of the Fourteenth Century (Including the Forme of Cury)* (London: Published for The Early English Text Society by the Oxford University Press, 1985), 172.
86 Pegge, *Forme of Cury*, no. XIX.
87 Constance B. Hieatt, 'Making Sense of Medieval Culinary Records', in *Food and Eating*, ed. Carlin and Rosenthal, 104.
88 John M. Manly and Edith Rickert, eds., *The Text of the Canterbury Tales Studied on the Basis of All Known Manuscripts*. Vol. 4. *Text and Critical Notes, Part 2* (Chicago: University of Chicago Press, 1940), 139–47.
89 Urban T. Holmes, *Daily Living in the Twelfth Century Based on the Observations of Alexander Neckam in London and Paris* (Madison: University of Wisconsin Press, 1952), 88.
90 See Scott Russell, 'Dubbel Vision: Step-by-Step Recipes for Recreating Six Legendary Belgian Beers', *Brew Your Own Magazine*; http://www.byo.com/component/k2/item/576-dubbel-vision (accessed 16 June 2013); Harry T. Peck, *Harper's Dictionary of Classical Antiquities* (London: Harper and Brothers, 1898).
91 Andrew Dalby, *Cheese, a Global History* (London: Reaktion, 2009), 81.
92 See Global Price and Income History Group, 'English Prices and Wages, 1209–1914 (Gregory Clark)', available at http://gpih.ucdavis.edu/Datafilelist.htm#Northwest (accessed 16 June 2013).

7

Early Modern Childbirth and Herbs – The Challenge of Finding the Sources

Nicky Wesson

Introduction

My initial research was undertaken with the aim of establishing which herbs early modern women used in childbirth. Herbs are little used in childbirth in England today and, as a medical herbalist and childbirth advisor, I looked for information from the past that might prove of value now. However, as researchers have discovered, this task is almost impossible because so few clues remain as to whether herbs were actually used. In this chapter, I discuss the beliefs and fears of early modern women around childbirth, some religious influences on acceptable practices, and also I consider evidence from books and recipes for the recommendation and use of herbal remedies, in particular for pain relief. I consider some reasons why the evidence might be exceptionally hard to obtain and suggest further research possibilities.

Childbirth and archival sources

According to historians, evidence for what happened in childbirth in early modern England is hard to establish. Pollock says that there is 'no document extant which supplies a complete description of childbirth in early modern England',[1] and that to uncover evidence means combing personal papers, diaries and autobiographies, although these are rare documents for pre-Civil War England, especially those compiled by women.[2] Wilson believes that direct documentation of the lives of poor women is particularly scant.[3] Much of our information about giving birth, as Gowing reflects, comes from literary and prescriptive sources including the midwifery manuals which began to be published in the vernacular from the middle of the sixteenth century.[4] Although focusing on an earlier period, Europe in the Middle Ages, Gibson remarks that 'it is the privy space of the birthing room that is silence for the historian', and argues for an interdisciplinary lens to gain oblique information, including records of saints' lives and miracles, romance narratives, ballads, legal documents and letters.[5]

She sees these sources as showing remarkable consistency in childbirth practices. Such an approach, drawing on a variety of sources, is also appropriate in considering the early modern period.

However, Cressy, in considering the ceremonies of the life cycle, reflects that the bulk of documentation in early modern England was generated by men, confined to the viewpoints of fathers, ministers, doctors and scribes.[6] Even where, unusually, we do have documentary evidence from women who attended births, these women have little to say. Pollock has noted that Lady Grace Mildmay (c. 1552-1620), who wrote about her medical practice in her diary, made no detailed references to births attended and did not comment on her own daughter's birth.[7] Lady Margaret Hoby (1571-1633), who also attended births, revealed little more, for example:

> In the morning at six o'clock I prayed privately, that done, I went to a wife in travail of child about whom I was busy till one o'clock, about which time, she being delivered and I having praised God, I returned home and betook myself to private prayer.[8]

Rare and graphic accounts of the pain of labour, such as that experienced by Alice Thornton (1626-1707), remain much quoted.[9] Few historians have considered the aspect of herbal medicine in relation to childbirth, except to dismiss the possibility that herbs, or indeed any of the animal or mineral preparations, could have any beneficial or adverse effect on labour beyond the psychological, being 'ineffective remedies'.[10] Some have argued that herbs could be effective abortifacients and were often used as such.[11]

In this chapter I discuss some reasons why there may be a lack of records of childbirth practices, and consider recommendations for herbs for easing childbirth which can be found in printed medical advice and recipe collections. My findings suggest that, although recipes for pain in childbirth are relatively scarce, pain could have been relieved by the use of selected herbs, and recipes for relieving afterpains may have been tacitly understood as being also effective for labour pain. In addition, some widely recommended herbs may have been effective in preventing sepsis.

The church and childbirth

The influence of the Church on attitudes to the 'pain and peril' of childbirth was pervasive. Prior to the seventeenth century, the Catholic Church had acknowledged women's anxiety about forthcoming labours, and supplied spiritual and tangible comfort ranging from specific saints, masses and the sacrament to holy girdles, stones, relics and amulets or charms, many of which would be lent out to women by their churches and monastic houses.[12] According to the Bible, women were destined to suffer in childbirth as retribution for Eve's transgression in tempting Adam. 'Unto the woman he said "I will multiply thy sorrow and thy conception; in sorrow thou shalt bring forth children"'.[13] Thus, women were taught that their suffering would not only atone for Eve's sins but bring them personal redemption and salvation. It is no longer easy to appreciate the extent to which religious beliefs permeated people's lives, but this teaching was powerful and persistent and lasted until Queen Victoria began to alter public opinion by accepting chloroform for her labour pain.[14]

The Church also widely assumed responsibility for the regulation of midwives. This was intended to protect the spiritual rather than the physical well-being of mother and baby – there was no recognized training or qualification for midwives.[15] From 1512, representatives of the Church were permitted to grant licences for practitioners of medicine and surgery, followed shortly by midwifery licences. The bishops who issued the licences were concerned as to the character and experience of midwives, and sought testimonials as to their calibre. However, their main aim was to eliminate unreformed, superstitious practice and to ensure that sick or dying babies who were baptized by midwives while still in the birthing chamber, and occasionally before they had been fully delivered, were directed into the right faith. The licensing system lasted until 1642, the content of the oath that midwives swore in front of their bishops remaining remarkably consistent over the years.[16]

Religious works did recognize the potential hazards of childbirth. *The Monument of Matrones*, published in 1582 and one of the earliest and largest devotional works for women, contains 38 prayers for childbirth, 17 to be said in labour, particularly in a difficult labour or on death.[17] The Church also acknowledged that midwives might use herbs in pregnancy and childbirth, though not necessarily in an approved way. Part of the midwives' oath includes the declaration that they will not use any herb, medicine or potion to cause a miscarriage or abortion. The oath sworn by Eleanor Pead, midwife, in front of Matthew, Archbishop of Canterbury, in 1567 (the earliest existing oath), included mention of herbs which should not be used:

> in such time of necessity, in baptising any infant born, and pouring water upon the head of the same infant, I will use pure and clean water, and not any rose or damask water, or water made of any confection or mixture; and that I will certify the curate of the parish church of every such baptising.[18]

Midwives were expected to inform the Church of alternative practices such as sorcery, witchcraft and incantations.[19] Although midwives may not have been prosecuted as witches to the extent that has been believed,[20] they were tried, particularly in Scotland where the licensing system was not in existence. Some of the prosecutions show that attempts at the removal of pains in childbirth were made by use of charms. Agnes Sampson was a Scottish 'witch' who, in 1590, admitted administering magical words to take away the pains of women in childbirth.[21] In 1632, Allie Nisbet of Hilton, also in Scotland, was accused of having 'taken the pains off a woman in travail, by some charms and horrible words... and laid them on another woman who straight away died'.[22]

By 1588, the oath sworn by Margarete Parrey, a midwife and widow, of St Magnus in London, included clear instructions on secrecy:

> ITEM that ye shal be secrete and not open anye matter appertayninge to your office... unlesse necessary or grete urgent causes shall constreyne you soe to doe.[23]

The teachings on the necessity and positive benefit of childbirth pain, and a midwife's sworn obligation to keep her business secret except in the direst emergencies, combined to create a culture where advice on, and use of, pain relief could be perceived as problematic. If midwives and other women kept such knowledge, if it existed, secret, then this would have further reduced the range of records on which we can draw to examine the use of herbs in childbirth.

The birth

Many preparations were made for the birthing chamber – the couple's bedroom or another room depending on the degree of affluence of the expectant families. There appears to have been a kind of system of exchange and loan that applied at all levels of society for such aids as charms, prayer girdles, eagle-stones and 'mydwyves chaires'.[24] Midwives also carried some of these things with them to be lent to their neediest clients.[25]

Customarily when labour started, the midwife, who might be some distance away or with another woman, would be sent for. As she travelled to help, the father called on neighbours and other women to attend the birth, and these women, known as God-sibs or gossips, might be as many as ten in number. They could include relations and members of the elite classes who might have particular interest or expertise in birth.[26] Men were excluded from the birthing chamber.[27] On her arrival, the midwife would take charge, remove her rings and bracelets, don an apron and see to the mother. One of her roles was to supply easily digested food, broth and 'caudle', the celebratory drink which was powerfully associated with childbirth.[28] According to Cressy, the midwife would have clysters, purges, poultices, liniments, ointments and herbal infusions to relieve the woman in labour, and part of her job was to apply these – anointing, bathing and lubricating.[29] Some midwives brought a collapsible birthing stool or chair with them, although these tended to fall from favour in the later part of the seventeenth century with the rise of the man-midwife who preferred to deliver his ladies in bed.[30] Following the birth, the baby was washed in wine or warm water to which milk infused with mallow (*Althaea* spp.), salad oil or butter was added. He, or she, was dressed in the softest old linen and wrapped in swaddling bands before being presented to the father with the words, 'See Father – here is your child, God give you much joy with it or take it speedily to His bliss'.[31]

Birth could, and did, proceed without any intervention or assistance. Remarkably, some women gave birth in the same room where others slept without disturbing them at all.[32] Many authors of the midwifery manuals urged midwives not to meddle with mothers – not to be pushing and pulling, or urging them to push before they wanted to or needed to – and pain may have been caused by unwarranted interventions. Allowing birth to take its course can be difficult, and particularly distressing examples are those where the outcome might have been better if left to nature. For example, Margaret Clerk, who went into labour in 1700, was delivered of a son, but her husband wrote 'when everybody had run into my room to bring me the good news, she fell into fainting fits'.[33] A physician and two surgeons were summoned, who deduced that the placenta was stuck to her uterus and tried to remove it manually. They were 'too hasty in their operations, by which she lost a great deal of blood'.

Margaret screamed in agony for a full hour before death came at 11 am, four hours after her son was born.[34]

The level of pain and complications experienced in childbirth may have been connected with bodily health. Contemporaries in both England and France noted that poor country women were more likely to have an easier birth than affluent town-dwellers who got less light and exercise and ate a more refined diet.[35] Although rickets was described as a new disease, the first child deaths from the disease being notified in the London Mortality Bills of 1630–34,[36] it was thought that the rickety pelvis was responsible for obstructed labours which led to the death of both mother and child, following days of agony.

There does not seem to be a record of the way that people responded to these deaths. Sharon Howard believes that the physician and midwife were seen as God's instruments, and that while it was sinful to place too much faith in them alone, it was equally wrong to reject them or fail to take care of one's bodily health.[37] Speculation that pregnancy would have been a time of personal anxiety about death has been voiced by Laurence and others.[38] McQuay, in examining the detailed parish records of Shipton-under-Wychwood in Oxfordshire (a particularly complete set), found that for the period 1565–1665, a total of 52 women died in or around childbirth out of 4,090 confinements, a maternal death rate equivalent to 1,270 per 100,000 births.[39]

Women's writing on fears of giving birth

Mortality rates from all causes were considerable in women of childbearing age, and women who had direct experience of other women's births must have been anxious for their own lives. Some mothers wrote explicit instructions to their husbands on the care of their existing children should they die in childbirth.[40] Although strong religious beliefs may have given women acceptance of God's will in calling them or their children to be with Him, women must still have felt apprehension about the suffering they might expect, even if it was not readily articulated.[41] The ability to bear pain was a key consideration. For example, Elizabeth, Countess of Bridgewater (b. 1626), who died in 1663 is quoted by Linda Pollock. She prayed:

> I beg of thee to have compassion on me, in the great paine I am to feele, in the bringing forth of this child and I beseech thee, lay no more on me, then thou wilt enable me to bear.[42]

Undoubtedly, the things that women had seen and experienced influenced the degree of apprehension that they felt. Alice Thornton, who as an unmarried woman watched her sister give birth with difficulty (and die within a fortnight of the birth), is often quoted on her fifth labour:

> But loe! it fell out contrary, for the childe staied in the birthe, and came crosse with his feete first, and in this condition conteinued till Thursday morning between two and three o clocke, at which time I was upon the racke in bearing my childe with such exquisitt torment, as if each lime were divided from the other, for the space

of two houers; when att length, beeing speechlesse and breathlesse, I was by the infinitt providence of God, in great mercy delivered.[43]

Midwives' diaries and inventories

Harley has made an impassioned plea for archivists to look out for midwives' diaries and, indeed, anything relating to childbirth.[44] By 1994, he had found only three diaries – from London, Kendal and Whitby – none of which, perhaps for the reasons already discussed, contain much information beyond times, dates and names of the babies delivered and details of their father's occupations. Catherina Schrader's memoirs (1693–1740)[45] contain gripping and sometimes horrifying accounts of women giving birth, although she said little about her medicines. The Kendal midwife's diary does contain a list of ingredients for two recipes for an unspecified purpose at the back.[46] Many of the ingredients were resinous and not native to England and would need to have been purchased, most likely from an apothecary. Evenden says that traces of equipment for making and storing medicines have been found in inventories of midwives and their relatives. She notes that Samuel Hartlib (c. 1600–62) wrote of an unnamed midwife who discovered a miraculous 'Spanish Roote' which when applied to the birth passage, enlarged it so that the child was instantly brought forth. However, she would not disclose the name or source of the remedy to anyone.[47] This secrecy appears to have been a hallmark of the midwife. Later midwives in different countries display the same reticence – Schrader maintains it even in her diary, which is otherwise full of detail, for example 'fomented woman over a bath of mother herbs',[48] 'bled a bucketful of blood, I gave her a little something: the flooding abated'.[49] Shorter also describes a German midwife who refused to divulge her secrets to a doctor.[50]

Legal and other records

For midwives who did not carry their own remedies, *The Compleat Midwife* recommended, 'You ought to give orders for things to be had from the Apothecaries'.[51] It is likely that apothecaries also supplied medicines direct to women for childbirth. Pelling has given examples from the prosecutions of the College of Physicians in the sixteenth and seventeenth century. These provide records of medical practitioners, such as James Blackborne (fl. 1611), who specialized in women's conditions including providing remedies to ease the pain of childbirth. However, although known for this type of provision, Pelling adds that it is possible some of these practitioners treated women by proxy, so that others actually provided care and administered medicaments.[52]

Direct testimony recorded in courts of law can provide convincing evidence that women used remedies in cases of problems of labour. An example comes from testimony relating to a prosecution for infanticide, quoted by Laura Gowing. In this testimony, Sissily Linscale deposed that Ann Linscale (her cousin) was giving birth and she was:

crying out back and body, and the said Ann sent her the said Sissily, for Elizabeth Agarr... then the said Agarr went to the said Ann, and seeing her ill, she went from that house to her owne house, and came back with a bottle and paper, and made Ann Linscale drink that in the bottle and she took something out of the paper and cowled it up into lumps and made the said Ann Linscale swallow them. Upon this she the said Ann Linscale was delivered of a child which had a little life in it then.[53]

This testimony suggests that some women not only had both liquid and dry medicines but also that they were already prepared. In this case, the child died, and such events likely leading to prosecution may provide us with further records of the activities of women, albeit not always specifying the nature of the treatments offered.

Obstetric textbooks

Much information about the herbs recommended in labour comes from the obstetric or midwifery manuals, although other suggestions can also be found in herbals and general medical books. A summary of the history of obstetric text books in sixteenth- and seventeenth-century England is provided by the work of Audrey Eccles,[54] and midwifery texts are also covered in Elaine Hobby's chapter in this book.

There is some evidence for women owners and readers of midwifery texts. Anne Crompton of Breightmet, in the parish of Bolton, left a 'Midwives Book' valued at 1s 6d in 1681.[55] Elizabeth Sleigh and Felicia Whitfield's 'Collection of medical recipes' contains the briefest mention of childbirth, 'My Lady Graces receipt to hasten a woman's labour',[56] and also includes a list of books.[57] Dated 12 May 1647, the list includes Jacques Guillemeau's (1550–1613) book – the only secular book apart from four French books, in around 40 devotional works.

Remedies for childbirth

Remedies sought to assist with childbirth were not necessarily plant-based. They were sometimes magical (human intervention intended to alter the natural order of the world), and an example is an eagle stone such as the one kept by the Dean of Christchurch – a natural phenomenon whereby a hollow pebble contains an internal projection which breaks off, so that the pebble rattles when shaken – which was highly prized as a powerful aid to childbirth. Lord Conway described in considerable detail his attempts to buy one to assist his pregnant wife.[58] There were many other aids to childbirth which employed the significance of colour, magic or number, often placed in direct contact with the body, and not necessarily herbal. For example, Rivière mentions the use of:

> the Eyes of an Hare taken in the month of March which are carefully to be taken out and dried entire with Pepper. Let one of these with Pepper be so tied to her

Belly that the Sight of the Eye may touch her belly: and it will bring forth the Child, be it alive or dead. Which being done take away the Eye lest it bring forth the womb itself.[59]

Any analysis of herbal remedies can only be approximate as recipes include those for application prior to the onset of labour, as well as those for women in labour. Although there are often separate sections for enabling the birth of a dead child, recipes can also be found for bringing forth the child, dead or alive. It was difficult for attendants to determine whether the baby was still alive, and there was often advice on how to determine foetal death from external signs. Some recipes have instructions that relate to the severity of the condition, but in most instances, recipes follow one after the other with no indication as to which is best in what circumstance or how to decide when one had failed.

Herbal remedies for childbirth in midwifery manuals

Recommendations for the use of herbs in labour were surveyed from a number of advice books.[60] These were examined for their recommendations for easing childbirth. Looking at the manuals, which differ widely in the number of suggestions that they make, around 130 different things are suggested – not all of them plant-based. For example, drinking women's milk is recommended by six books, and animal substances such as hen's or bull's gall, and occasionally chemicals such as vitriol and sulphur are included. About 120 remedies are based on herbs which are to be administered in a variety of ways, both outwardly and inwardly. For example, Paré recommends an ointment that is to be applied prior to birth in 'a truss or girdle of most thin and gentle dog-skin, which also being annointed with same unguent, may serve very necessarily for the better carrying of the infant in the womb'.[61]

Ruf [Rueff] (1500–58) recommends a sternutory (agent to promote sneezing) in the *Expert Midwife*:

> But if it shall happen that the birth is hindred by siccicity, drinesse, or a straitnesse of the necke or privie pas-sages of the Matrix, a little quantity of sneesing-powder and Pepper is to be blowne into the nostrills of the labouring-woman with a quill; also her mouth is to be kept close, and her breath to be kept in, and sternutation of sneesing is to be provoked, whereby the breath being driven downward, may thrust and depress the infant to the nethermost parts.[62]

The *Expert Midwife* also recommends a bath:

> afterward let her use this bath or fomentation, the bath, I say, reaching up so high that it may come over her belly: Take Marish-Mallowes, the herbe and root, sixe handfulls of other Mallowes, Camomile, Melilot, Parsley, of each foure handfulls, Lineseed, Fenegreke, of each two handfulls; let all these things be boiled in water, in which let the labouring woman sit or sometimes apply Sponges dipped in the same warme to her belly and backe.[63]

Herbs might also be administered via a pessary to help bring down the child, as suggested by Eucharius Rösslin: 'One should moisten wool in rue juice/ and shove the wet wool into the woman's genitals'.[64] A gentler application can be found in the *Expert Midwife*:

> Also wee shall use this Pessary, which you shall make the lenghth and bredth of a finger of pure wool, and shall cover it over with silke, which you shall orderly use dipped in the juyce of Rue, or herbe-Grace, in which Scamonie is dissolved.[65]

Fumigation was another method of applying herbs:

> And if this does not help then one should come to the woman's aid/ with smoke to the genitals/ of myrrh and galbanum and castoreum/ you should put all of these together/ with cow bile/ Take a dram's weight of these things you have put together/ and lay it on a small ember/ and let the smoke go up under the woman.[66]

Plasters were also applied, generally from the navel to the genitals, as described by William Sermon (bap. 1629, d. 1680):

> by applying a Plaister of Galbanum to the Navell, I cured a Seamans wife in the City of Bristol, who just after her being brought to bed, had convulsion fits, strange cold sweats, and wholly deprived of her speech for the space of twelve hours.[67]

Ointments were also applied internally to the cervix:

> An oyntment for the Midwifes hands
> Oyl of Hempseed, one ounce and a half, Oyl of Castor half an ounce, Gall. Moschafe half a scruple, Laudanum one scruple. Make of this an oyntment, with which, let the Midwife often anoint the neck of the womb.[68]

Mostly, however, medicines were taken inwardly as pills or drinks:

> Take of the Gum Bdellium, Myrrh of the seed of Savine, Storax liquida, that is Stactes, Castorem, Agaricum, of each halfe a scruple Diagridion sixe graines, temper them with the pulpe of Cassia newly extracted as much as may suffice and make Pills of them as being as a Pease: Both these medicines procuring a speedy birth, are approved almost of all skilful Physicians, and are in use.[69]

> If you cannot have the said Borax, then take two scruples, or forty grains of Date-stones powdred very fine, and drink in in Cinamon-Water; or for want of that, in a draught of good Hypocras. The weight of a crown of the powder of the leaves of Cretan dittany, drank in Cinamon-water, worketh the same effect.[70]

On examination, some of the manuals recommended many different herbs and some far fewer: leading is *The Ladies Companion* with 57, *Expert Midwife* (47), *The Rose Garden* and *Child-birth, or, the Happie Deliverie* (both 44), *Compleat Midwife* (33), *Midwives Book* (20), *Queens Closet* (10) and Paré, *The Works* (8). However, taking the number of remedy references overall, there were some clear favourites. Excluding the carriers or exipients such as different types of wine, and sweet almond oil (usually used externally but sometimes prescribed to be taken), there are eight which head the list. Cinnamon (*Cinnamomum* spp.) leads with 35 mentions, saffron (*Crocus sativus*) has 26, myrrh (*Commiphora* spp.) 19, mugwort (*Artemisia vulgaris*) 16, savin (*Juniperus sabina*) 11, the birthworts (*Aristolochia* spp.) had nine overall, Cretan dittany (*Origanum dictamnus*) seven, and pennyroyal (*Mentha pulegium*) six mentions. Some of these herbs are reputed abortifacients and are claimed to have a long history of helping women to rid themselves of unwanted pregnancies. McLaren has detailed at length many of the occasions where these herbs were used, and lists ergot (*Claviceps* spp. of fungi), pennyroyal and savin as being most frequently employed.[71] Shorter also noted that saffron – the stigmas of the *Crocus sativus* – which has also been used as an emmenagogue (used to bring on the menses) was used by the Egyptians in 2200 BCE in an oil which was rubbed onto the abdomens of women who were having difficulty in labour.[72] The interesting herbs are cinnamon and myrrh which are not generally recognized as being emmenagogic, and are discussed further later in this chapter.

Household recipes

Recipe books were collections of handwritten recipes, both medicinal and culinary, that were amassed by households and subsequent owners – often women. As such, they might be expected to contain recipes to help women in labour. Childbirth was a relatively frequent occurrence that recipe collectors might be involved in directly, as mothers, but also as birth assistants. However, it is apparent from examination of some of the recipe books at the Wellcome Library for the History of Medicine in London that childbirth recipes can be low in number; there are commonly just one or two recipes in each book. Some recipes are written illegibly or are presented in an unusual way. In a Staffordshire collection, the Jerningham Family Receipt Book contains a recipe for 'forcing away the Child dead or alive'. This recipe is set about with asterisks and numerals and mentions a 'pouder hastning the Birth. It is a great Secret for the purpose, And brings away the Child whether alive or dead, as also the afterbirth'.[73] The powder could have been from a variety of sources, including plants or fungi, for example ergot, a fungus which grows on rye and can stimulate uterine contractions.[74]

The scarcity of these childbirth recipes might reflect the way in which recipe books were constructed and used, as they were often public documents in the sense that they could be viewed by family, friends and others. Thus, there would have been less likelihood of including recipes which were considered inappropriate (for pain in childbirth) or secret (as above). Anne Stobart has uncovered a number of recipes relating to childbirth in her study of seventeenth-century domestic medicine.[75] Her sources included 11 printed medical advice books and 11 archive folders of recipe books dated from the late sixteenth century through to the end of the seventeenth century. Amongst a total of 6,513 medical recipes, 128 (just under 2 per cent of the total) recipes treated some aspect of childbirth. These recipes represented about one-fifth of all recipes relating to reproductive matters (such as menstrual disorders, fertility and male reproductive problems).

Conditions for which recipes were provided included miscarriage (1) and premature labour (1), women in labour – reasons for use in childbirth were generally not specified – although some recipes were for 'hard travell' (17), to 'provoke throwes' [contractions] (3), to provoke contractions with a dead child (16), to 'ease' childbirth (5), for those who 'cannot be delivered' (4), for 'fainting' (9), for the 'after birth' (4), to deliver the afterbirth (3), for 'broken child' (1), for flood or looseness after labour (3) and for 'afterpains' (21). Some recipes fall into two or more categories. Recipes mentioned preparations of some individual herbs and spices including cherry (*Prunus* spp.) water (3), cinnamon (2), saffron (2), balme (*Melissa officinalis*) water (2), and other recipes included preparations such as 'The Lord Chesterfield's excellent powder'. Some items included the virtues of herbs such as comfrey (*Symphytum officinale*), contra yerva,[76] motherwort (*Leonurus cardiaca*) and saffron.

It is clear that, to some extent, a wide range of childbirth-related conditions are catered for by these recipes. However, only three of these recipes specifically mention pain in the title: one is for pain of the heart associated with fainting fits, another relates to a 'paine in the bottome of the belly with a bearing down and fulnes like to the mother', and the only one that refers to labour pain directly is the recipe 'to make women haue a quicke and speedie deliuerance of their children and without paine or at the least very little'.[77]

Significantly, there are a large number of recipes for afterpains. These are sharp pains felt as the uterus contracts back to its pre-pregnancy size. They are even felt acutely after the birth as the baby feeds, and their intensity grows with each subsequent pregnancy, so that a woman who has given birth several times may find them as severe as labour pain, although shorter in duration. In one family, 'A Water for Afterthrowes' was copied out on three occasions.[78] The afterpains are painful but not injurious and it is possible that some herbs would also work to relieve pain in labour. Could it be that these recommendations were understood to work for labour pain as well?

Pain-killing herbs were certainly known in the early modern period. An example of a preparation known to ease pain is *Unguentum Populeon* (poppy ointment), which includes fresh buds of black poplar (*Populus nigra*), violet (*Viola* spp.) leaves [petals], and venus navil [pennywort] (*Umbilicus rupestris*) combined with tops of young bramble (*Rubus fruticosa*) bush, leaves of black poppy (*Papaver* spp.), mandrake (*Mandragora officinarum*), henbane (*Hyoscyamus niger*), nightshade (*Atropa belladonna*), lettice (*Lactuca sativa*), the greater and lesser houseleek (*Sempervivum* spp.) and burdock (*Arctium lappa*).[79] This recipe from Gideon Harvey (c. 1637–1702) includes a striking number of plants containing tropane alkaloids which can affect the central nervous system. Applied as an ointment and absorbed through the skin and mucosal membranes, this ointment would undoubtedly have had powerful narcotic, sedative, analgesic and antispasmodic actions.[80] Further work is needed to consider the use of such herbs. Meanwhile, it is apparent that some of the recommended herbs might have other benefits.

Cinnamon and myrrh

Rivière wrote of cinnamon: 'And in the first place it is common among the women to give the groaning wife a spoonful or two of Cinnamon water'.[81] Gideon Harvey took a similar view to Culpeper over what he considered to be exploitation of the people

– although by apothecaries rather than physicians – and wrote *The House Apothecary and Family Physitian*, in which he compared the College of Physician's recipe for cinnamon water and showed how to make a much better-quality product at home.[82]

Cinnamon is not widely prescribed in Western herbal medicine at present, although it features in a number of clinical texts consulted, including those concerned with the use of essential oils. The phytochemicals identified in cinnamon bark are essential oil of which there is up to 4 per cent in the bark, which contains cinnemaldehyde (about 60–75 per cent), cinnamyl acetate, cinnamyl alcohol, cuminaldehyde, eugenol and methyl-eugenol. The bark also contains tannins consisting of polymeric tetrahydroxyflavandiols, cinnzelin and cinnzelonal, and coumarin.[83] Wren notes that cinnamon has been used for thousands of years and cites four biblical references. He states that its actions include the following properties: hypotensive (lowers blood pressure), spasmolytic (reduces spasm), and inhibits cycloxygenase and lipoxygenase enzymes of arachidonic metabolism (anti-inflammatory).[84] Bone provides evidence for the use of cinnamon in treating uterine haemorrhage, menorrhagia (excessive menstrual bleeding) and for antispasmodic activity. It is not contra-indicated in pregnancy. It is anti-fungal, and cinnamon extract has demonstrated analgesic activity.[85] Conway recommends it for dysmenorrhoea (painful periods).[86] Reid shows that *Cinnamomom cassia*, which is similar and also recommended in the midwifery manuals, is used for the same indications in Chinese traditional medicine.[87] Hili, a research chemist, and colleagues have examined many essential oils from plants for their antimicrobial, antifungal and antibacterial properties and found that the essential oil of cinnamon bark is effective in inhibiting *Escherichia coli, Staphylococcus aureus, Pseudomonas aeruginosa, Schizosaccharomyces pombe, Saccharomyces cerevisiae* and *Torulopsis utilis*.[88] Interestingly, Lawless has noted that oil of cinnamon leaf stimulates contractions in childbirth.[89]

Overall, cinnamon can be seen as antimicrobial, antispasmodic, stimulating of uterine contractions and valuable in the case of uterine haemorrhage. Made to Gideon Harvey's recipe, it would be likely to retain sufficient volatile oil to effect these actions.[90] Cinnamon is an imported spice that might not be expected to reach the poor, but McLaren says that members of the upper orders frequently assumed the task of providing for lying-in women the potions that they might need, so that the assumption that expensive spices were only employed by a tiny elite is not necessarily true.[91]

Myrrh, like cinnamon, has strongly antiseptic properties. Although it is now largely used for the treatment of wounds and infections, particularly those of the mouth, its essential oil is recognized as having an effect on the uterus.[92] It is used in Ayurvedic medicine to treat female disorders and in Chinese traditional medicine to treat menstrual block.[93]

It is interesting that two herbs with powerfully antiseptic properties are among those most frequently mentioned in the midwifery texts. They both seem to have properties which act upon the uterus, and they would also protect against infection. Women undoubtedly did suffer from puerperal sepsis or childbed fever, commonly recognized as likely to be fatal on the fifth day after delivery.[94] However, although the need for asepsis was not recognized, it does seem possible that there was an appreciation of the benefits of the antimicrobial properties of some herbs. The Kendal midwife's recipes mentioned above are full of gums and resins, most of which have antiseptic properties.[95]

If the continual anointing of the privities that so disturbed the man-midwives was as universal as implied, one might expect the infection rate and consequent mortality rate to be overwhelming, but Lawrence indicates that the evidence suggests that infection was not a major cause of death.[96] Much more work is required to substantiate the possibility that herbs like cinnamon and myrrh did have useful properties in the context of early modern childbirth, both in pain relief and reducing infection.

Conclusion

Some historians have been dismissive of the value of herbal and other medicines in the past. Although there is still much to be learned about plant medicine, growing bodies of evidence demonstrate that herbs can have therapeutic effects, and it is regrettable that we are apparently unable to readily access much of the valuable information about childbed herbs that may have been used by early modern women. This investigation initially aimed to determine which herbs were used in childbirth in early modern England by considering various sources of advice in print and manuscript medicinal recipes. During the course of the research it became evident that recipes to assist in childbirth were under-represented in comparison with those dealing with the antenatal and post-partum period. This was not a consequence of any ideas of modesty or inhibition about the use of herbs for female complaints, since it was quite possible to find out how to promote menstrual flow, deal with excessive menstrual bleeding, and how to cope with problems following the birth. It gradually became clear that there were reasons why midwives and others might conceal information about childbirth practices, and it began to seem that knowledge regarding the use of herbs in childbirth might be hard to obtain because it was deliberately and effectively withheld from the public domain.

It cannot be proved that women used herbs for pain in childbirth – yet it seems that pain-killing herbs were well known for other complaints – and labour could be very lengthy and extraordinarily painful. It may be that oblique sources such as court depositions can be examined for evidence of the use of remedies in childbirth. Recommendations for post-partum pain may have been acceptable in a culture where religious beliefs dictated that the pain of childbirth was pre-ordained as an opportunity for a woman's salvation and personal redemption. Although the midwives of early modern England could teach us much, we currently need to identify more evidence from which to learn.

Recommended reading

Cressy, David. *Birth, Marriage, and Death: Ritual, Religion, and the Life-Cycle in Tudor and Stuart England.* Oxford: Oxford University Press, 1997.

Gelis, Jacques. *History of Childbirth: Fertility, Pregnancy and Birth in Early Modern Europe.* Oxford: Polity, 1991.
Gowing, Laura. *Common Bodies: Women, Touch, and Power in Seventeenth-Century England.* New Haven, CT: Yale University Press, 2003.
O'Dowd, Michael J. *The History of Medications for Women: Materia Medica Woman.* New York: Parthenon Publishing Group, 2001.
Wilson, Stephen. *The Magical Universe: Everyday Ritual and Magic in Pre-Modern Europe.* London: Hambledon and London, 2000.

Notes

1. Linda A. Pollock, 'Childbearing and Female Bonding in Early Modern England', *Social History* 22, no. 3 (1997): 289.
2. Linda A. Pollock, *With Faith and Physic: The Life of a Tudor Gentlewoman, Lady Grace Mildmay, 1552–1620* (London: Collins and Brown, 1993), 1.
3. Adrian Wilson, 'The Ceremony of Childbirth and Its Interpretation', in *Women as Mothers in Pre-Industrial England: Essays in Memory of Dorothy Mclaren*, ed. Valerie A. Fildes (London: Routledge, 1989), 95, 81.
4. Laura Gowing, *Common Bodies: Women, Touch, and Power in Seventeenth-Century England* (New Haven, CT: Yale University Press, 2003), 150. See also ch. 4 in this book for a literary analysis of early-modern midwifery manuals.
5. Gail M. Gibson, 'Scene and Obscene: Seeing and Performing Late Medieval Childbirth', *Journal of Medieval and Early Modern Studies* 21, no. 1 (1999): 10.
6. David Cressy, *Birth, Marriage, and Death: Ritual, Religion, and the Life-Cycle in Tudor and Stuart England* (Oxford: Oxford University Press, 1997), 16. See also Thomas G. Benedek, 'The Changing Relationship between Midwives and Physicians During the Renaissance', *Bulletin of the History of Medicine* 51, no. 4 (1977): 551; Robert Schuckner, 'The English Puritans and Pregnancy, Delivery and Breast Feeding', *History of Childhood Quarterly* 1, no. 4 (1974): 640.
7. Pollock, *With Faith and Physic*, 11, 107.
8. Antonia Fraser, *The Weaker Vessel: Woman's Lot in Seventeenth-Century England* (London: Mandarin, 1993), 503.
9. Sharon Howard, 'Imagining the Pain and Peril of Seventeenth-Century Childbirth: Travail and Deliverance in the Making of an Early Modern World', *Social History of Medicine* 16, no. 3 (2003): 367–82.
10. Audrey Eccles, *Obstetrics and Gynaecology in Tudor and Stuart England* (London: Croom Helm, 1982), 88.
11. Edward Shorter, *Women's Bodies: A Social History of Women's Encounter with Health, Ill-Health, and Medicine* (New Brunswick, NJ: Transaction Publishers, 1991), 183. See also John Riddle, *Eve's Herbs: A History of Contraception and Abortion in the West* (Cambridge, MA: Harvard University Press, 1997).
12. Cressy, *Birth, Marriage, and Death*, 22.
13. Genesis 3:16.
14. Michael J. O'Dowd, *The History of Medications for Women: Materia Medica Woman* (New York: Parthenon Publishing Group, 2001), 282.
15. Thomas R. Forbes, 'The Regulation of English Midwives in the Sixteenth and Seventeenth Centuries', *Medical History* 8, no. 3 (1964): 235–44.

16 Ibid.
17 Colin B. Atkinson and William P. Stoneman, '"These Gripping Greefes and Pinching Pangs": Attitudes to Childbirth in Thomas Bentley's *The Monument of Matrones* (1582)', *Sixteenth Century Journal* 21, no. 2 (1990): 197.
18 John Strype, *Annals of the Reformation and Establishment of Religion, and Other Various Occurrences in the Church of England, During Queen Elizabeth's Happy Reign*, 3 vols (Oxford: Clarendon Press, 1824), vol. I, 243.
19 Stephen Wilson, *The Magical Universe: Everyday Ritual and Magic in Pre-Modern Europe* (London: Hambledon and London, 2000), 173.
20 David Harley, 'Historians as Demonologists: The Myth of the Midwife-Witch', *Social History of Medicine Bulletin* 3, no. 1 (1990): 1-26.
21 Ibid., 14.
22 Wilson, *Magical Universe*, 177.
23 James Hitchcock, 'A Sixteenth-Century Midwife's License', *Bulletin of the History of Medicine* 41, no. 1 (1967): 75-6.
24 Pollock, 'Childbearing and Female Bonding', 289.
25 Doreen Evenden, *The Midwives of Seventeenth-Century London* (Cambridge: Cambridge University Press, 2000), 85; Cressy, *Birth, Marriage, and Death*, 51.
26 Cressy, *Birth, Marriage, and Death*, 22; Nicky Wesson, 'The Experience of Childbirth for Early Modern Women', *MIDIRS Midwifery Digest* 15, no. 2 (2005): 151-7.
27 Cressy, *Birth, Marriage, and Death*, 55.
28 Alan Davidson, *The Oxford Companion to Food* (Oxford: Oxford University Press, 1999), 146. Caudle was a hot drink made from ale, occasionally wine, thickened with strained egg yolks, sweetened with honey or sugar, spiced and gently heated until the eggs thickened.
29 Cressy, *Birth, Marriage, and Death*, 61.
30 Eccles, *Obstetrics and Gynaecology*, 93.
31 Cressy, *Birth, Marriage, and Death*, 62.
32 Gowing, *Common Bodies*, 153-4.
33 Pollock, 'Childbearing and Female Bonding', 291.
34 Ibid., 291.
35 Jacques Gelis, *History of Childbirth: Fertility, Pregnancy and Birth in Early Modern Europe* (Cambridge: Polity Press, 1991), 152; Alice Clark, *Working Life of Women in the Seventeenth Century*, 3rd ed. (London: Routledge, 1992), 267.
36 Layinka Swinburne, 'My Little Lord's Legs: Lay Treatment of Rickets in Early Modern England' (paper presented at conference on Recipes in Early Modern Europe: The Production of Medicine, Food and Knowledge, Wellcome Unit for the History of Medicine, Oxford, 13 February 2004).
37 Howard, 'Imagining the Pain and Peril', 373.
38 Anne Laurence, *Women in England, 1500-1760: A Social History* (London: Weidenfeld and Nicolson, 1994), 77-9.
39 T. A. I. McQuay, 'Childbirth Deaths in Shipton-under-Wychwood, 1565-1665', *Local Population Studies* 42 (1989): 54-6. These rates are similar to those determined by Schofield using indirect techniques. See Edward A. Wrigley and Roger S. Schofield, *The Population History of England 1541-1871* (Cambridge: Cambridge University Press, 1981).
40 Adrian Wilson, 'The Perils of Early Modern Procreation: Childbirth With or Without Fear?', *Journal for Eighteenth-Century Studies* 16, no. 1 (1993): 6.
41 Ibid., 6, argues that as very few women wrote about their fears, few felt them.

42   Pollock, 'Childbearing and Female Bonding', 291.
43   Howard, 'Imagining the Pain and Peril', 367–82; Alice Thornton, *The Autobiography of Mrs. Alice Thornton of East Newton, Co. York*, ed. Charles Jackson (Durham: Andrews for Surtees Society, 1875), 84.
44   David Harley, 'English Archives, Local History, and the Study of Early Modern Midwifery', *Archives (British Records Association)* 21, no. 92 (1994): 151.
45   Hilary Marland, ed., *Mother and Child Were Saved: The Memoirs (1693–1740) of the Frisian Midwife, Catharina Schrader* (Amsterdam: Rodopi, 1987).
46   Elizabeth Thompson, *The Diary of a Kendal Midwife: 1669–1675*, ed. Loraine Ashcroft (Carlisle: Curwen Archives Trust, 2001), 56–7. According to Loraine Ashcroft, the recipe ingredients included (with her clarifications in brackets): Cloves, Calamus aprus [acorus?], Labdanum [gum], Spike [Spikenard or Spike lavender], Basil, Cinamon, Storax, Calamint, Benjamin [Benzoin – oleo-gum-resin], White Sandars, Marjoram, Storax liquida, Camphor, Gum dragon [Gum Tragacanth], Gum Arabic, Rosewater, Muske, Civet and Cipres [Cypress?].
47   Evenden, *Midwives*, 82.
48   Marland, *Mother and Child Were Saved*, 55.
49   Ibid., 79.
50   Shorter, *Women's Bodies*, 29.
51   Evenden, *Midwives*, 82.
52   Margaret Pelling, *Medical Conflicts in Early Modern London: Patronage, Physicians, and Irregular Practitioners 1550–1640* (Oxford: Clarendon, 2003), 217, 220.
53   Gowing, *Common Bodies*, 152.
54   Eccles, *Obstetrics and Gynaecology*, 11–15.
55   Harley, 'English Archives', 145–54.
56   Elizabeth Sleigh and Felicia Whitfeld, 'Collection of Medical Receipts, with Some Cookery Receipts 1647–1722', Western MS 751, Wellcome Library, London, f. 22.
57   Ibid., f. 80 (inverted).
58   Marjorie H. Nicholson, ed., *Conway Letters: The Correspondence of Anne, Viscountess Conway, Henry More and Their Friends, 1642–1684* (New Haven, CT: Yale University Press, 1930), 8.
59   Lazare Rivière, *The Practice of Physick in Seventeen Several Books*, trans. Nicholas Culpeper, Abdiah Cole and William Rowland (London: Printed by Peter Cole, 1655), 519.
60   These included (1) Thomas Chamberlayne, *The Complete Midwife's Practice Enlarged* (London: Printed for Obadiah Blagrave, 1680); (2) Nicholas Culpeper, *A Directory for Midwives or, a Guide for Women, in Their Conception, Bearing, and Suckling Their Children* (London: Printed by Peter Cole, 1651); (3) Jacques Guillemeau, *Child-birth, or, the Happie Deliverie of Women* (London: A. Hatfield, 1612); (4) Rivière, *Practice of Physick*; (5) Eucharius Rösslin, 'The Rose Garden', in Wendy Arons, *When Midwifery Became the Male Physician's Province: The Sixteenth Century Handbook: The Rose Garden for Pregnant Women and Midwives* (London: McFarland, 1994); (6) Jakob Ruf [Rueff], *The Expert Midwife, or an Excellent and Most Necessary Treatise of the Generation and Birth of Man* (London: Printed by E. Griffin for S. Burton, 1637); (7) William Sermon, *The Ladies Companion or the English Midwife* (London: Edward Thomas, 1671); (8) Jane Sharp, *The Midwives Book, or, the Whole Art of Midwifry Discovered*, ed. Elaine Hobby (New York: Oxford University Press, 1999); (9) *The Queens Closet Opened* (London: Nathaniel Brook, 1655).

61 Ambroise Paré, *The Works of That Famous Chirurgeon, Ambroise Parey*, trans. Th. Johnson (London: Printed by Mary Clark and to be sold by John Clark, 1678), 545.
62 Ruf, *Expert Midwife*, 84.
63 Ibid., 97.
64 Arons, *When Midwifery Became*, 64.
65 Ruf, *Expert Midwife*, 86.
66 Arons, *When Midwifery Became*, 63.
67 Sermon, *Ladies Companion*, 122.
68 Chamberlayne, *Complete Midwife's Practice Enlarged*, 299.
69 Ruf, *Expert Midwife*, 85.
70 Chamberlayne, *Complete Midwife's Practice Enlarged*, 292.
71 Angus McLaren, *Reproductive Rituals: The Perception of Fertility in England from the Sixteenth to the Nineteenth Century* (London: Methuen, 1984), 89–111.
72 Shorter, *Women's Bodies*, 182.
73 A late seventeenth-century remedy book among the Jerningham family papers and which appears to be the work of a specialist, an apothecary or physician rather than a collection of family remedies, and from the appearance of the handwriting it was compiled over a number of years. Mrs E. Newman, personal communication, 24 August 2004. 'Medical Recipe Book, Late Seventeenth Century', The Stafford Family Collection, Jerningham Papers, D641/3/H/3/1, Staffordshire Record Office, Stafford.
74 O'Dowd, *History of Medications for Women*, 15–20.
75 I am grateful to Anne Stobart for details of recipe titles drawn from her recipe database compiled for Anne Stobart, 'The Making of Domestic Medicine: Gender, Self-Help and Therapeutic Determination in Household Healthcare in South-West England in the Late Seventeenth Century', unpublished PhD thesis, Middlesex University, 2008.
76 Maud Grieve, *A Modern Herbal: The Medicinal, Culinary, Cosmetic and Economic Properties, Cultivation and Folklore of Herbs, Grasses, Fungi, Shrubs and Trees with All Their Modern Scientific Uses*, ed. C. F. Leyel, repr. 1931 ed. (London: Peregrine Books, 1976), 219, lists contrayerva as *Dorstenia contrayerva*, a root supplied from South America.
77 Stobart, 'Making of Domestic Medicine', recipe database.
78 Ibid.
79 Gideon Harvey, *The Family Physician, and the House Apothecary* (London: T. Rooks, 1676), 97–8.
80 Gazmend Skenderi, *Herbal Vade Mecum* (Rutherford, NJ: Herbacy Press, 2003), 239, says that mandrake is antispasmodic and and antisecretory; R. C. Wren, *Potter's New Cyclopaedia of Botanical Drugs and Preparations*, ed. Elizabeth M. Williamson and Fred J. Evans, 2nd ed. (Saffron Walden: C. W. Daniel, 1988), 28, 49, 142, 149, 169, 222, 223, says, for example, that poppy is narcotic, analgesic and antispasmodic; henbane is antispasmodic, anodyne and sedative; nightshade or belladonna is narcotic and sedative.
81 Rivière, *Practice of Physick*, 519. The first use of cinnamon found by Elaine Hobby is in the 1545 edition of *The Byrth of Mankynde*, where it is substituted for the senna that had been previously recommended by Rösslin (in the 1540 version) (personal communication).
82 Harvey, *Family Physician*, 22–3.
83 Wren, *Potter's New Cyclopaedia*, 77–8.

84 Ibid.
85 Kerry Bone, *A Clinical Guide to Blending Liquid Herbs: Herbal Formulations for the Individual Patient* (St Louis, MO: Churchill Livingstone, 2003), 149–50.
86 Peter Conway, *Tree Medicine: A Comprehensive Guide to the Healing Power of Over 170 Trees* (London: Piatkus, 2001), 160.
87 Daniel P. Reid, *Chinese Herbal Medicine* (Wellingborough: Thorsons, 1987), 116.
88 Pauline Hili, C. S. Evans and R. G. Veness, 'Antimicrobial Action of Essential Oils: The Effect of Dimethylsulphoxide on the Activity of Cinnamon Oil', *Letters in Applied Microbiology* 24, no. 4 (1997): 269–75.
89 Julia Lawless, *The Encyclopaedia of Essential Oils* (Shaftesbury: Element, 1992), 83.
90 Harvey, *Family Physician*, 22.
91 McLaren, *Reproductive Rituals*, 49.
92 Lawless, *Encyclopaedia of Essential Oils*, 135.
93 Mark Blumenthal, Alicia Goldberg and Josef Brinkman, eds., *Herbal Medicine: Expanded Commission E Monographs* (Austin, TX: American Botanical Council, 2000), 273–4.
94 Gelis, *History of Childbirth*, 246.
95 William C. Evans, *Trease and Evans' Pharmacognosy*, 14th ed. (London: W. B. Saunders, 1998), 289.
96 Laurence, *Women in England*, 79; McQuay, 'Childbirth Deaths': 55.

8

Testamentary Records of the Sixteenth to Eighteenth Centuries as a Source for the History of Herbal Medicine in England

Richard Aspin

Introduction

The documentary sources for the history of herbal medicine in early modern England and Wales are varied and potentially voluminous. At the same time, however, they are widely scattered, often elusive and frequently ambiguous or frustratingly reticent and imprecise. In an age when use of healing herbs was presumably ubiquitous and entirely unremarkable, the occasions for recording such use or alluding to the practice of herbal medicine and its associated epiphenomena – raw materials, apparatus, and so on – were few: the practice did not, apparently, offend the civil or ecclesiastical authorities and thus come to the attention of the law; it was not contentious in the eyes of the medical establishment and so did not for the most part elicit opprobrious comment from that quarter;[1] and herbal knowledge and expertise were largely matters of oral transmission and practical craft skills that had no need for written instruction manuals. It must, on the whole, be the case that the practice of herbal medicine was so integral to everyday life in the three centuries between 1500 and 1800 that it made an equivalent claim on the attention of contemporaries – and thus attained a similar level of visibility in the historical record – as other routine domestic activities such as the preparation of food and the management of children.

Over the course of the three centuries under discussion, the quantity of both printed and manuscript books treating of healing herbs that were produced in England increased exponentially; however, it is arguable that this had more to do with wider social and economic developments such as the growth of the book trade and the rise of literacy than with any fundamental shift in the place of herbal medicine in English popular culture. Besides, it is difficult to assess how such books were used or what part they played in herbal medical practice. Certainly, they rarely contain the sort of practical information that would have been required for a practitioner without access to a body of received knowledge and expertise. Even handwritten medical recipe compilations were often, it seems, produced as much to record a network of personal and family relationships, or to mark significant events like marriages, as to provide a body of herbal and medical knowledge or a guide to practice.[2]

It appears that, from the early seventeenth century, lay people in England began to compile manuscript collections of medical recipes in significant numbers.[3] The recipes were largely based on herbal ingredients and were prescribed for a range of general and specific diseases and complaints. But these collections were not obviously practical manuals, let alone repositories of herbal knowledge, per se. Herbals had been printed in English from the early sixteenth century: the first printed illustrated herbal in English, *The Grete Herball* of 1529, was translated from a French work, but it was little more than a regurgitation of inherited medieval lore and contained no specifically English elements. William Turner's (c. 1508–68) monumental *New Herball* was published in three parts between 1551 and 1568 and represented the foundation of a specifically English herbal tradition in print, albeit one that relied heavily on contemporary continental authorities.[4] Between Turner's work and publication of John Parkinson's (c. 1567–1650) *Theatrum botanicum* in 1640, the tradition was consolidated by the introduction of geographically specific data referring to English localities and growing conditions, most notably in John Gerard's (c. 1545–1612) *Herball*, which appeared in 1597 and was subsequently revised. By the seventeenth century, works such as these would have already been the prime source of objective information about healing herbs available to a literate audience;[5] indeed, manuscript compilations frequently import recipes from published sources more or less verbatim.[6] Evidence of ownership and use of such printed texts can shed light on the extent and nature of lay engagement with herbal medicine in our period, but surviving copies are scattered amongst myriad libraries, and any audit and analysis of copy-specific data of the sort required to build up a general picture of such engagement would be a daunting task.[7]

In order to attempt to build up as comprehensive a picture as possible of the place of herbal medicine in the early modern period, it is therefore necessary to seek evidence in the types of archives that were produced for quite other purposes than recording knowledge and practice as such. This chapter investigates one potentially rich source, the records of the administration of probate. Following an overview of testamentary records – principally wills and probate inventories – examples are given of the kind of information which can be gleaned from these sources. But, finding and interpreting this information is not without its difficulties, and the chapter concludes by discussing some of these methodological challenges.

Wills and the process of probate

The surviving records of the various ecclesiastical probate jurisdictions of early modern England constitute a rich and varied store of information and insight on the history of the everyday. This body of primary documentation has not, until recently, been much used by historians of health and medicine, although that is beginning to change as the focus of scholarly attention has moved away from medical elites towards the experience of typical practitioners and their patients, and as access to the probate records is improved by the publication of lists and indexes.[8]

The Church courts of England and Wales had jurisdiction over testamentary affairs from, at latest, the thirteenth century, until the Principal Probate Registry was established in 1858. Wills had been drawn up by kings and other members of the nobility from an even earlier period but by the fourteenth century it seems that the ecclesiastical courts had obtained a near monopoly of inspecting, validating and executing wills – the process known as probate – and the proportion of the population making wills increased more or less continuously, as far as we can tell, over the next four centuries, albeit never beyond a minority of the total. The legal and administrative framework governing probate also grew more complex over time, leading to the generation of more and more fulsome records. This is not the place to enter into any detailed discussion of this framework and its ramifications, which have been sufficiently described elsewhere.[9] Suffice to say that, by the sixteenth century, the Church courts were producing, or demanding, broadly three types of record that are now of particular interest to social and economic historians: wills and registered copies of wills; inventories of goods and chattels; and executors' and administrators' accounts.[10]

Wills are formal records of the wishes of property-owners in respect of the disposal of their property after death. They were usually dictated to a scribe and tended to follow a fairly standard form during our period, beginning with details of the testator's personal circumstances, moving through their wishes for the distribution of their estate and ending with the nomination of executors. Within this basic model, the contents can vary enormously, with some wills merely transferring an undifferentiated estate to a single heir, whilst others might go into minute detail over the distribution of personal and household effects. Occasionally a will was not scribed in the presence of the testator but written down (usually) after his death to record his last wishes as spoken before witnesses. The courts recognized such nuncupative wills, and they make up a significant minority of the total.[11] In the event of a property-holder dying intestate, or a will being in some way defective or inoperative, the court could award letters of administration usually to a widow or next of kin.

The Church courts had jurisdiction over the disposal of personal property only – movable goods, credits and leaseholds – but not real estate, that is freehold and copyhold land and buildings. The latter was subject to the laws of inheritance, which varied from place to place and were a matter for the common law, although over time the likelihood of testators including dispositions of real estate in their will increased.[12]

Original wills were normally kept by the probate registry of the relevant court and, in addition, copied into a register book. A certified copy might be made for the executor(s). In order for probate to be granted, an inventory of the deceased's personal possessions was demanded, to ensure that executors and administrators did not defraud the estate, and these were also filed in the registry. These documents also tended to follow a common form, beginning with the name and status of the deceased, then moving on to identify the appraisers and, finally, listing goods and chattels, first movables and lastly cash and credits. Beyond that, the level of detail can vary a great deal, both as a result of the size and wealth of the estate and the inclinations and assiduousness of the appraisers.[13]

Accounts were the last documents to be drawn up during the probate process, being required from executors and administrators to justify their expenses: they were normally produced about a year after probate was granted. These expenses might include funeral costs, debts paid on the estate to creditors, and provision for children. It has been argued that accounts provide a more accurate and realistic perspective on the wealth of estates and distribution of money than wills and inventories, which after all record intentions and ideal positions rather than what actually happened.[14] This may be true for general economic and social analysis but, for current purposes, accounts are probably the least useful of the three categories of document under discussion: not only are they rather few in number but they do not generally specify personal or household items, or detail bequests.

Who made wills and why?

We do not know how many early modern wills survive, let alone how many were originally made, but it is evident from the published indexes of wills that there was a steady growth in the proportion of the population making wills from the mid-sixteenth to the early seventeenth century: the rate of increase then appears to level out, merely keeping in broad line with the growth of national population for the remainder of that century.[15] If, as has been suggested, some two million English and Welsh wills survive in some form for the period from the mid-sixteenth to the mid-eighteenth centuries, then a sizeable minority of the adult population is implicated.[16]

This large minority is, of course, not at all representative of the adult population as a whole, being biased in favour of three broad subsets of the national population: the male, the relatively wealthy and the elderly. Within this predictable overarching generalization, however, analysis of surviving wills has revealed interesting patterns of variation and nuance. Whilst the number of married women who made wills is understandably extremely small, spinsters and particularly widows are well represented, rising from perhaps 15 per cent to some 25 per cent of all testators over the course of our period.[17] Likewise, by no means all testators were wealthy, even though the indigent are obviously entirely absent. Will-making was driven by personal and family circumstances as much as by wealth, and even those of modest means might have good reason to want to control the disposition of their property or to ensure their inheritance. Finally, illness and death came unpredictably and at any age in early modern England: it is not so much the elderly who are over-represented as testators but those who were ill and dying.[18]

Fewer probate inventories than wills survive, perhaps a million for England and Wales for the entire period of ecclesiastical jurisdiction, and this implies that many fewer were drawn up in the first place.[19] Despite there being a statutory requirement for executors or administrators to exhibit an inventory of the deceased's goods and chattels before the court in order that probate could be granted, this clearly did not lead to universal inventory-taking and, during the eighteenth century, the practice seems to have more or less died out.[20] The geographical distribution of inventories, as represented by their numbers in the various record offices, is more variable than wills, and they are rarely encountered outside the period between about 1580 and 1720.[21] Beyond that, the degree to which they are representative of the general adult population is presumably similar to the case with wills described above. An analysis of inventories from the archdeaconries of Cornwall and Canterbury, based on a random sample of some 4,000 items for each archdeaconry for the period 1600 to 1750, suggests that inventories presented in these courts were broadly representative of the second through to the sixth deciles of the population by wealth and status: in other words, the top 10 per cent and bottom 40 per cent of the population are largely absent, the former presumably because their wills were proved in the Prerogative Court of Canterbury – the superior court for the ecclesiastical province of Canterbury before which wills of the wealthiest inhabitants of the province were typically proved – the latter because they had insufficient property to dispose. This population represents a somewhat wider spread that that normally understood by the term 'middling sort', including as it does some wage-earners as well as a proportion of the gentry.[22]

Probate accounts are much the least common of the three main types of testamentary record. Only some 43,000 survive and they are heavily concentrated in just a handful of counties.[23] After 1690, they more or less peter out entirely. These accounts are associated principally with indebted or encumbered estates, or the administration of estates of those who had died intestate. And it is evident that they were required differentially for high value estates, and so are very far from representative of the generality of early-modern testamentary business.[24]

Survival and distribution of testamentary records

Before the creation of the Principal Probate Registry in 1858, probate was administered for the most part by local Church courts, either at the diocesan or sub-diocesan level.[25] In addition, the two archbishops' courts, known respectively as the Prerogative Courts of Canterbury and York, claimed jurisdiction over the disposal of estates lying in more than one diocese within their respective provinces. During the Commonwealth period (1653–60), the Prerogative Court of Canterbury briefly exercised a monopoly of probate throughout England and Wales.[26] Ideally the Church courts constituted a hierarchy of jurisdictions that provided for probate to be administered at the appropriate level, broadly according to the value or geographical distribution of the estate. However, it is clear that if this was indeed the general pattern of administration, then there were enough exceptions to the rule to make prediction of the court before which any given will was presented a somewhat hazardous exercise: courts were jealous of their rights and seem to have had a natural tendency to try to extend them, whilst testators for their part might have a preference for a particular court, perhaps by dint of its prestige.

After 1858, the extant records of the various ecclesiastical probate jurisdictions were transferred to the new Principal Probate Registry and district probate registries until, from the 1950s, most of the surviving records of the Church's testamentary administration were transferred to public record repositories: the records of the Prerogative Court of Canterbury and the Surrey courts, which had been held in the Principal Probate Registry in Somerset House, were the last to be transferred, in 1970.[27]

The pattern of distribution of these records in national and local record offices has been influenced by the many vicissitudes of historical chance over the centuries. Clearly, the systematic registration, or official copying, of wills had a significant impact on the likelihood of record survival, but it is not the only, or even necessarily the most important, factor governing the pattern of record distribution. Apart from the variable frequency of record survival generated by differential practice between courts, the most significant influence on record survival was undoubtedly the quality of care and storage that the records enjoyed in the period before the creation of the civil probate registries in 1858 and, to some extent, subsequently when conditions often remained sub-optimal.[28] Occasionally, single events caused catastrophic loss, such as the destruction by enemy action in 1942 of all probate records for the diocese of Exeter that were held in the Exeter probate registry.

Value of testamentary records for the history of herbal medicine

The particular value of testamentary records for our purposes – as indeed for many other investigations into the history of everyday life in the early modern period – is that they constitute one of the few bodies of documentation that sheds extensive light on the lives, activities and material conditions of the 'middling sort'. It is not always easy to establish the class status of compilers of manuscript recipe books, the principal genre of document that has been used hitherto to illuminate the role of herbal medicine in contemporary health care and household culture, but it is almost certain that they were largely drawn from the upper strata of society, at least during the earlier part of our period.[29] Besides, since so many recipe books, such as the extensive collection in the Wellcome Library, have been removed from their original context and have thus lost much of their early provenance, it is often difficult to localize them or even identify their compilers and users. No such impediments are presented by testamentary records.

All three main types of testamentary record have value for documenting the history of herbal medicine, although the more common categories of wills and inventories are potentially the more helpful sources. Wills vary considerably in the amount of detail they convey, but it is fairly common to find dispositions of a range of personal and household effects, including clothing, books, furniture and utensils. Books are rarely identified in ways that would satisfy a modern librarian, and are often described as much by their physical appearance as their content, but, amongst the more common Bibles and prayer books, medical books, particularly herbals and occasionally even handwritten recipe books, are mentioned.[30] It is highly unusual for perishable products to be included in wills, except in the form of gross quantities held in store by farmers or merchants. The household economy and its activities can, however, be inferred to some degree from the identification of kitchen and other utensils. It is quite common to find weights, measures, scales, beams, pestles and mortars (see Figure 8.1) among the bequests described in early modern wills, as well as the more frequent pots, pans, posnets and skillets. Less common are stills and alembics – relatively expensive pieces of apparatus used for the distillation of liquors, whether for culinary, medical or alchemical purposes. Their presence is by no means necessarily indicative of professional medical practice: John Browne, innholder of the Cock at Chelmsford, bequeathed to his daughter Margaret his 'tin stillatory lymbeck to make aquavite' in his will of 1573.[31] On the other hand, another Essex testator, John Evered, almost certainly was in the business of medicine, as he bequeathed to John his son 'all [his] books whatsoever they be English or Latin, two stills, one limbeck, two brass mortars,[his] scales great and small, [and] a great mortar of marble stone' in 1586.[32]

These relatively specialist kitchen or medical implements were frequently qualified in ways that would perhaps have been unnecessary for more familiar items of furniture, clothing or equipment, presumably the better to ensure that beneficiaries and executors could identify them correctly: thus Thomas Stallon of Latton, Essex, described in his will his 'brazen mortar and iron pestle' and 'great scales with an iron beam and leaden weights' among the items he bequeathed to his son John.[33]

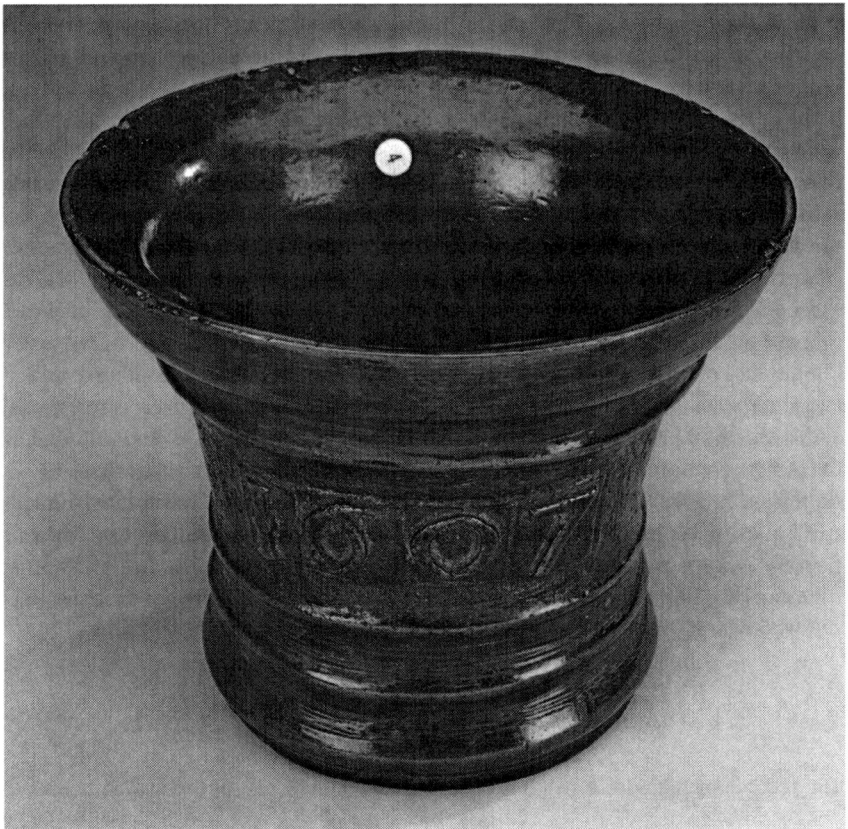

Figure 8.1 Bronze mortar dated 1607, made in England. An example of a category of relatively high-value kitchen utensil occasionally found described in wills or inventories. Credit: Wellcome Library, London.

Clearly, inventories generally provide more information about household contents and their monetary value than wills, but the latter can have the unique quality of conveying the more intangible values – associational or sentimental – that testators might attach to their possessions, or suggest via the details of a bequest something of the nature of the relationship between a testator and legatee that would otherwise remain invisible. When Joyce Penrose of Ledbury bequeathed her still to her cousin, Alice Brainch, in 1663, she was presumably doing more than just identifying a relatively high value piece of household equipment for disposal to a relative, but making a deliberate choice of a particular individual who would value it and use it to best effect.[34]

Inventories record the movable goods and chattels, as well as cash, debts and leases, of the deceased. An analysis of 1,372 Glamorgan domestic inventories from the period 1600–1750 by Alun Withey reveals that some 11 per cent record the presence of a pestle and mortar, and some 3 per cent of a still. Comparative percentages from a small sample of inventories from Montgomeryshire – a poorer and less populated county – give only 2 per cent and 0.2 per cent respectively.[35] The sizeable differential between more and less developed regions of the country is confirmed by Overton et al. in their analysis of Kentish and Cornish inventories of the same period: the presence of a still among household effects is recorded in 7.5 per cent and 1.5 per cent of inventories respectively.[36] There is precious little evidence of the presence of herbs or other perishable ingredients in these inventories, presumably because they were either of insufficient value to record or held in insufficient quantities, but it is reasonable to assume that the kitchen equipment identified was put to dual use, that is to say to prepare both foodstuffs and medicines. Few households would have had the wherewithal or desire to maintain a medicinal closet as reconstructed for example from the inventories of Elizabeth Freke (1642–1714), but we must suppose that the skills and knowledge required to convert raw produce into food were also deployed to make basic medicines, using for the most part the same utensils and techniques.[37] The absence of firm lines of demarcation between both the culture of food preparation and the manufacture of basic infusions and tonics, as well as between professional and lay medical practice, at least in the earlier part of our period, is demonstrated by the terms of some of the bequests in wills from Elizabethan Essex abstracted by F. G. Emmison. In 1592, the surgeon, John Ammat of West Horndon, left his instruments and books to his brother, Thomas, but his 'lymbeck' was bequeathed to a Mistress Bentley.[38] Another surgeon, Robert Turner of Great Dunmow, left to 'widow Aylet at the Swan [his] best brass mortar with pestle and Philippe [sic] More her daughter [his] still wholly as it standeth'.[39]

Using and interpreting testamentary records

The records of the administration of probate constitute one of the largest bodies of documentation pertaining to the everyday lives of the propertied classes in early modern England and Wales. Why then have they not been more extensively exploited by social historians and indeed academic historians of all sorts? The answer lies in the nature of the records and the limitations of the standard means of access to their content. It is a truism to state that archives are organized for the administrative purposes of their producer rather than the convenience of later historians. The ecclesiastical authorities needed, above all, to record and track testators, to ensure that executors carried out their obligations, debts were paid, minors protected and ultimately their own fees settled. A secondary consideration was to safeguard jurisdictional rights by insisting on their claims to oversight, which were very largely geographically based. Consequently, the surviving records of probate lend themselves more readily to research by family historians and biographers and, to a degree, by local historians than by others. In addition, the conventional means of access to the content has been by name and place indexes, partly because these are the easiest finding aids to compile, but also because both creators and past users of the records have found such tools of most use.

Efficient exploitation of this documentation by other sorts of historians thus depends upon improving and extending the means of access to its content. The local finding aids available within the repositories where probate records are held are variable but often include name and place indexes at least. The earliest such indexes to be published date to the later nineteenth century but for a long time they were limited to recording names of testators, place of residence and date the will was proved.[40] More recent indexes have included occupation, which provides a means of identifying particular demographic groups – spinsters, for instance, or surgeons – but is not a particularly effective tool for selecting a subset of testamentary records for evidence of an activity like herbal medicine that presumably crossed occupational and gender boundaries. Was the practice more widespread among women than men, among lay people than professionals, or, come to that, among country-dwellers rather than townspeople, or the richer sort rather than the more modestly set up? Supposition might lead to a focus on a particular demographic or geographic group but, short of an exhaustive analysis of a large body of records selected more or less at random, the answers must remain beyond reach.

Systematic analysis of the contents of probate records depends, of course, on the sort of time-consuming work that is normally beyond the capacity of an individual researcher except in respect of a circumscribed geographical and date range.[41] Typically, such work has been a collective enterprise, depending as it often does on transcription or calendaring of documents prior to analysis of the contents. Architectural and topographical historians have led the way, with perhaps the most notable example being the heroic efforts of the late Marion Herridge on behalf of the Surrey Domestic Buildings Research Group.[42] Another group is the Ledbury Wills Group, whose transcriptions can be found online via VCH Explore, the website of the Victoria County History.[43] Other transcripts of local probate records can be found via this site, but, although they provide a necessary foundation for analysis of the contents, much more work needs to be done to allow the records to reveal their secrets to historians asking questions about the prevalence of herbal medical knowledge and practice in the early modern period. Since there have been relatively few analyses of the contents of large quantities of wills or inventories for evidence of such knowledge or practice per se, medical historians must normally depend on the efforts of others who have reason to record the contents systematically for other purposes.[44]

158   *Critical Approaches to the History of Western Herbal Medicine*

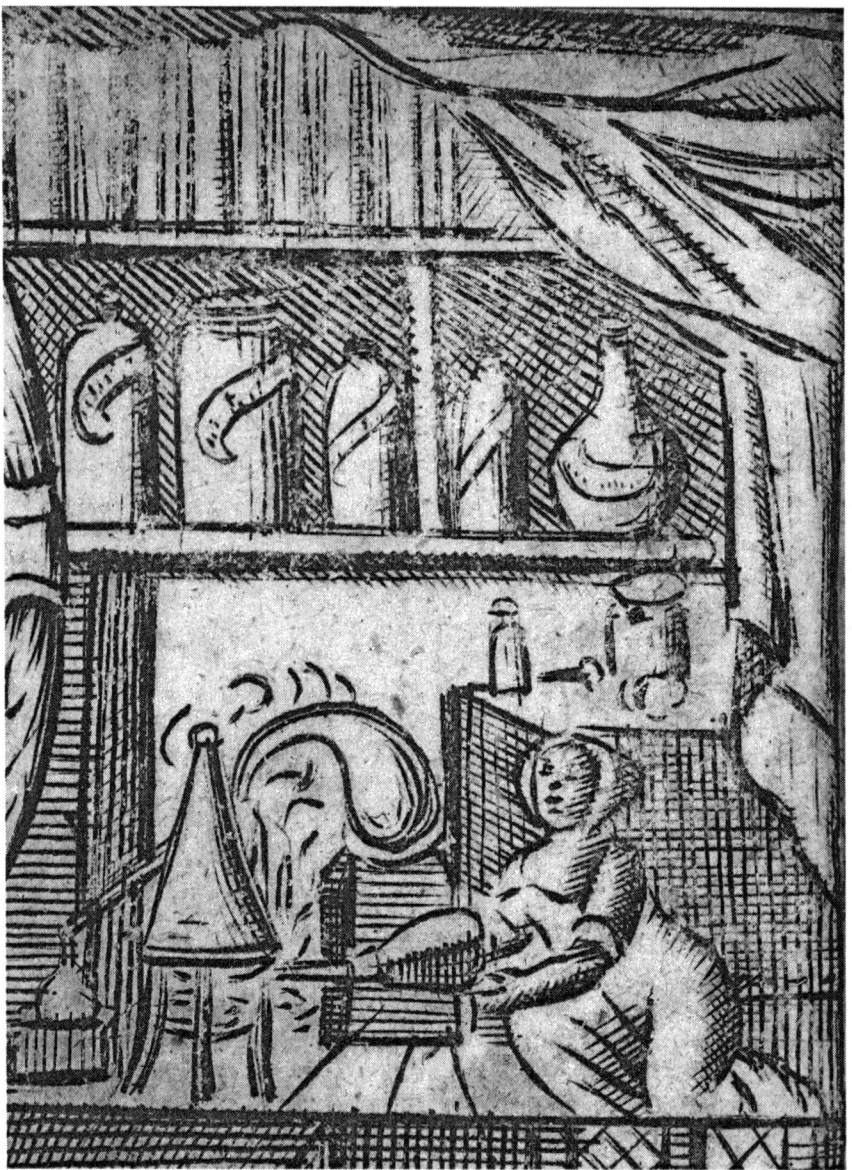

Figure 8.2 Illustration of a woman using a still. Illustration from J. S., *The Accomplished Ladies Rich Closet of Rarities: Or, the Ingenius Gentlewoman and Servant-Maids Delightful Companion* (London: Printed by W. and F. Wilde, for N. Bodington and J. Blare, 1691), scene opposite title page. Credit: Wellcome Library, London.

One such study by Overton et al., on a large sample of Cornish and Kentish inventories, analyzes the early modern household as a locus for economic activity. The status or occupation of the subjects of the inventories – gentleman, yeoman, husbandman, widow, and so on – was recorded as well as a detailed catalogue of the items of household production equipment. The data were used to define production categories – farming, dairying, mining, and the like – and to correlate utensils and the activity they implied with occupation and status groups. The making of herbal medicines did not often require specialist equipment but relied on the use of more or less standard kitchen utensils. The one exception to this rule was distilling, which demanded relatively expensive apparatus, principally a still or alembic, a specially constructed vessel in which the heated liquid for distillation was placed and from which its vapour was extracted (see Figure 8.2).[45]

Overton et al. do not identify the status of the decedents in whose inventories stills occur, but one would guess they are found disproportionately among the effects of the well-to-do. Pestles and mortars, which are not mentioned at all by the authors, were presumably more widely distributed, but along with other items of standard kitchen equipment do not seem to be deemed indicative of a particular production category. This is fair enough in as much as such tools had multiple uses, but it is also clear that the authors do not conceive of the production of medicines existing outside the traditional professional context of apothecaries and druggists.[46] The foregoing proves that it is generally insufficient for medical historians to rely upon the research outputs of economic historians working with testamentary records to provide the raw material for their more focused investigations, let alone rely upon interpretation of the data by non-specialists. However, provided the original data is systematically and comprehensively recorded and can be recovered, it does not much matter that published outputs provide only a partial picture. The important requirement is for large-scale data capture that is discipline-neutral, so that it can be used and reused to shed light on all sorts of research questions.

Even in the hands of specialists, data extracted from testamentary records needs to be handled with care. Testators might mention recipe books, mortars and alembics in their wills, but it is not obvious how these items were employed or how large a part they occupied in the life of the testator or their household. Besides, some dispositions of particularly valuable or important personal or domestic effects might be made informally – both wills and inventories might ignore heirlooms and particular bequests – and thus remain hidden from the scrutiny of both probate court and posterity. Assessors were primarily concerned with the valuation of property and had less interest in describing objects in detail. Kitchen utensils were typically of low monetary value, but behind the routine entries of pots and pans in a probate inventory lies a world of practice, craft and knowledge on which these records are silent, and about which we can only speculate without corroborating evidence. Rare is the testamentary document that explicitly reveals something of the 'biography' of a particular utensil: thus in his will of 1593, Henry Collen of Woodham Ferrers bequeathed to his daughter Anne a 'great brass pot and a limbeck which [he] used to distil aquavite in'.[47]

It follows that testamentary records speak to us most eloquently when used in conjunction with literary and other sources. The bequest by Elizabeth Okeover

(1629–c. 1671) of her 'resate books' in her will of 1670 acquires meaning and resonance alongside surviving manuscript recipe books that are, if not the very books that Elizabeth cites, at least testimony to her role as a lay medical practitioner.[48] Without the evidence of the manuscripts, her bequest would indicate a singular concern for a rather unusual genre of book but only hint at the evident extent of her engagement with medicine. Conversely, manuscript recipe books, whether or not their owners and compilers can be clearly identified, are often frustratingly resistant to interrogation: who scribed them, what status did they have as household or personal possessions, how carefully did their owners try to ensure their preservation and continuing utility after their death – these and other questions might be illuminated by the supporting evidence of testamentary dispositions.[49]

Conclusion

The surviving records of the Church's testamentary jurisdiction in England and Wales provide perhaps the richest body of documentation available for the study of the lives of large sections of the general population during the early modern period. Patchy and variable in distribution and content as they are, testamentary records nevertheless expose to view something of the personal, family, social and economic lives of individuals who would otherwise be largely invisible to posterity. But, beyond the familiar difficulties occasioned by patchy record survival and poor condition of documents or illegibility of early modern handwriting, testamentary records present their own particular challenges to effective exploitation by historians. The sheer complexity of the ecclesiastical jurisdictional map makes it no easy task to predict where any individual will might be proved:[50] finding aids are primarily designed to identify individual testators and are much less aimed at assisting enquiries that relate to locations, occupations or groups in general. Modern indexes, often published, have gone some way to redress this deficiency, but with so much of the richness of the records embedded within the details of the texts, only systematic recording of individual data elements from wills and inventories will allow social and economic, and indeed medical, historians to exploit them effectively. The use of relational databases to store and link these data elements has been shown to provide a key to unlock the full potential of the records. Much more work needs to be done – indeed it has in truth scarcely begun – but enough has been achieved and revealed to mark a clear way forward for the systematic exploitation of these records to illuminate the pre-modern past.

Recommended reading

Arkell, Tom, Nesta Evans, and Nigel Goose, eds. *When Death Us Do Part*. Oxford: Leopard's Head Press, 2000.

Camp, Anthony J. *Wills and Their Whereabouts*. 4th ed. London: A. J. Camp, 1974 (and subsequent editions).

Gibson, Jeremy S. W. *Wills and Where to Find Them*. 4th ed. Chichester: Phillimore for the British Record Society, 1974.
Overton, Mark, Jane Whittle, Darron Dean, and Andrew Hann. *Production and Consumption in English Households, 1600–1750*. London: Routledge, 2004.

Notes

1   Licensed members of the College of Physicians, founded in 1518, had a statutory monopoly of the practice of physic within seven miles of London, and the College pursued illicit practitioners with some vigour, but herbal medical practitioners who fell foul of the College authorities were typically arraigned for deficient knowledge of herbs, or for straying into practice beyond their competence, rather than for any fundamental objection to the epistemological foundations of medical herbalism. See Margaret Pelling, *Medical Conflicts in Early Modern London: Patronage, Physicians, and Irregular Practitioners 1550–1640* (Oxford: Clarendon, 2003). The burden of the complaint about herb women by the apothecary Thomas Johnson, that they were 'ignorant and crafty', is the same, quoted by Juanita Burnby, 'The Herb Women of the London Markets', *Pharmaceutical Historian* 13, no. 1 (1983): 5–6.
2   Sara Pennell, 'Material Culture, Micro-Histories and the Problem of Scale', in *History and Material Culture: A Student's Guide to Approaching Alternative Sources*, ed. Karen Harvey (London: Routledge, 2009), 182–3. See also Pennell's introduction to the Primary Source Microfilm collection of Wellcome manuscript recipe books, Sara Pennell, ed., *Women and Medicine: Remedy Books, 1533–1865: From the Wellcome Library for the History and Understanding of Medicine, London* (Reading: Primary Source Microfilm, Thomson Gale, 2004).
3   Manuscript recipe compilations are widely distributed among research libraries and record repositories; many remain in private hands, and they appear not infrequently at auction. One of the largest institutional collections is held by the Wellcome Library in London: a total of some 75 seventeenth-century examples have recently been digitized and indexed for consultation on-line. See Wellcome Library, 'Finding Recipe Manuscripts Online', http://wellcomelibrary.org/using-the-library/subject-guides/food-and-medicine/finding-recipe-manuscripts-online/ (accessed 16 June 2013).
4   For more on Turner, see ch. 11 in this book.
5   *The Grete Herball* (Southwark: Peter Treueris for L. Andrewe, 1529); John Gerard, *The Herball or, Generall Historie of Plantes* (London: Edm. Bollifont for John Norton, 1597); John Parkinson, *Theatrum botanicum: The Theater of Plants, or, an Herball of a Large Extent* (London: Tho. Cotes, 1640); William Turner, *A New Herball* (London: Steven Mierdman [1551]); William Turner, *The Seconde Parte of William Turners Herball* (Cologne: Arnold Birckman, [1562]).
6   See, for example, the Recipe Book of Elizabeth Bulkeley, [1627], Western MS 169, Wellcome Library, London, which begins with recipes culled from Gerard.
7   A recent inventory of women who owned printed herbals is given in Rebecca Laroche, *Medical Authority and Englishwomen's Herbal Texts, 1550–1650* (Farnham: Ashgate, 2009): Appendix B lists 24 individuals, of whom 15 are attested by surviving books, from a sample of 140 actual volumes in American libraries.

8   An obvious exception is a recent work investigating the changing role of professional medical care at the end of life in the seventeenth century. See Ian Mortimer, *The Dying and the Doctors: The Medical Revolution in Seventeenth-Century England* (Woodbridge: Royal Historical Society/Boydell, 2009).
9   Notably in Tom Arkell, Nesta Evans and Nigel Goose, eds., *When Death Us Do Part* (Oxford: Leopard's Head Press, 2000).
10 The surviving records of the Church courts are now held for the most part in the network of county record offices throughout England. The main exceptions to this rule are the records of the two higher or Prerogative courts of Canterbury and York, held in the National Archives and the Borthwick Institute respectively, and the records of the Welsh courts, which are all in the National Library of Wales. See Anthony J. Camp, *Wills and Their Whereabouts*, 4th ed. (London: A. J. Camp, 1974) and Jeremy S. W. Gibson, *Wills and Where to Find Them*, 4th ed. (Chichester: Phillimore for the British Record Society, 1974).
11 Nigel Goose and Nesta Evans, 'Wills as an Historical Source', in Arkell et al., *When Death Us Do Part*, 47–9.
12 Tom Arkell, 'The Probate Process', in Arkell et al., *When Death Us Do Part*, 7–8.
13 See, for example, the sample inventories transcribed in Arkell et al., *When Death Us Do Part*, 370–80.
14 Amy Erickson, 'Using Probate Accounts', in Arkell et al., *When Death Us Do Part*, 103–4.
15 Goose and Evans, 'Wills', 38–43.
16 Ibid., 39, citing Amy Erickson.
17 Ibid., 46–7.
18 Ibid., 44–6.
19 There is some evidence that inventories were sometimes destroyed by ecclesiastical registries: Camp, *Wills*, xviii.
20 Jeff and Nancy Cox, 'Probate 1500–1800: A System in Transition', in Arkell et al., *When Death Us Do Part*, 25–7. Cox and Cox do, however, point to evidence that inventory-taking continued to be more common than the survival of inventories among probate records suggests, since personal representatives continued to have an interest in protecting themselves from claims against the estate made in the common law courts. Such unexhibited inventories might survive among estate or solicitors' papers.
21 Tom Arkell, 'Interpreting Probate Inventories', in Arkell et al., *When Death Us Do Part*, 72–3. In addition to particular counties such as Devon and Essex being poorly served by surviving inventories, there are few pre-1660 survivals for the Prerogative Court of Canterbury.
22 Mark Overton et al., *Production and Consumption in English Households, 1600–1750* (London: Routledge, 2004), 22–31. The authors do, however, insist that these proportions should be treated with caution as far as the country as a whole is concerned in view of the wide variation in regional coverage of inventories.
23 Mortimer, *Dying and the Doctors*, 2.
24 Ibid., 5–9.
25 At the micro level, the pattern of jurisdictions was immensely complex, with some 250 separate courts throughout the kingdom. Maps of the jurisdictions can be found in Gibson, *Wills*.
26 See Christopher J. Kitching, 'Probate During the Civil War and Interregnum', *Journal of the Society of Archivists* 5, no. 5-6 (1976): 283–93, 346–56.

27 Camp, *Wills*, xxxii–xxxv.
28 Ibid., xxxii–xxxiii. Elsewhere, Camp mentions the loss of thousands of wills from the Archdeaconry of Richmond, Yorkshire, which disappeared in transit between Lancaster and Richmond in 1748; ibid., 60.
29 The obvious prerequisite of literacy immediately narrows the potential pool of compilers. Moreover, the ability to write was less widespread than reading knowledge alone, especially among women. See Andrew Wear, *Knowledge and Practice in English Medicine, 1550–1680* (Cambridge: Cambridge University Press, 2000), 40, n. 74. It is noteworthy that where the owners of surviving manuscript compilations of the first half of the seventeenth century can be identified, they are usually members of the nobility and higher gentry.
30 It is likely that the 'physic and medicine books' bequeathed by Dame Frances Powlett, widow of Sir Edward Waldegrave, to her daughters in 1599 were manuscript compilations, especially as she also mentions her 'still waters and medicines belonging to surgery and physic', indicating that she was a lay practitioner. See Frederick G. Emmison, *Elizabethan Life: Wills of Essex Gentry and Merchants Proved in the Prerogative Court of Canterbury* (Chelmsford: Essex County Council, 1978), 37. Elizabeth Okeover left her 'resate books' to her sister in her will of 1670. See Will of Elizabeth Okeover (registered copy), Prerogative Court of Canterbury wills, PROB 11/335, f. 195 (National Archives, Kew), quoted in Richard Aspin, 'Who Was Elizabeth Okeover?', *Medical History* 44, no. 4 (2000): 539. Rebecca Price Brandreth bequeathed 'two receipt books in folio written by [her]self' in her will of 1740. Madeleine Masson and Anthony Vaughan, eds., *The Compleat Cook, or Secrets of a Seventeenth-Century Housewife* (London: Routledge and Kegan Paul, 1974), 345.
31 Frederick G. Emmison, ed., *Essex Wills. The Bishop of London's Commissary Court, 1569–1578*, vol. 9 (no. 127) (Chelmsford: Essex Record Office, 1994), 19. Another Essex testator, Thomas Freman of Sible Hedingham, even describes himself as an 'acqua-vitae maker' in 1589, see Frederick G. Emmison, ed., *Essex Wills: The Bishop of London's Commissary Court, 1587–1599*. Vol. 11 (no. 137) (Chelmsford: Essex Record Office, 1998), 95.
32 Frederick G. Emmison, ed., *Essex Wills: The Bishop of London's Commissary Court, 1578–1588*, vol. 10 (no. 129) (Chelmsford: Essex Record Office, 1995), 70.
33 Emmison, *Essex Wills, 1587–1599*, 228.
34 Will of Joyce Penrose, PROB 11/316, transcribed in Victoria County History (VCH), VCH Explore, 'Ledbury Wills and Inventories 1621–1640', http://www.victoriacountyhistory.ac.uk/explore/items/ledbury-wills-and-inventories-1621-1640 (accessed 16 June 2013).
35 Alun Withey, *Physick and the Family: Health, Medicine and Care in Wales, 1600–1750* (Manchester: Manchester University Press, 2011), 100–3. Rather similar ratios to seventeenth-century Glamorgan appear to be indicated for the 445 inventories from Elizabethan Surrey transcribed and indexed by Marion Herridge: some 37 of these mention a pestle and mortar and a further 60 a mortar alone, with eight mentioning a still. D. M. Herridge, ed., *Surrey Probate Inventories, 1558–1603*, vol. 39, Surrey Record Society Publications (New Series) (Woking: Surrey Record Society, 2005).
36 Overton et al., *Production and Consumption*, 37. The authors do not report the frequency of pestles and mortars.
37 Elaine Leong and Sara Pennell, 'Recipe Collections and the Currency of Medical Knowledge in the Early Modern "Medical Marketplace"', in *Medicine and the Market*

in England and Its Colonies, c. 1450–c. 1850, ed. Mark S. R. Jenner and Patrick Wallis (Basingstoke: Palgrave Macmillan, 2007), 134–5.
38 Emmison, *Essex Wills, 1587–1599*, 5.
39 Frederick G. Emmison, ed. *Essex Wills: The Archdeaconry Courts, 1591–1597*, vol. 6 (no. 114) (Chelmsford: Essex Record Office, 1998), 205.
40 The earliest seems to have been *A Calendar of Grants of Probate and Administration and of Other Testamentary Records of the Commissary Court of the Venerable the Dean and Chapter of Westminster… 1504–1858* (London, 1864). This was the sole product of an ambitious scheme to print calendars of all the records of the Principal Probate Registry, which foundered on the sheer scale of the records. Camp, *Wills*, xxxiii.
41 Perhaps the outstanding example of such an individual project is the series of volumes by F. G. Emmison, entitled *Essex Wills*, covering the period 1558 to 1603 and published in 11 volumes between 1982 and 1998. The volumes include not only abstracts of the wills proved in the commissary and archdeaconry courts but, in addition to person and place indexes, detailed subject indexes that allow interrogation of the contents of individual wills.
42 This group was founded in 1970 to study and record details of domestic architecture in the county. One of their earliest publications was Joan Holman and Marion Herridge, eds., *Index of Surrey Probate Inventories: 16th–19th Centuries* (Epsom: Domestic Buildings Research Group, 1986), which records almost 6,000 Surrey probate inventories from various courts. Marion Herridge later transcribed the earlier inventories in Herridge, *Surrey Probate Inventories*. In addition, a useful guide to resources for the study of probate records is given by Jean Manco, 'Using Wills and Probate Inventories in Building History', http://www.buildinghistory.org/wills.shtml (accessed 16 June 2013).
43 VCH Explore, 'Ledbury Wills' (note 34). There are 422 documents dating from the mid-sixteenth century to 1700 available online which are transcribed from originals held in the Herefordshire Record Office and the National Archives.
44 An example of such work is that of Anthony Buxton who has analyzed the surviving probate inventories of seventeenth-century Thame in Oxfordshire using a relational database. See Antony Buxton, 'Furnishings and Domestic Culture in Early Modern England', http://podcasts.ox.ac.uk/people/antony-buxton (accessed 16 June 2013). Mortimer also used a relational database to analyze the contents of probate accounts that had been originally recorded by Peter Spufford. See Mortimer, *Dying and the Doctors*, 6.
45 Anne Stobart has, however, warned against the automatic assumption that mention of a still in an inventory necessarily implies active distillation: some 25 per cent of the stills mentioned in the same Cornish inventories analyzed by Overton et al. seem to have been in poor condition or otherwise out of regular use. Anne Stobart, 'The Making of Domestic Medicine: Gender, Self-Help and Therapeutic Determination in Household Healthcare in South-West England in the Late Seventeenth Century' (unpublished PhD thesis, Middlesex University, 2008), 182–3. See also Stobart's Appendix 4.4.
46 It is perhaps indicative that the authors appear to consider the presence of a still to be evidence of the production of alcoholic spirits, which is of course not necessarily the case. Overton et al., *Production and Consumption*, 58.
47 Emmison, *Essex Wills, 1587–1599*, 73.
48 Recipe Books of the Okeover Family, c. 1675–c. 1725, Western MSS 3712 and 7391, Wellcome Library, London. See Aspin, 'Elizabeth Okeover', 540.

49 It is, however, surely exceedingly rare to find such a careful description of handwritten recipe books in a will as given by Rebecca Price Brandreth in 1740: 'two receipt books in folio written by myself... both of the said books being bound with leather and on the inside Lidds of each of them is mentioned that they were written in the year 1681 by Rebecca Price (that being my maiden name)'; quoted by Pennell, 'Material Culture', 185.

50 Kent, for instance, enjoyed six separate probate jurisdictions (seven if the Prerogative Court of Canterbury is included). Overton et al., *Production and Consumption*, 29.

Part Three

Focusing on One Individual: Biographical and Other Textual Sources

Introduction

Susan Francia and Anne Stobart

Scholars have painstakingly revealed the lives and contributions of medical writers and medical practitioners, sometimes those of less well-known individuals in the classical period.[1] The availability of authoritative source texts is key for an understanding of the contribution of such individuals to medical theory and practice and, for example, Lily Beck has provided a recent acclaimed transcription of the key text of Dioscorides.[2] Accurate translations of texts in context are essential, and John Wilkins and others have brought us improved editions of some other classical texts.[3]

Biographical studies have provided much of the past literature about the history of medicine, and it is generally acknowledged that many earlier works focused on significant individuals known for their key contributions or discoveries.[4] In more recent times, studies in medieval and early-modern medical history have extended to consider the lives of other medical individuals, such as the detailed study of an 'ordinary' doctor in seventeenth-century London by Harold Cook.[5] Other studies have considered the lives of individuals noted for their role in medical matters, including women of status such as Margaret Hoby and Grace Mildmay.[6] Further developments in the study of the history of medicine have brought the patient and their family into greater focus, many biographical studies drawing on diaries and letters to illustrate the everyday world of illness and medical treatment.[7]

Researchers have also considered the attitude of writers from the Renaissance onwards in relationship to nature as one based on the superiority of people, individually and collectively, thus progress only being possible once mastery over nature is established.[8] Despite the continuing significance of herbs in the *materia medica* of the early modern period, changes in understandings of the body and nature were laying the basis for major developments and the form of modern medicine as we know it today. Thus, although earlier persons who figure large in the history of herbal medicine may have been considered, it is their role in the development of modern medicine and science that has provided the focus of interest rather than herbal aspects. Some individuals may have been less well researched or, as Tobyn has pointed out in his chapter on Nicholas Culpeper, they may have been excluded and regarded as not being part of the mainstream of medicine.

This section re-examines selected individuals and their contributions to herbal history. Our first two contributors examine famous figures in ancient medicine. John Wilkins focuses on Galen, one of the giants of ancient medicine, though many translations of his work have not been updated since the early nineteenth century and only part of his work has been translated into a language other than Latin. This chapter discusses Galen's *Simples*, analyzing issues of translation, and discussing Galen's own approach to pharmacology. Other texts are also identified which may be used to access much of Galen's understanding of drugs based on medicinal plants.

Alison Denham and Midge Whitelegg also deal with a well-known historical figure in the history of ancient medicine, Dioscorides, who emphasized the importance of botanical study in medical practice. By analyzing the text of *De materia medica* and selected subsequent translations and interpretations, they focus on issues relating to Dioscorides' experience of plants and the accurate identification of medicinal plants. They also discuss unresolved questions surrounding Dioscorides' life, and explore the transmission of written herbal knowledge.

Our next two contributors look at the early modern era. Marie Addyman revisits the life and work of William Turner in the sixteenth century, celebrated today largely for his contribution to botanical plant identification. In doing so, she shows that in his lifetime Turner was designated 'the father of English physic', and that throughout his life he thought of himself as a physician. Although Turner has largely been seen as irrelevant to modern medicine, this author argues that his work in establishing accuracy in medicine provided an unacknowledged basis for all subsequent practice.

Jill Francis looks at John Parkinson, known to us as a gardener, apothecary and writer of the late sixteenth and early seventeenth centuries. She analyzes his contributions to the history of herbal medicine and to gardening, focusing on his two famous works: *Theatricum botanicum* and *Paradisi in sole*. Parkinson's herbal was one of the last in the genre of great herbals but it is his gardening book, rather than the herbal, which reveals more about his methods of working and his attitudes to the world in which he lived.

Notes

1 Vivien Nutton, 'Scribonius Largus, the Unknown Pharmacologist', *Pharmaceutical Historian* 25, no. 1 (1995): 5–9. For lists of biographical medical sources, see W. F. Bynum and Helen Bynum, eds., *Dictionary of Medical Biography*, 5 vols (Westport, CT: Greenwood Press, 2007); Leslie T. Morton and Robert J. Moore, *A Bibliography of Medical and Biomedical Biography*, 2nd ed. (Aldershot: Scholar Press, 1994).
2 Dioscorides, *Pedanius Dioscorides of Anazarbus: 'De materia medica'*, trans. Lily Y. Beck (Hildesheim: Olms, 2005). A further revised edition is now available (2011).
3 John Wilkins, 'The Contribution of Galen, *De subtilitante diaeta* (On the Thinning Diet)', in *The Unknown Galen*, ed. Vivian Nutton (London: Institute of Classical Studies, University of London, 2002), 47–55; also Mark Grant, ed., *Galen: On Food and Diet* (London: Routledge, 2000).
4 Constantinos C. Frangos, 'Towards a Realistic Approach to Medical Biography', *Journal of Medical Biography* 18, no. 1 (2010), 1.
5 Harold J. Cook, *Trials of an Ordinary Doctor: Joannes Groenevelt in Seventeenth-Century London* (Baltimore, MD: Johns Hopkins University Press, 1994).
6 Joanna Moody, *The Private Life of an Elizabethan Lady: The Diary of Lady Margaret Hoby 1599–1605* (Stroud: Sutton, 1998); Linda A. Pollock, *With Faith and Physic:*

The Life of a Tudor Gentlewoman, Lady Grace Mildmay, 1552–1620 (London: Collins and Brown, 1993). For further examples of women's autobiographies and analysis, see Sharon Seelig, *Autobiography and Gender in Early Modern Literature: Reading Women's Lives, 1600–1800* (Cambridge: Cambridge University Press, 2006).

7   Perhaps most well known are the medical concerns of Samuel Pepys in his diary. See Claire Tomalin, *Samuel Pepys: The Unequalled Self* (London: Viking, 2002). See also Joan Lane, '"The Doctor Scolds Me": The Diaries and Correspondence of Patients in Eighteenth-Century England', in *Patients and Practitioners: Lay Perceptions of Medicine in Pre-Industrial Society*, ed. Roy Porter (Cambridge and New York: Cambridge University Press, 1985), 204–48.

8   Nathaniel Wolloch, *History and Nature in the Enlightenment: Praise of the Mastery of Nature in Eighteenth-Century Historical Literature* (Farnham: Ashgate, 2010).

9

Galen's Simple Medicines: Problems in Ancient Herbal Medicine

John Wilkins

Introduction

Galen (c. 130–c. 200 CE) and Hippocrates (c. 460–c. 357 BCE) are two of the giants of ancient medicine. Galen is perhaps the greater, for while all of his works are the product of one mind, the Hippocratic corpus has a relationship to Hippocrates which is now impossible to divine. When it comes to access to their medical works, however, the situation is reversed. Most Hippocratic texts are available in a modern language, whereas only parts of Galen's work have been translated into a language other than Latin. Many of them, indeed, have not been edited since the 1820s. In pharmacology and medical botany, Galen and Hippocrates are joined in importance by Dioscorides (c. 40–c. 90).[1] Yet while Dioscorides can be read in a 'modern' edition of the early twentieth century[2] and in an English translation of the twenty-first century,[3] Galen's pharmacology languishes in the early nineteenth-century vulgate text of Kühn, with no translation into a modern language. Kühn's text, in fact, is the standard work of reference, with identification by volume number and page number.[4] Not only is a Latin translation difficult for many to read; the Greek text on which it is based is also woefully inadequate. This textual obscurity, which is sometimes referred to by translators,[5] is in urgent need of remedy, in order to make the treatise available to medical historians and twenty-first century practitioners.

In this chapter I begin with an account of the 11 books of Galen's *On Simple Medicines* (hereinafter *Simples*), and of its transmission to us from antiquity. In the second section, I identify Galen's preoccupations as a medical writer which have shaped his approach to pharmacology. In the third section, I give an overview of the treatise, with examples from the first five books of some theoretical points, and brief samples from the catalogues of simples, which occupy the last six books. And in the last section, I suggest that much of Galen's understanding of drugs can be learnt from other treatises which have been translated into English and other modern languages. These are the treatises *On the Elements According to Hippocrates, On the Natural Faculties, On Mixtures, On the Powers of Foods* and *On Maintaining Good Health* (or *Hygiene*),[6] all of which are likely to be of great relevance to historians interested in herbal medicine.

Galen is the great medical authority of antiquity, writing in the second and early third centuries CE, some 600 years after his Hippocratic predecessors, but working broadly within their system of humours. Galen famously has four humours, blood, phlegm, yellow bile and black bile, but these four are found in only one Hippocratic treatise, *The Nature of Man*.[7] By Galen's time, however, four seems to have been the accepted number of humours among physicians who followed the Hippocratic tradition (other 'schools' such as the Methodists did not). Galen is *the* text to read, both for his interpretation of Hippocrates and his incorporation of important developments in the intervening centuries (the 'Hellenistic period'), such as the studies of Herophilus (fl. 335–280 BCE) and Erasistratus (c. 304–259 BCE) on anatomy and physiology and of Dioscorides on medical botany. Galen is not the only medical writer of the period, but he is the most prolific (his texts accounting for some 10 per cent of all ancient Greek writing) and the most systematic, ordering and classifying his books in impressive bibliographical treatises.[8] He is also a polemical writer against the rival medical schools of the Empiricists and the Methodists, most of our knowledge of which derives from Galen's partisan attacks. Along with system and polemic, Galen's work is characterized by a firm insistence on logic to deduce the true cause of a phenomenon from an apparent cause, and an equal emphasis on experiment, to ensure that a claim has been properly tested and not merely passed on in ignorance. In addition, in many of his works he is the authoritative first-person controller of the narrative.[9]

This chapter sets out to clarify the aims and importance of Galen's principal text on pharmacology, of which the full title in Kühn's standard edition is *Galen, On the Mixture and Power of Simple Medicines*,[10] after some preliminary comments on how to access this work and how to assess the work of Galen in general.

The text of *Simples*

Editions

Classical texts from antiquity have, since the invention of printing, been 'edited'. This primarily means that all available manuscripts, or a selection, have been studied and evaluated to produce a reliable text. The Greek or Latin text might be provided with a translation and a commentary on the content, but the quality of the text is the key issue. The 'best' editions become standard works of reference until replaced by something 'better'. *Simples* is most readily found in the nineteenth-century vulgate text of all Galen's works, *Claudii Galeni opera omnia*, edited by Kühn. This edition prints Galen's Greek text with a Latin translation underneath, and is a mixture of earlier editions (Chartier of the seventeenth century and the Basle edition of the sixteenth) and emendations by Kühn and his associates. Kühn was Professor of Therapy at the University of Leipzig: he illustrates the need in the early nineteenth century for a full text of Galen to clarify and facilitate the eclectic use of ancient medicine made in the medicine of the time. Kühn's edition is to be found in university and other libraries and online at the Bibliothèque interuniversitaire de médecine (BIUM) in Paris, where all early printed editions of Galen can be found, from the first Aldine edition of 1525 onwards.[11]

In the centuries between Galen's writing of the work in the late second century CE and its reception in Kühn's edition, it was transmitted through late antiquity, quoted and excerpted by such authors as Oribasius (c. 320–c. 400 CE) and Paul of Aegina (died after 642 CE), translated into Syriac for Eastern Christian use in the sixth century and into Arabic for the Islamic world in the ninth, and preserved in Greek in Byzantium and other scholarly centres, possibly including some in southern Italy. Later, in the thirteenth century and beyond, Latin translations were made in the West, and Greek manuscripts returned to the West and were copied in the late Middle Ages and early modern periods. Venice played a particularly important role in the fifteenth and sixteenth centuries. The manuscripts acquired many accretions and modifications from scholars and their clients with particular requirements, both intellectual and practical. The prescriptions in the last six books of *Simples* were more copied than the first five theoretical books, and additions were made from the numerous copies of Dioscorides that were also transmitted in this period.[12] It appears that practical users of the lists of drugs and their strengths outnumbered those demanding the theoretical section. The text that finally came into the first printed edition (the Aldine) and ultimately into Kühn's vulgate edition thus has many accretions.

Petit shows that there are broadly two manuscript traditions, one transmitting the whole text and the other the classification of drugs alone (books 6–11).[13] Most of the manuscripts are comparatively late (twelfth to thirteenth century and fourteenth century) and are contaminated with additions from the tradition of Dioscorides, which is itself complex and transmitted in different orders (by affinity in Dioscorides' ordering, alphabetically for some later readers).[14] Partly because of this complexity, *Simples* has not been edited or translated in the Galen series edited in the Berlin Academy for a century (the Corpus Medicorum Graecorum)[15] and in Paris for the past 20 years (the Budé series).

This is partly to be explained by the total rejection of Galen's humoral physiology by the mainstream medical practice of today and partly because pharmacology is a technical area about which philologists in classics feel uneasy – principally because of its specialized vocabulary and theoretical underpinning. It is not a coincidence that a number of Galen's philosophical treatises have been translated, as well as a number of physiological and anatomical texts.[16] But the pharmacological texts have not been translated. *Simples* is the most fundamental of these texts, but they include also *Compound Medicines According to Place* and *Compound Medicines According to Kind*, along with *On Antidotes* and *Theriac to Piso*. Reference to texts and translations of Galen has been made much easier by Hankinson's *Cambridge Companion to Galen*, in which can be found appendices of titles, editions and translations, along with a bibliography.[17]

I am in the process of translating the *Simples* treatise. The translation is part of a research project directed by Philip van der Eijk for Cambridge University Press, which, ultimately, it is hoped, will translate all of Galen's works into English. The first volume is planned to include the newly discovered *On How to Avoid Distress*,[18] along with *On Diagnosis and Treatment of the Affections of the Soul* and *That the Faculties of the Soul Follow the Mixtures of the Body*, thus a focus on psychological and philosophical approaches once more. The series is planned to contain varying levels of annotation and commentary, according to topic and editorial wishes. The project targets as its highest priority those treatises that have a good modern text, normally one in the Corpus Medicorum Graecorum series in Berlin.

Simples is not in this category. There is no edited text and it will take years to prepare one. There is an urgent need for a provisional translation that can be revised once a modern edition becomes available in a decade or so. The interim Greek text that I am using is based on Kühn's text and on one of the manuscripts studied by Caroline Petit. Why is the need urgent? It is now some 150 years since the early developments in biomedicine which led to major challenges to Galen's humoral system in medical science and to the reduction of interest in Galen in classical studies. The time has now come for medical historians to reassess Galen's pharmacology, and for those practitioners who use holistic approaches to be able to reassess Galen's theories and categories.

Problems for the translator

Peter Singer, the translator of one of the texts that I shall be discussing at the end of this chapter, *On the Thinning Diet*, identifies basic difficulties in translating Galen:

> Complete consistency in translation – even of 'technical terms' – has not been possible. The term *dynamis*, for example, is sometimes 'faculty', sometimes 'property', occasionally 'power'; it is not possible to confine oneself to a single term without an intolerable strain on the normal parameters of English usage.... The word 'state'... regularly translates the Greek *diathesis* ('condition' being reserved for *hexis* and 'constitution' for *kataskeue*); but no other term than 'state' presented itself for the translation of *schesis* (which Galen actually describes as meaning the same as *diathesis*).[19]

In addition, there are many difficulties in identifying botanical and zoological names in antiquity. Singer has a footnote on plant names, in which he identifies five difficulties.[20] First, he has used a lexicon and made adjustments 'on the basis of what seems plausible'. However, the lexicon of Liddell, Scott and Jones is notoriously unreliable for plant names[21] and it seems to me that we need a stronger criterion than plausibility. Second, different contexts make an identification of a plant from its ancient name and given properties hazardous. Third, a different system of categorization leads to an ancient name covering various species while ancient differentiation may be gathered under one modern (Linnaean) species. Fourth, there is no necessary correlation between a modern name and an ancient one (carrots, for example). Finally, Singer suggests that ecological changes have impacted on plants and animals.

It seems to me that Singer correctly identifies some important problems. And he notes that they are much more severe in pharmacological texts. For the present purpose, we need to match them more closely with two key areas of interest. One is Galen's own methodology for identifying plants which have medical properties. I shall return to this below. And the second is to use the help of specialists in ancient botany, in particular Jacques André and Suzanne Amigues.[22] André's work is that of a careful philologist, who has assessed the contradictory scholarship on ancient lexicography and botany, while Amigues is an editor of Theophrastus (c. 370–c. 287 BCE). Her final volume gives a glossary of Greek plant names in Theophrastus based on a lifetime of philology and botanical fieldwork.

What is needed, therefore, in the accessible version of the text that I am preparing, are a number of principles. For example, consistent identification of technical terms, such as 'constitution', *dynamis* and *energeia*,[23] is needed. Plants must be clearly identified. In two recent translations of Galen's treatise on nutrition, the translators leave their readers in exactly the same position Galen was in when he set out to write the treatise. In his section (1.13) on the primitive wheats, 'einkorn, emmer and rice-wheat', according to Grant; and 'einkorn [tiphe], emmer [olyra] and emmer [zeia]', according to Powell, Galen finds it hard to distinguish each plant. Galen's sources were the doctors Diocles (died c. 312 BCE) and Mnesitheus (fourth century BCE), and Dioscorides, along with personal observation and talking to farmers, using their spelling and dialect.[24] In a useable English translation we surely need the Greek term and the Linnaean or other modern term. A herbal practitioner is not going to be able to use a translation of *Simples* that does not lay all the available information clearly on the page. The reader needs to know where the identification of a plant or drug is possible and where not – and where it is uncertain.

There is also the matter of guidance for the reader. What kind of introduction is needed? Many elements could be included: how *Simples* fits in the corpus (after *Elements and Mixtures* and before *Nutrition* (*De alimentorum facultatibus*)); the key characteristics of the treatise, and the key claims; how the treatise resembles, or does not resemble, the other work of Galen; how it differs from *Mixtures* and *Nutrition*. Further key points could include the use of anecdotes; reused material from *Mixtures*; alphabetical ordering of drugs; criticism of predecessors; polemic; and Galen's emphasis on collecting data, but not pushing forward boundaries in this particular work. And what is Galen's approach to pharmacology in general: he had huge supplies of cinnamon and theriac (*On the Avoidance of Grief*);[25] he emphasized properties and not superstition; and the importance of compounds rather than isolating and refining properties.

Understanding the context of Galen

The time has come for medical historians to reassess Galen's pharmacology, and for those practitioners who use holistic approaches to be able to reassess Galen's theories and categories.

One challenge to this reassessment is the recent work of the medical historian David Wootton in *Bad Medicine*.[26] Wootton's attack on the Galenic system is narrowly focused on the development of the microscope and the use of blood-letting, but it rests on the central assumption that in Galen's time there was no experimentation, no consideration of the individual patient, and blind acceptance of tradition at the expense of experiment and proof. This may be an accurate description of some practice in the eighteenth and early nineteenth centuries, but it is far from the principles of Galen for whom extensive research, experimentation and logical deduction are the keys to accurate understanding. Wootton also concentrates on therapy, which for Galen in his discussion of preventive medicine constitutes only half of the medical art. The other half of Galenic medicine is preventive, in which the doctor monitors a person's health but need not intervene as long as the patient remains healthy. This will best be achieved if the person follows the six 'necessary activities' (later known as Galen's 'non-naturals'), which are discussed below. Galen's treatise on preventive medicine (*De sanitate tuenda/On Maintaining Good Health*) has been translated into English (albeit imperfectly),[27] as has Galen's treatise on nutrition (*De alimentorum facultatibus/On the Powers of Foods/On the Properties of Foodstuffs*).[28] It is thus possible to study Galen's approach to preventive medicine, prior to the need for therapy. As regards therapy, the theory on which *Simples* is based, that is *On the Elements according to Hippocrates*, *On the Natural Faculties* and *On Mixtures*, have all been edited and translated, as has *On the Therapeutic Method*.[29]

Modern readers are thus able to study Galen's theory of drugs (the content of the first five books of *Simples*) without difficulty, and the properties of drugs themselves can be partly studied in the translations of the treatise on nutrition. Galen explains in that treatise and in *On the Natural Faculties* that he understands a drug as an agent producing change in the body, in distinction from a food, which sustains the body but does not alter it. He has adopted a basic Hippocratic tenet.

It is most desirable to read Galen's pharmacology as a coherent system of thought, based on observation, experiment and long experience and research. Even if a reader disagrees with it, he or she will be able to reflect on current assumptions and preoccupations in a self-critical way. We, as much as Galen, need help with basic questions about the relationship between human beings and the natural world, the relationship between food and medicine, and the status and nature of knowledge in medicine – not to mention the dialogue between medical science and the past.

Galen's approach to medicine

Galen's pharmacology sits within a medical system that had been developed over many centuries, from the pioneering Hippocratic doctors through the Hellenistic courts of the Ptolemies in Egypt, Seleucids in Antioch, Attalids in Pergamum, and Mithridates in Bithynia to the complex medical world of the Roman Empire. Physicians at those courts had developed botany and pharmacology under royal patronage to help to protect kings against assassination by poison.[30] Galen in his turn was physician to the emperors Marcus Aurelius (188–217 CE) and his successors and has much to say about the universal remedy of kings against poison, theriac, in his *On Antidotes* and *Theriac to Piso*.

Galen's claims to authority, though, are based less on patronage and more on his extraordinary industry and ability to cover nearly all areas of medicine. He wrote bibliographical books on his own books and their order of composition and publication: he was extraordinarily learned. He was the doctor who could extend the medicine of Hippocrates and small city states to the world of knowledge of the Roman Empire.[31] In

Simples, as we shall see below, he reviews predecessors and acknowledges some debts. Many, though, are incorporated silently. Galen envisages that his readers will already have seen earlier treatises on the elements and humours, especially his own *On the Elements According to Hippocrates*, *On the Natural Faculties* and *On Mixtures*. Here, too, he sets out how drugs introduce change, in contrast to food which nourishes but otherwise maintains a steady state.

There are, however, shared properties between Galen's drugs and foods. Garlic appears in both categories, for example. When it comes to therapy, therefore, Galen envisages that the patient will have exhausted the possibilities of healthy living in a stable state and is in need of a more drastic change (see below on what Galen has to say about preventive medicine and about nutrition).

Ideally, following these principles will keep the patient away from the doctor's surgery, though advice will still be needed on occasion for the patient about his or her individual nature, and about any misleading indications which may lead the patient astray. In these treatises, Galen uses his trademark guides of logic (how to reach a true conclusion; how to distinguish a true cause of an effect from an apparent cause) and personal observation to give the most authoritative account.

In addition, preventive medicine and nutrition give more power to the patient, allowing him or her to lead a daily life that remains in balance and in accord with Galen's natural principles. Galen seems to have been a very competitive, controlling figure who strove to outshine all his peers, but despite this, could countenance the independence of the patient.

If, however, disease occurs, normally through an imbalance in the humours of the body, then pharmacological intervention will be needed. To understand drugs, Galen moves away from patient-centred healing to the generally agreed properties of plants, animals and minerals. Galen sets out at the beginning of *Simples* his principles, and what underpins them: see below. There follows extensive discussion of theoretical issues, for example on the compound properties of many simple drugs.

Later, he reviews his best sources of information and other predecessors. Dioscorides is highlighted.[32] Galen rejects popular stories and superstitions (Dioscorides retains some of these) but does not fully eliminate social factors, as we shall see. In comparison with the nutritional treatise, however, there is little anecdotal and investigative material. Properties are known and documented.

Once the simples are understood, Galen's readers can go on to his treatises on compound medicines, antidotes and theriac, the last of which may be of doubtful authenticity.[33]

On Simple Medicines

I begin with four entries in Galen's list of simples to illustrate the text under discussion, from antirrhinum to *achrades* (wild pears), from Book 6:[34]

> Antirrhinum. *Antirrhion* or *antirrhinon* [*Misopates orontium* (L.) Raf., according to Amigues] has a fruit similar to the snout of a heifer. It is ineffective for healing.

> In itself it has a similar power to the *boubonion*, but in much reduced form, so you will learn about it from that plant.[35]

> Clivers (Goosegrass). *Aparine* [*Galium aparine* L., according to Amigues]. Some call it *philanthropos* others *omphakokarpos* [Dioscorides 3.90]. It is moderately cleansing and drying. It also has a certain fineness of particles.[36]

> The leaves and the branches of the Pear, *apion* [*Pyrus communis* L., according to Amigues], are harsh, but the fruit has a certain watery sweetness. Consequently the mixture is clearly uneven according to its parts, having a certain earthy quality and a watery quality, and accordingly a certain coldness and a certain good mixture. For this reason when eaten they are good for the mouth of the stomach and reduce thirst. When used as a plaster, they dry and cool moderately, as I know myself from gluing a wound with them when no other drug was available.

> So-called Wild Pears. *Achrades* [*Pyrus amygdaliformis* Vill., according to Amigues] are both more astringent and more drying than other pears and for this reason, also glue larger wounds and avert discharges.[37]

The first five books of *Simples* are somewhat rhetorical and philosophical, trying to isolate guiding principles in pharmacology. The last six are prescriptive.

A number of studies of Galen's pharmacology are available. An overview is provided in Vogt.[38] Amongst the others, Fabricius traces the authors that Galen has used in his work and the ideas that he draws from them. This is in a sense a commentary on Galen's own account in *Simples* and related works. From a more therapeutic perspective, Harig has studied the concept of intensity in Galen: for many drugs, the strength of the property is given as part of the general description. Most useful, probably, is Debru's edited collection of essays on logic, definition, pharmacological method and practice and Galen's most famous drug theriac (the treacle of the early modern period).[39] Topics covered include science and magic, Galen's use of Hippocratic texts on pharmacology, Galen's use of Dioscorides and his redefinition of the relationship between pharmacology and medicine by tying drugs closely to their physiological impact; efficacy and error; the use of Galen in the sixteenth century; and the Paracelsians on Galenic medicine. Also important is the joint article by Scarborough and Nutton,[40] which explores the introduction to the *De materia medica* of Dioscorides and concludes that Dioscorides is a better pharmacologist than Galen. Galen himself may have agreed with that, for he certainly made use of Dioscorides' work and is much less likely to criticize him than many of his predecessors.

Galen's system is a natural, holistic system, based on the balancing of the four humours. Notions of balance in the body are therefore central, and with symmetry and proportion these are important ideas to bring to medicine in the twenty-first century. Galen's own focus is on the 'mixtures' of properties of drugs, which he discusses in the treatise of that name, and their powers (*dynameis*), as in the longer title of the treatise. What is the power or *dynamis* of a drug? Galen has this to say in the first book:

> A simple drug has that name because it is the opposite of a compound, and the part that coincides with its nature is pure. The 'power' [*dynamis*] is an active cause:

sometimes it works actively [*energeia*] and at others potentially. The property working actively [*energeia*] is the property of heating with fire and cooling with ice, while working potentially would be the property of heating with pellitory, castor and similar drugs, and cooling with henbane, mandrake and related drugs. That for something to be a power [*dynamis*] it is purifying in the class of purifying drugs, emetic in the emetics, provoking to sneeze among the sneezing drugs, to cough among the coughing drugs, and according to each of the other actions the name for what creates that effect – almost no one will deny. But what the essence [*ousia*] of this power [*dynamis*] might be, some have supposed that it cannot be known, such as the Sceptic philosophers and among the doctors the so-called Empiricists. Those who claim it can be known have differed amongst themselves also. Some refer to the size, shape and positions of particles and channels; others to heat and cold and wetness and dryness, each according to their own teaching, as I demonstrated in the treatise on the *Elements According to Hippocrates* – that it is from the hot and the cold and the dry and the wet that the body of all other things and of animals is created. We will locate these essences [*ousiai*] of powers [*dynameis*] in all other matter and in drugs in particular. This was what I demonstrated in the third book of *Mixtures*. And the person who wants to follow what I am now saying should be trained in that treatise. For it is the case that everything that needs to be known about drugs in general has been said in that treatise. And on this occasion I shall say nothing new in this whole class of treatment. But what was said for drugs as a whole in that book I will now work through in detail in this one.[41]

In the first and subsequent books, Galen applies these general principles (which, as he says, are not new) to particular substances. A good example is the discussion of olive oil, which identifies the many confusing phenomena that might present themselves:

It is sufficient, I think, in the first place to investigate the most important oil and the one called 'oil' by all people. The fruit from which this oil [*elaion*] comes is alone called the olive [*elaia*] and the tree also is called *elaia*. And this is named simply and foremost oil [*elaion*], and all the others by metaphor and analogy.

And of this properly termed oil [*elaion*] which is the concern of our whole argument at the present time, there are many differences according to age, when it is either new or like must or at its best or old. And according to the method of preparation when it is straight and simple and on its own, or is made with salt. Then there is a difference according to the fruit itself, when it is ripe or unripe. Then there are changes brought about by technique, when they keep it as it was when originally prepared, or it has been clarified.[42] No few other authors have written about clarification, and I will do so in the following pages. I studied to test out the power of all these oils, and what I detected in each case I will relate later. But now I first want to conclude the task I set myself. The majority of doctors are not right to think that drugs cannot be tested nor arguments made about their powers.

It is necessary to test only those drugs that are unmixed and free from all acquired properties. The starting point is the case of the best state of the body; and then those with a bad mixture; then in this way to the simple diseases as was defined in the book before this and in the third book of *On Mixtures*, and to argue by always distinguishing the accidental from what is first and foremost and of itself.

Some doctors make a mistake not only in these respects but also in their opinions about medical conditions. To go straight to olive oil, nearly all agree that it is a cure for fatigue [*kopos*], but they are not of the same opinion over what sort of condition fatigue is. For one says that it is a dryness of the joints which have lost their moisture through movements; another adds that it concerns the muscles, and another in opposition to them says it is much moisture and tension and heat, when a flow rushes up to vigorously moving parts. Another holds not the mass of fluids responsible but their quality alone, claiming that with immoderate movement there arises a certain liquefaction of fat and soft flesh, a certain part of which is breathed out and part is retained in the body and because this is acrid [*drimu*] and irritant it produces an olive-oil-like condition. Consequently even if there is agreement on the curing of fatigue with olive oil, the dispute over the state of the body does not allow any secure argument on the power of olive oil.[43]

Before the alphabetical list of simples begins in Book 6, Galen has a number of points to establish, not least that he will use alphabetical order.[44] These points are of interest since Galen here, and elsewhere, justifies the writing of yet another treatise, often because others have made mistakes or generated confusion. At the same time, he does not necessarily acknowledge all of his debts. It is therefore essential to establish what he has got from previous books,[45] when he does acknowledge these, just as it is to emphasize what he has done by way of experiment, autopsy and clinical practice. Galen's review of previous works is a most valuable survey of earlier pharmacology.[46]

Taking his lead from the first of the Hippocratic *Aphorisms*, Galen declares that he has no time for Egyptian and Babylonian plant names,[47] nor for particular or figurative names as other authors have. He then turns to the grammarian Pamphilus of Alexandria:

> Now Pamphilus,[48] who compiled the work on plants, is clearly writing about his subject matter as a grammarian. He has not seen the plants which he is describing nor has he tested their power [*dynamis*]; rather, he has trusted without testing what all previous writers have said. This author has thus written books with pointless additions of a host of names to each plant and then description of a plant, which has been changed from human shape. Then he has added certain incantations, libations and fragrant offerings over the removal from the ground of these plants, and other such trivial magic touches. Now Dioscorides of Anazarbus wrote in five books of material useful for all, derived not only from plants but also from trees, fruits, juices and liquids and mentioning in addition all the mined minerals and the parts of animals. He seems to me to have produced a treatise on the materials of drugs in the most complete form of all. For many things have been written well about them in earlier authors but no one has written comparably about all materials, unless someone were to press the claims of Sextius Niger[49] the Asclepidean.[50] And indeed in this case, everything is well said, with the exception of the argumentation on causes. It is necessary for anyone who wishes to become

skilled in these materials to read this work, and also the works of Heracleides of Tarentum[51] and Crateuas[52] and Mantias.[53] These authors did not write uniformly like the two previous authors, and did not bring everything into one collection, as Dioscorides did, but they wrote separately, if it so chanced, about the preparation and testing of drugs. Thus Heracleides of Tarentum wrote in one place on purging or drugs for drinking or drugs for flushing out, as did Mantias; and just on remedies ready to hand, as did Apollonius;[54] or drugs according to place, as did Mantias. The majority of uses for drugs was discussed by the ancient doctors in their treatises on therapy, and the same is true of nearly all more recent medical writers. There are many statements by Hippocrates, by Euryphon, by Dieuches, by Diocles, by Pleistonicus, by Praxagoras and Herophilus,[55] and there is no ancient author who did not contribute to the art of medicine something greater or smaller on the knowledge of drugs, without the magic or trickery that Andreas[56] later displayed. Thus anyone who has time to spend with useful books written on drugs has many by ancient authors, as I have said, and no small number by more recent authors right up to those linked with Pamphilus and Archigenes.[57]

Galen's method in *Simples* is to summarize properties and degree, rather than demonstrating these in the entry (which is the method in *Nutrition*). He is also less inclined to identify names than in *Nutrition*.[58] In *Simples*, some entries are much more substantial than others, however. The first two,[59] on *abrotonon* (*Artemisia arborescens*, L., according to Amigues) and *hagnos* or *lugos* (*Vitex agnus-castus*, L., according to Amigues), are substantial, the former referring to comments in Dioscorides and Hippocrates, and the latter referring to the Thesmophoria festival at which women sat on twigs of this plant to signify an absence of conception. As I have mentioned above, Galen orders the drugs alphabetically rather than by medical properties and effectiveness. But effectiveness is a significant organizing principle that he chooses elsewhere, in *On the Powers of Foods* and *On the Thinning Diet*, for example. In the first, the most calorific and the most helpful in their passage through the body are given priority; in the second, those most able to cut through thick humours, especially phlegm, starting with alliums, are selected.

Galenic texts related to *Simples*

Galen makes clear at the beginning of *Simples* that the treatise contains nothing new. It is largely a reassessment of a discussion on drugs set out in his Book 3 of *Mixtures* in which distinctions between drugs and foods are made and properties defined and discussed.

A health adviser interested in maintaining a patient in good health would also benefit from reading *On Maintaining Good Health* and *On the Powers of Foods*. In the former, Galen sets out his programme for healthy living which is designed to reduce the incidence of disease considerably. Only if the patient lives unwisely and invites premature aging, or if the patient suffers some outside attack, will drugs be needed.[60] Normally, a doctor's task is to monitor a patient's nature from birth so as to ensure that at all stages of life that person is able to live 'according to nature' and in equilibrium with his or her environment. Galen promotes six activities necessary for health. These are: breathing and the environment; food and drink; movement and rest; sleeping and waking; filling and emptying (that is the balancing of the humours in the body); and mental well-being. These activities are not original to Galen, but like much of his work they are adapted from predecessors and put into a comprehensive programme. The doctor will thus in Galen's system be able to build a healthy programme for the patient based on the patient's daily activity at work, in the city streets, in the gymnasia and baths, and in their home environment. Needs will vary according to age, with foods and exercise adjusted for young and old. Older people, for example, whose body heat is less, are in need of foods that thin the humours – wild birds rather than pork and garlic, and onions rather than cereals and pulses.

But a healthy life ought to produce a healthy old age. Galen thus sets out systematically how the natural organism of the patient can live healthily in the city. If problems arise, normally brought about by imbalances in the body through excessive work or unwise exercise, then adjustments to food, exercise and sleep can be made. There is lengthy discussion of fatigue or *kopos* in the treatise (often brought on by excessive exercise, which is a major preoccupation), which shares some of the discussion of olive oil in *Simples* mentioned above. Certain kinds of inflammation produced by fatigue are particularly threatening to health, and should best be addressed by blood-letting, but, says Galen, there are always alternative therapies based on foods and drugs for those not suited to, or afraid of, blood-letting. Geriatric conditions may also call for drug treatments, including the expensive theriac, which stimulates many failing elderly bodies, but is extremely expensive since it is composed of some 40 ingredients, some of them imported from the Indian Ocean.

Lifestyle, well-being and leading a balanced life are the preoccupations of *On Maintaining Good Health*, which constitutes Galen's programme of preventive medicine. It can be followed by the ordinary person living in a Greek or Roman city. The ordinary person can do so if he is educated and aware, but some will often need the advice of standard professionals, if not a physician: these may be wet nurses for mothers, trainers for youths, gymnastic trainers and masseurs for adults. Galen assumes, as often, that the person he refers to is a man, and that he will ideally be wealthy enough to support himself without daily employment, for this is one of the causes of ill health. Employers do not consider the health needs of their workers (whether imperial civil servants or manual workers) sufficiently and cause them to work too hard, eat at the wrong time and possibly miss the baths in the afternoon, another road to unbalancing the humours. The treatise is closely related to two other treatises, *On the Powers of Foods* and *On the Thinning Diet*, which are also available in translation.[61]

On the Powers of Foods also reflects Galen's desire to shine in the culture of the Roman Empire by giving as wide and knowledgeable a survey of nutrition as he can, ranging from the edges of empire in Spain and Syria to enquiring of farmers in the fields of Thrace what they call their staple grain and what type of plant it is. Indefatigable and ever curious, Galen presents himself as the master of medical knowledge.[62] The treatise on nutrition, like *Simples*, draws on the distinction made in

Natural Faculties and *Mixtures*, that a food is assimilated into the body as nourishment whereas a drug has an impact on the body and produces change. Many of the foods in the nutrition treatise appear also in the lists of *Simples*, though with interesting differences of emphasis. The nutritional treatise, of course, classifies according to nourishment given, and orders foods accordingly, starting with the most nutritious. Arguments are given to help identify properties and to distinguish active from inactive agents. Neither principle is that followed in the pharmacology, where the order is alphabetical, rather than botanical or zoological, and little argument appears in the lists of drugs. Rather, it is implied that properties are well-established and not in dispute. The concerns of the two treatises come close together in the second book of *On the Powers of Foods* which deals with plants other than cereals and pulses, the nourishing content of Book 1. Many of these green plants are said to have little or no nutritional value (by which Galen means the equivalent of our calorific value), but to have pharmacological properties which produce change in the body. These changes may aid or impair digestion, but they indicate the proximity of nutrients and drugs in Galen's system. His least nourishing plants are garlic and the alliums, which are, however, the first to be chosen in the treatise *On the Thinning Diet* since their sharp juices are the best among all foods at cutting through the thick humours, particularly of phlegm.

The grape-hyacinth is a good example of a food which has pharmacological properties:

> Purse-tassels are from the same class as the above-mentioned. For their root is eaten apart from the leaves, but sometimes the shoot is also eaten in spring. In itself it has an obvious sharp, harsh property, due to which it somehow stimulates appetite in the relaxed *stomachos* [cardia].[63] Nor is it unfavourable for those who need to cough anything up from the chest and lung, even though the substance of the material is rather thick and viscid. Its pungency counteracts the thickness, since it naturally cuts viscid, thick things, as was stated in my *On Drugs*. So that if they are twice-boiled they are more nutritious, but are now no use for those who need to cough material up, since they have got rid of everything pungent. In this case it is better to eat them with vinegar, together with oil and fish sauce.[64]

On the Thinning Diet, which I referred to above, reorders the lists of foods, starting with those that have the greatest thinning quality, and concluding with the least, such as beef and pork.[65] Like the nutritional volume, this is a work which is accessible to the layman with care – there is little technical and theoretical discussion and the remedies lie in the standard diet rather than in exotic imports – but for the practitioner it fits into theories of humoral balance and the need to cut through phlegm, in the blood in particular. This treatise is the next stage up from the nutritional treatise, in focusing on those with an inappropriate accumulation of a thick humour. Galen would probably advise the practitioner to read it with *On Good and Bad Juices*. If these approaches are not successful, then a simple or compound drug will probably be needed.

Conclusion

Once the vernacular translation using the vulgate text and one of the better manuscripts has been produced, herbal practitioners and other researchers will be able to discern what Galen's detailed approach to scientific knowledge is and evaluate its claims and potential. This is one response to Wootton's attack on Galen and Hippocrates, which belongs more appropriately to their reception today rather than to their own works. A second response is to repeat that pharmacology was not a first line of defence in ancient medicine. Wootton assumes that therapy was the aim of medicine, but Galen's prior method is, of course, healthy living by the patient which should be able to reduce the incidence of disease considerably, so that drugs will not be needed. A final point for Wootton is that while Galen did advise bloodletting in some cases, especially in serious fevers, his several treatises on the subject insist on careful and not general use, especially if the patient has any reservations. Wootton sometimes makes it appear that bloodletting is the first remedy chosen by Galen, whereas in fact it was likely to be one of the last, along with surgery.

Like his predecessors, Galen depended on centuries of human interaction with plants, animals and minerals. He had not tested medical materials with double blind trials, of course, but he had subjected many of them to testing, and he had weeded out much magical material in his predecessors, including Dioscorides. At every opportunity, as a matter of principle, he subjected his knowledge to logical methods to identify properties and causes.

Recommended reading

Debru, Armelle, ed. *Galen on Pharmacology: Philosophy, History, and Medicine: Proceedings of the Vth International Galen Colloquium, Lille, 16–18 March 1995.* Leiden: Brill, 1997.
Gill, Christopher, Tim Whitmarsh, and John Wilkins, eds. *Galen and the World of Knowledge.* Cambridge: Cambridge University Press, 2009.
Hankinson, R. J., ed. *The Cambridge Companion to Galen.* Cambridge: Cambridge University Press, 2008.
Singer, P. N., ed. *Galen: Selected Works.* Oxford: Oxford University Press, 1997.
Wootton, David. *Bad Medicine: Doctors Doing Harm since Hippocrates.* Oxford: Oxford University Press, 2006.

Notes

1   For more on the Hippocratic texts, see ch. 2 in this book; on Dioscorides, see chs 2 and 10.
2   Max Wellmann, ed., *Pedanii Dioscuridis Anazarbei De materia medica libri quinque*, 3 vols (Berlin: Weidmann, 1906–14).
3   Pedanius Dioscorides, *Pedanius Dioscorides of Anazarbus De materia medica*, trans.

Lily Y. Beck, 2nd revised and enlarged ed., vol. 38, Altertumswissenschaftliche Texte und Studien (Hildesheim: Olms, 2011).
4   Galen, *Claudii Galeni opera omnia*, ed. Carolus G. Kühn (Leipzig: C. Cnobloch, 1821–33). The first page of *On Simple Medicines*, for example, is referred to as 11.379. A number of Galen's treatises have come to light since Kühn's text was published: see Vivian Nutton, ed., *The Unknown Galen* (London: Institute of Classical Studies, University of London, 2002); Véronique Boudon-Millot and Jacques Jouanna, eds., *Galien. Tome IV. Ne pas se chagriner* (Paris: Belles Lettres, 2010).
5   Mark Grant, ed., *Galen: On Food and Diet* (London: Routledge, 2000), 12, writes: 'Not wanting to stray far from Galen's words, I have tried to strike a balance between the literal and what can be read comfortably'. He also alludes to the vulgate Latin translation reprinted in the nineteenth century in 'the twilight of Galen's long period of predominance' and observes, 'what Galen writes is surprisingly accessible to the modern reader'. So there is hope, but a rather fearsome weight of history and the past.
6   Editions and translations respectively: Arthur J. Brock, ed., *Galen. On the Natural Faculties* (Cambridge, MA: Harvard University Press, 1916); Phillip De Lacy, ed., *Galen: On the Elements According to Hippocrates*, vol. 5, part 1, Corpus Medicorum Graecorum (Berlin: Akademie Verlag, 1996); Robert M. Green, *A Translation of Galen's Hygiene: (De sanitate tuenda)* (Springfield, IL: Charles C. Thomas, 1951); Owen Powell, ed., *Galen: On the Properties of Foodstuffs* (Cambridge: Cambridge University Press, 2003); P. N. Singer, ed., *Galen: Selected Works* (Oxford: Oxford University Press, 1997).
7   Jacques Jouanna, ed., *La nature de l'homme/Hippocrate*, vol. I, parts 1, 3, Corpus Medicorum Graecorum (Berlin: Akademie-Verlag, 1975).
8   *On My Own Books* and *On the Order of My Own Books* in Singer, *Galen: Selected Works*.
9   Laurence M. Totelin, 'And to End on a Poetic Note: Galen's Authorial Strategies in the Pharmacological Books', *Studies in History and Philosophy of Science Part A* 43, no. 2 (2012): 307–15.
10 See further C. Petit, 'Theorie et pratique: connaissance et diffusion du traité des *Simples* de Galien au Moyen Age', in *Fito-zooterapia antigua y altomedieval: Textos y doctrinas*, ed. Arsenio Ferraces Rodriguez (Coruña: Universidade da Coruña, 2009), 79–95.
11 See Bibliothèque numérique Medic@, Histoire de la santé, http://www.bium.univ-paris5.fr/histmed/medica.htm (accessed 9 June 2013).
12 See Petit, 'Theorie et Pratique'; Marie Cronier, 'Recherches sur l'histoire du texte du *De materia medica* de Dioscoride' (unpublished PhD thesis, University of Paris IV-Sorbonne, 2007).
13 Petit, 'Theorie et Pratique'.
14 John Scarborough and Vivian Nutton, 'The Preface of Dioscorides' Materia Medica: Introduction, Translation and Commentary', *Transactions and Studies of the College of Physicians of Philadelphia (5th series)* 4, no. 3 (1982): 187–227.
15 'Galen of Pergamum: The Transmission, Interpretation and Completion of Ancient Medicine', http://cmg.bbaw.de/ (accessed 17 June 2013).
16 See Brock, *On the Natural Faculties*; Ian Johnstone and G. H. R. Horsley, eds., *Method of Medicine/ Galen*, 3 vols, Loeb Classical Library (Cambridge, MA: Harvard University Press, 2011); Margaret T. May, ed., *Galen, On the Usefulness of the Parts of the Body*, 2 vols (Ithaca, NY: Cornell University Press, 1968).

17 R. J. Hankinson, ed., *The Cambridge Companion to Galen* (Cambridge: Cambridge University Press, 2008), 391–403.
18 Discovered in Thessaloniki in 2006: see Boudon-Millot and Jouanna, *Ne pas se chagriner*.
19 Singer, *Galen: Selected Works*, xliv. A *dynamis* in Greek signifies an ability to do something or a potential to do something. It is a complicated scientific term discussed by Aristotle, Galen and many others. The best modern analogy is electricity: the power is potentially there to run a device, but may not be activated in all cases, until it is switched on.
20 Ibid., 403. For more on the identification of plants from ancient names, see also ch. 10 in this book, which focuses on carrot and other plant identifications.
21 Henry G. Liddell, Robert Scott and H. Stuart Jones, *A Greek-English Lexicon: A Supplement*, 9th ed. (Oxford: Clarendon Press, 1968); John E. Raven, *Plants and Plant Lore in Ancient Greece* (Oxford: Leopard's Head Press, 2000).
22 Suzanne Amigues, ed., *Théophraste: recherches sur les plantes*, 5 vols (Paris: Les Belles Lettres, 1988–2006); Jacques André, *Les noms de plantes dans la Rome antique* (Paris: Les Belles Lettres, 1985).
23 The activated as opposed to the potential property of a drug.
24 John Wilkins, preface to Powell, *Properties of Foodstuffs*, ix–xxi; John Wilkins, 'Galen and Athenaeus in the Hellenistic Library', in *Ordering Knowledge in the Roman Empire*, ed. Jason König and Tim Whitmarsh (Cambridge: Cambridge University Press, 2007), 69–87.
25 Boudon-Millot and Jouanna, *Ne pas se chagriner*.
26 David Wootton, *Bad Medicine: Doctors Doing Harm since Hippocrates* (Oxford: Oxford University Press, 2006).
27 This is Green, *Galen's Hygiene*.
28 Grant, *On Food and Diet*; Powell, *Properties of Foodstuffs*.
29 De Lacy, *Galen: On the Elements*; Brock, *On the Natural Faculties*; Johnstone and Horsely, *Method of Medicine*.
30 On the doctors at the royal courts, see Galen's list below, and Jean-Marie Jacques, ed., *Oeuvres. Tome 2: Les thériaques, fragments iologiques antérieures à Nicandre* (Paris: Les Belles Lettres, 2002), xiii–xlviii.
31 See Christopher Gill, Tim Whitmarsh and John Wilkins, eds., *Galen and the World of Knowledge* (Cambridge: Cambridge University Press, 2009); Wilkins, 'Galen and Athenaeus'; Wilkins, preface to Powell, *Properties of Foodstuffs*; and Totelin, 'Galen's Authorial Strategies'.
32 See Cronier, 'Recherches sur l'histoire', and Dioscorides, *De materia medica*, 2011.
33 See Nutton, *Ancient Medicine*, 395.
34 Galen, *Opera omnia*, 11.834.
35 The entry, 4.119 for *boubonion*, 'groin plant', comes under beta: it is also identified with the Attic Aster ('Aster Attikos'). It works as a plaster or when tied to the affected part. Liddell, Scott and Jones, *Greek-English Lexicon*.
36 Antirrhinum and *aparine* are discussed in Dioscorides, 4.130. Amigues suggests that the antirrhinum offers little, with an insignificant root (noted by Theophrastus). Dioscorides has magical uses for antirrhinum which Galen omits (*historeitai*): it is an antidote for poisons if an amulet is carried, and it seduces if in oil of lily.
37 My translation, as are all translations from *Simples* in this chapter.
38 Sabine Vogt, 'Drugs and Pharmacology', in Hankinson, *Cambridge Companion*, 304–22.

39 Armelle Debru, ed., *Galen on Pharmacology: Philosophy, History, and Medicine: Proceedings of the Vth International Galen Colloquium, Lille, 16-18 March 1995* (Leiden: Brill, 1997). See also Cajus Fabricius, *Galens Exzerpte aus älteren Pharmakologen* (Berlin: De Gruyter, 1972); Georg Harig, *Bestimmung der Intensität im medizinischen System Galens: Ein Beitrag zur theoretischen Pharmakologie, Nosologie und Therapie in der Galenischen Medizin* (Berlin: Akademie-Verlag, 1974).
40 Scarborough and Nutton, 'The Preface of Dioscorides'.
41 Galen, *Opera omnia*, 11.380-81. According to Liddell, Scott and Jones, *Greek-English Lexicon*, pellitory [*purethron*] is *Anacyclus pyrethrum*, henbane [*huoskuamos*] is *Hyoscyamus niger*, mandrake [*mandragora*] is *Mandragora officianalis*, although the latter is *Mandragora autumnalis* Bertol. according to Amigues.
42 Literally 'whitened'.
43 *Simples*, Book 2 (7-10) in Galen, *Opera omnia*, 11.484-6.
44 Galen, *Opera omnia*, 11.792.
45 See Fabricius, *Galens Exzerpte*.
46 The most useful studies are John Scarborough, *Pharmacy and Drug Lore in Antiquity: Greece, Rome, Byzantium* (Farnham: Ashgate, 2010); Jacques, *Oeuvres. Tome 2. Les thériaques*.
47 The dependence of Greek medicine on Egyptian and Babylonian predecessors may have been much more extensive than appears from the self-confident works of the Hippocratic writers and of Galen. Galen rejects non-Greek names because they make identification of plants even more complicated. Some Egyptian botany also included superstitious incantations, which Galen mentions with derision.
48 This, and the following notes, give references to encyclopaedia entries on the previous authors mentioned. Pamphilus: Christine F. Salazar, ed., *Brill's New Pauly: Encyclopaedia of the Ancient World: Antiquity*, English ed. (Leiden: Brill, 2002-10), 10.412; Paul T. Keyser and Georgia Irby-Massie, eds., *The Encyclopaedia of Ancient Natural Scientists: The Greek Tradition and Its Many Heirs* (London: Routledge, 2008), 606-7.
49 Sextius Niger was an important influence on Dioscorides also.
50 On Asclepiades of Bithynia see Salazar, *Brill's New Pauly*, 2.96-8; Keyser and Irby-Massie, *Encyclopaedia*, 170-1.
51 Salazar, *Brill's New Pauly*, 6.173-4; Keyser and Irby-Massie, *Encyclopaedia*, 370-1.
52 Salazar, *Brill's New Pauly*, 3.920-1; Keyser and Irby-Massie, *Encyclopaedia*, 491.
53 Salazar, *Brill's New Pauly*, 8.255; Keyser and Irby-Massie, *Encyclopaedia*, 525.
54 Apollonius (Mys?); see Salazar, *Brill's New Pauly*, 1.882; Keyser and Irby-Massie, *Encyclopaedia*, 111.
55 Galen's list includes many of the important doctors of the fourth century BCE between Hippocrates and the great Hellenistic theorist, Herophilus, on whom see Heinrich Von Staden, *Herophilus: The Art of Medicine in Early Alexandria* (Cambridge: Cambridge University Press, 1989).
56 On Andreas at the court of the Ptolemies, see Salazar, *Brill's New Pauly*, 1.680-1; Keyser and Irby-Massie, *Encyclopaedia*, 77-8.
57 Galen, *Opera omnia*, 11.793-6. On Pamphilus and Archigenes, see Salazar, *Brill's New Pauly*, 1.989-90.
58 Of the primitive wheats mentioned above (einkorn, emmer and rice wheat), *zeia* and *olyra* are not a problem in *Simples*; and *tiphe* is not mentioned at all. Their identification is a huge problem in *On the Powers of Foods* for two reasons: cereals are the major providers of calorific nutrition (*trophe*); and identification is high on the agenda there.

59 Galen, *Opera omnia*, 11.798–810.
60 Green, *Galen's Hygiene*, 5.1.
61 *On the Powers of Foods*, see Grant, *On Food and Diet*, and Powell, *Properties of Foodstuffs*; *On the Thinning Diet*, see Singer, *Galen: Selected Works*.
62 See Wilkins, 'Galen and Athenaeus'; Totelin, 'Galen's Authorial Strategies'.
63 The upper part of the stomach, where it meets the oesophagus.
64 Powell, *Properties of Foodstuffs*, 111.
65 See John Wilkins, 'The Contribution of Galen, *De subtilitante diaeta* (On the Thinning Diet)', in *The Unknown Galen*, ed. Vivian Nutton (London: Institute of Classical Studies, University of London, 2002), 47–55; and for a translation, see Singer, *Galen: Selected Works*.

10

Deciphering Dioscorides: Mountains and Molehills?

Alison Denham and Midge Whitelegg

Introduction

In 1492, Niccolò Leoniceno (1428–1524), Professor of Medicine at Ferrara in Italy, justified his critique of Pliny's *Natural History* by saying that the texts of ancient writers must be interpreted with care because 'the health and life of men depend on it'.[1] He was engaged in editing classical texts for use by medical practitioners prescribing herbs, but the problem remains the same for herbalists and historians today: how can we evaluate classical herbal texts and learn from the authors without compromising safe practice?

We have recently discussed the transmission of written herbal knowledge, using *De materia medica* by Pedanius Dioscorides (c. 40–c. 90 CE) as a starting-point.[2] Our book sought to address the lack of a coherent description of the history of Western herbal medicine from classical times up to the present day. A particular focus was to examine the transmission of knowledge about herbs through the centuries through the bibliographic evidence that may support clinical use for a selection of 27 plants. Such a project has relevance to Western herbal practitioners, helping to consolidate their tradition and inform their clinical prescribing, as there are few studies of the past transmission of herbal knowledge. We sought to review clinical usage in addition to considering the identity of the plants under discussion.[3] Many issues arose in the interpretation of the texts, and in this chapter we explore some further issues and make suggestions on the interpretation of the text of *De materia medica*. Some issues appear straightforward, whilst others provide a challenging complexity, hence the 'mountains and molehills' of our title.

De materia medica was published towards the end of the first century CE, but there remains debate on the date. Our main interest here is to establish the context in which Dioscorides worked, his sources and his experience, as well as the contribution he made in terms of plant identification. We look at the question of Dioscorides' service as a doctor in the Roman army, and propose that he may not have travelled as widely as claimed by other authors. However, Dioscorides was undoubtedly concerned with the identification, quality and sourcing of medicinal plants, and we use the text of Pliny's *Natural History* to discuss this.

Researchers in the history of natural history have sought to trace the evolution of botanical thought, and this has led to comparisons between the texts of Pliny (c. 24–79 CE) and Dioscorides which were written around the same time in the late first century CE. Stannard argues that Pliny (Gaius Plinius Secundus) had substantial influence on later medicine, in that his work was used by medieval writers.[4] An edition of his *Natural History* was printed in Venice in 1469 and Nauert argues that Pliny was used by Renaissance humanist scholars who were endeavouring to translate or prepare new Latin editions of Greek texts including that of Dioscorides.[5]

Ogilvie gives an account of the development of botanical study in Europe, in particular the changing concepts and language needed to study and describe plants,[6] and in this chapter we show the endeavours of some Renaissance authors to engage with the identification of medicinal plants. The correct identification of medicinal plants was an issue for Dioscorides, for Renaissance authors and remains a problem today for herbal practitioners. The importance of Dioscorides is that he prefigured later practitioners in his emphasis on the significance of botanical study to clinical practice.

Methodology and sources

Sources for the study of herbal medicine in the classical period are generally overlaid with the interpretations of later writers and translators. We evaluate aspects of the life of Dioscorides and sources for this information, and consider the publication date of *De materia medica*. The later focus of our chapter is on the identification of the medicinal plants with a review of extracts from the texts relating to specific plants which illustrate some of the challenges in interpretation of the text. The choice of plants is immense but our selection illustrates some of the relevant issues for a plant which it is relatively easy to be certain about: elecampane (*Inula helenium*), in addition to two plants which have been particularly difficult to confirm in terms of identification: wild carrot (*Daucus carota*) and hyssop (*Hyssopus officinalis*). The original manuscript of *De materia medica* was written in Greek and the version used here is the translation into English by Lily Beck which is based on the standard Greek edition by Max Wellmann.[7] Riddle gives a comprehensive account of the versions and translations of *De materia medica*.[8] Touwaide argues that the use and reuse of different versions and excerpts is complex, and that there was contact between Christian, Islamic and Jewish authors in particular in Byzantium (now Istanbul), Italy and Spain.[9] However, versions through late antiquity and the medieval period are outside the scope of this chapter.[10]

The five volumes of *De materia medica* include 827 items: 651 plants and plant products, 87 animal products and 89 minerals (see Table 10.1). The text is written in a consistent and orderly fashion with plants grouped by type and by action.[11] For each entry, the name(s), botanical description and sources, therapeutic usage, medicinal preparations and warnings are given. The disease descriptions are brief, which suggests that the book was designed for use alongside another textbook on medical care.

Table 10.1 Items in *De materia medica*.

Volume	Total	Category	Number
I	129	Aromatic plants and spices	29
		Oils, unguents (34) resins (8) minerals (2)	44
		Trees, shrubs	56
II	186	Animal products, including honey	84
		Grains, beans	25
		Vegetables	49
		Herbs	28
III	158	Herbs, roots, seeds	155
		Birdlime, glues	3
IV	192	Herbs, roots	192
V	162	Minerals	89
		Wines	56
		Grapes, vinegars, water, oxymels	17
	827	All categories	827

Source: Dioscorides, *Pedanius Dioscorides of Anazarbus De materia medica*, trans. Lily Y. Beck (Hildesheim: Olms, 2005).

Biography of Dioscorides

Dioscorides is significant in the 'creation myth' of herbal medicine, as one of the key authors referred to in the herbal medicine curriculum.[12] Before considering the text, it is useful to consider this story and set him in context. Pedanius Dioscorides lived in the first century CE, and was born in Anazarbus in the Roman province of Cilicia. The site is near the village of Dilekkayam, north-east of Adana, in south-eastern Turkey. At that time, much of Asia Minor retained the Greek language and culture but formed part of the Roman Empire. The forename Pedanius suggests he had become a Roman citizen through an aristocratic sponsor named Pedanius. Scarborough and Nutton propose that Dioscorides studied medicine in the city of Tarsus, capital of Cilicia, as he dedicated his books to Laecanius Arius (fl. first century CE), a medical practitioner in Tarsus.[13] Scarborough and Nutton give the dedication as:

> At your insistence I have assembled my material into five books, and I dedicate my compendium to you in fulfilment of a debt of gratitude for your sentiments towards me: for you are naturally friendly to all men of culture, especially to our fellow professionals, and particularly to me. The attitude towards you of the excellent Laecanius Bassus is no small proof of your magnanimity, as I have

discovered from my association with you and from observing your enviable mutual friendship.[14]

Dioscorides' travels

We now turn to the widely repeated claim that Dioscorides observed medicinal plants during his travels as 'a Greek surgeon to Nero's army',[15] and question the certainty of this. Nero was Roman Emperor from 54 to 68 CE. In his Preface, Dioscorides criticizes earlier authors for their lack of care concerning botanical descriptions, and compares this with his own interest in the identification of medicinal plants. He states that:

> By contrast, I have had, almost from my earliest years, an unquenchable desire to know about the materia medica, and I have travelled a great deal. You are well acquainted with my *soldier's life*.[16] [our emphasis]

In contrast, Riddle translates the contentious phrase as a 'soldier-like life' and this small difference in phrasing has led to intense scholarly debate.[17] Riddle points out that many places referred to in *De materia medica* were trading cities or Greek settlements around the Mediterranean, to which Dioscorides was more likely to have travelled in a civilian capacity. Nutton also notes the distribution of these places but suggests that Dioscorides must have had some military service.[18] However, medical staff in the imperial Roman army had a variety of roles and we can draw no specific inferences about the activities of Dioscorides.[19] There was a substantial standing army in the provinces of the Roman Empire,[20] and six legions in the Roman East after 68 CE, as the Emperor Vespasian (9–79 CE) pursued a policy of bringing neighbouring client states into the Roman Empire.[21] To conclude, it appears that Dioscorides could have been attached to the Roman legions in Eastern Asia Minor or elsewhere in the empire, either in a civilian or military role, but it is unlikely that he travelled as widely as supposed.

Places named in *De materia medica*

Although it has been claimed that Dioscorides 'set out on extensive journeys within the Roman Empire',[22] we were only able to find one place in *De materia medica* where Dioscorides refers to personal experience. He says, 'all milk disturbs the bowel and the stomach wherever the pasture is scammony, or hellebore, or mercury, or clematis, as we personally witnessed in the Vestini Mountains'.[23] However, Dioscorides was undoubtedly concerned with the provenance of medicinal plants and fulfils the objective stated in his Preface of giving prominence to the quality of plant materials and their sources, such as 'the best [unguent] of iris smells only of iris and of nothing else. Such is the unguent of iris that is made in Perge of Pamphylia and that made in Elis of Acaia'.[24] Throughout his books, Dioscorides discusses places where plants grow

Table 10.2 Places given in *De materia medica* (number of mentions in the text).

A	Asia minor	67	E	Balkans, mainland Greece	30
	Cilicia	16		Achaea, Aetolia	7
	Galatia	9		Anticyra, Boeotia	2
	Asia	8		Macedonia	5
	Cappadocia	8		Boeotia	3
	Pontus	8		Illyria	3
	Lycia	4		Peloponnese	3
	Pamphylia	4		Arcadia	1
	Cyzicus	3		Attica	1
	Pisidia	2		Magnesia	2
	Caria	1		Megara	1
	Chalcedon	1		Messine	1
	Commagena	1		Thrace	1
	Phrygia	1	F	Islands	24
	Tralles	1		Crete	9
B	Italy	12		Cyprus	5
	Italy	1		Chios	4
	Liguria	2		Cos	2
	Sicily	2		Cyclades	2
	Vestini	2		Rhodes	1
	Apulia	1		Samothrace	1
	Campania	1	G	Africa	38
	Etruria	1		Egypt	20
	Istria	1		Ethiopia	7
	Ravenna	1		Libya, Cyrene	6
C	West	15		Cyrene	4
	Spain and Balearic islands	8		Mauretania	1
	Sardinia	2	H	East	52
	France and islands	1		Syria	18
	Gaul	1		Arabia	13
	Massilia	1		India	9
	Narbonne	1		Armenia	4
	Stoichos	1		Petra	4
D	North	5		Medea	3
	Bosforus (Crimea)	2		Phoenicia	1
	Colchis	2			
	Sarmatia	1			

Sources: Dioscorides, *Pedanius Dioscorides of Anazarbus De materia medica*, trans. Lily Y. Beck (Hildesheim: Olms, 2005); Nicholas G. L. Hammond, *Atlas of the Greek and Roman World in Antiquity* (Park Ridge, NJ: Noyes Press, 1981).

plentifully such as 'the wild cumin: it grows in very large quantities and quite vigorously in Carthage of Spain'.[25]

Table 10.2 lists places named by Dioscorides as given in the translation by Beck. The names have been confirmed[26] but may retain inaccuracies and will not correspond with modern borders. Most entries are for Asia Minor, mainland Greece and the Greek islands. Places are also given in Italy, the western Mediterranean, the Black Sea coast, the Mediterranean coast of Africa and the eastern Mediterranean from Syria down to Arabia. This supports Riddle's argument that the places could have been reached by sea by Greek traders.

Egypt is the most common place given, and Marganne asks what evidence there is to support the claim that Dioscorides visited Egypt.[27] She reviews the places from which Dioscorides states that plants originate and compares his text with that of Pliny's *Natural History*. For the 40 references she finds to products from Egypt, she argues that all of these references were to common plants, plants described by earlier authors such as Theophrastus (c. 370–c. 287 BCE) or plants described as of high quality if sourced from Egypt. She notes that Pliny includes more references to Egypt than Dioscorides, but is not thought to have visited Egypt, and so concludes that there is no direct evidence of a visit to Egypt by Dioscorides either. More recent scholarly work has found a long history of international trade in herbs and spices. For example, in discussing the plants used in the Hippocratic corpus, Totelin gives evidence of trade with Arabia, India, Egypt, Ethiopia and North Africa, and argues that continuous trade between Greece and Egypt had existed since the sixth century BCE.[28]

So, although Dioscorides was undoubtedly concerned with plant provenance, he may have travelled less widely than previously assumed. We now turn to the date of publication which has also been a source of scholarly debate.

Date of publication of *De materia medica*

The reason for interest in the date of publication of *De materia medica* is that it may help us to understand the text better. The specific date of publication is unknown but here we suggest a date after 79 CE using the reference in the dedication above to Laecanius Bassus (fl. first century CE) and the date of publication of Pliny's *Natural History*. We will discuss uncertainties over the dates of the sources used by Dioscorides and the date of the first definite citation of the work.

The reference to Laecanius Bassus in the dedication of *De materia medica* is significant since Laecanius Bassus was one of the two proconsuls of the Roman province of Asia.[29] The provincial capital was Ephesus where there remain the ruins of the Nymphaeum (fountain) of Gaius Laecanius Bassus. The inscription on the fountain states that he was governor of Ephesus in 78/79 CE.[30] Laecanius Bassus had previously been consul in Rome in 64 CE, and his family traded in olive oil.[31] This provides some dating evidence as the dedication implies that Dioscorides observed the friendship between his tutor and Laecanius Bassus.

Another important consideration in establishing the date of publication of *De materia medica* is that it is not listed as a source in Pliny's *Natural History*, which can be dated as Pliny died during the eruption of Vesuvius on 24 August 79 CE.[32] In his encyclopaedia of 37 books, Pliny lists authorities for each book, so, for example, for Book 23 he gives 20 authorities both Roman and Greek, and additionally 42 medical writers.[33] Certainly, the section in Book 22 on mushrooms must have been written after the death of the Emperor Nero in 68 CE as in discussing his mother, Agrippina, Pliny refers to 'yet another poison – her own son Nero'.[34]

Equally, Pliny does not refer to a medical work of prescriptions published before 48 CE by Scribonius Largus (fl. 40–50 CE), another doctor with a connection to the Roman army.[35] However, it is difficult to believe that Pliny would not have referred to such a substantial work as *De materia medica* if it was available to him, and this may suggest that the two men were working in different places at the same time. Wellmann argues that the Greek author Sextius Niger (fl. 0–40 CE) was a source for both Dioscorides and Pliny by comparing sections of each book with fragments of the text of Sextius Niger.[36] In later papers, Wellmann discusses the sources of Pliny and argues that a range of Greek sources were probably used by both authors.[37] The sources given by Dioscorides in his Preface are discussed by Scarborough and Nutton, and Marganne, but unfortunately no source can be unequivocally dated and thus cast light on a possible date of publication.[38] The topic of sources for *De materia medica* would benefit from further scholarship.

The first known citation of *De materia medica* is in the Hippocratic glossary published by Erotian (fl. 40–70 CE) in the first century CE.[39] This refers to the identification of wolfsbane. The sentence referring to the work of Dioscorides is placed within the text in an authoritative translation, and so should be part of the original text by Erotian. However, since the manuscripts used for the translation were copies themselves, it is possible that this could have been a *scholia* (explanatory note) inserted into the main text by a later copyist. This has been shown to occur with other texts.[40] The glossary of Erotian was dedicated to Andromachus. According to Galen (c. 130–c. 200 CE), Andromachus was imperial doctor to the Emperor Nero,[41] but there were two doctors called Andromachus, father and son, and either man could have been the dedicatee of Erotian. Using the evidence of the entry in this glossary, a publication date has been suggested for *De materia medica* of 60–78 CE.[42] However, in the light of the evidence for publication near or after the death of Pliny in 79 CE and around the time of the proconsulship of Laecanius Bassus in 79–80 CE, the question of the publication date remains open.

Plant descriptions and identification

Returning to our main theme, although we have suggested that Dioscorides may have travelled less than previously assumed, it is certain that he considered that identification of plants was important. He gives written plant descriptions for 142 out of the 155 plants in Vol. III, and 182 out of the 192 plants in Vol. IV. There are some evocative descriptions, but the extent of description varies and can be very brief in some cases. There are many plants, as shown later with hyssop, for which the description is given by analogy with other plants. Unfortunately, any illustrations in the texts are not necessarily helpful in identifying the plant being described by Dioscorides, as illustrations were added only in later editions.[43]

For some herbs we were able to identify very similar entries in Pliny, and the following example shows that rather than having seen the plant growing in the wild, the two authors could have used the same written sources. Dioscorides describes the white water lily (*Nymphaea alba*), and then:

> There is also another water lily that has leaves similar to the leaves of the above, but a root that is white and rugged, and a quince-yellow flower that shines and resembles a rose… it grows around Thessaly, by the river Peneios.[44]

Pliny describes the white water lily, and then 'There is another kind of nymphaea growing in the river Penius in Thessaly. It has a white root and a yellow head the size of a rose'.[45]

The significance of the comparison above with Pliny is that he is known not to have travelled to all the places given in his *Natural History*. Pliny was not a medical practitioner but a senior Roman administrator who served in the Roman imperial army in Germany (45–57 CE). During the reign of the Emperor Vespasian, he was Procurator, responsible for imperial revenue and expenditure, in northern Spain and, possibly, Africa and Gallia Narbonensis.[46]

Cautions in interpretation of *De materia medica*

Caution is needed in the use of *De materia medica*, as studies of individual herbs show there are recurring issues concerning botanical identification[47] and naming in Greek and Latin.[48] Even where the identification of the herb seems probable, it cannot be supposed that the herb has been in continuous usage in northern Europe over the last 2,000 years.[49] This is particularly a problem where historians uncritically repeat Latin binomials ascribed to the herbs in *De materia medica* by authorities such as André.[50] This gives a false impression of the quality of the evidence, and our cautions are equally expressed in a recent study of the plants given in the Hippocratic corpus.[51] Much scholarship in this area was undertaken between the late eighteenth and early twentieth century, and a full evaluation of the naming of the plants in *De materia medica* is urgently needed.[52]

Certainty in identification: Elecampane

Here we take elecampane to illustrate some aspects of identification and later transmission, with particular reference to the botanical description of the plant.[53] Dioscorides writes:

> It has leaves nearly resembling those of the narrow-leaved mullein but rougher and longish, – and they are stemless, – and a large and aromatic root, somewhat pungent and orange-tawny from which off-shoots are taken for planting just like

the off-shoots of lilies and arums. It grows in mountainous, thickly shaded and moist places. The root is dug up in the summer, and after it is cut up, it is dried.[54]

There is no mention of the flowers, but the leaves of elecampane are large and stemless and similar to the leaves of narrow-leaved mullein (*Verbascum niveum* var. *niveum* syn. *Verbascum angustifolium*).[55] *Inula helenium* and 25 other *Inula* spp. are included in the flora of Turkey.[56] The large aromatic root is indeed propagated by cutting sections, so there is nothing here which opposes the identification as *Inula helenium*.

Renaissance writers sought both to identify the plants written about by Dioscorides and to give fuller plant descriptions. Pietro Andrea Matthioli (1501–77) observes that elecampane was very commonly used in medicine but that the leaves in Italy were larger than described by Dioscorides. He refers to other Greek versions of the text of *De materia medica*, one of which refers to yellow flowers, and includes the text about this plant from Pliny.[57] Matthioli based his 1554 Italian version of *De materia medica* on the translation into Latin published by Jean Ruel (1474–1537) in 1516. His subsequent Latin edition was popular throughout the sixteenth century, and entries were updated and debated.[58]

Other authors, writing in Latin, built on the text of Dioscorides, such as Leonhart Fuchs (1501–66).[59] His description has a different wording, gives the name Enula campana and argues that this was the plant in the text of Dioscorides. He copied the location given in the text above by Dioscorides, adding that it was also planted in gardens everywhere.

Turning to later texts available in English, we find the work by Rembert Dodoens (1516–85) in which he gives a vivid description which reads as though from observation of a living specimen:

> Elecampane has great, broad, soft leaves, immediately springing uppe from the roote, not much differing from the leaves of white Mullein, but greater and larger, amongst which springeth up a thick hairy long stalke, commonly longer than a man, beset with leaves of the same sort, but smaller, of a light green colour above, but whitish underneath; at the toppe of the stalke there grow fair, large, yellow shining flowers like starres, and in figure like to Chrysanthemon or golde-flower but a great deal larger, and almost as large as the palme of one's hand.[60]

This version of Dodoens is the English edition translated by Henry Lyte (c. 1529–1607) from the French edition of 1578. In 1557 the text had been translated from the original Flemish into French and edited by the botanist Charles de l'Ecluse (1526–1609).[61]

In his *Herbal*, John Gerard (c. 1545–1612), in the version edited by Thomas Johnson (c. 1600–44) for publication in 1633, gives an accurate but differently worded description for elecampane which compares the leaves to 'those of great Comfrey, but soft and covered with a hairy downe, of a whitish greene colour, and more white underneath, slightly nicked in the edge', and gives places where it grows such as 'in an orchard as you go from Colbrook to Ditton Ferry, which is the way to Windsor'.[62] In 1640, John Parkinson (c. 1567–1650) briefly discusses the identity of the Helenium of Dioscorides, Theophrastus and Pliny, and then describes elecampane.[63]

The description given by Parkinson was copied exactly by Nicholas Culpeper (1616–54)[64] and continues to be seen today in modern editions.

We have considered elecampane because it provides a readily identifiable example, but many other plants are not so readily recognized.

Confusion in transmission: Wild carrot

Accurate identification of Dioscorides' plants has more often given cause for debate. While some plants, such as elecampane, may be immediately identifiable from the detail provided by Dioscorides, his text offers much opportunity for confusion. Two differing examples are illustrated here, using mainly Beck's text and opinions drawn from Renaissance writers: these are wild carrot and hyssop, where accurate identification is clear-cut and debatable, respectively.

Wild carrot is a study in complexity. For botanists, it is a plant of variable morphology including several subspecies which can hybridize with each other.[65] The various subspecies lead to debates about different names for plants which are quite similar in appearance and use. Following Beck's translation, wild carrot is initially well described by Dioscorides:

> Staphilinos agrios [*Daucus carota* var. *silvestris* and *D. carota* L.] Wild carrot and cultivated carrot
> 1. The wild carrot: but some call it ceras. It has leaves like those of the carrot but wider and somewhat bitter, an upright stem that is rough and that has an umbel like that of dill on which there are white flowers, and in the middle there is something small and purplish, as if it were nap on woollen cloth; the root is as thick as a finger, a span long, aromatic, and edible when boiled.... The cultivated carrot, which is more edible, is suitable for the same purposes, but it acts more weakly.[66]

A very clear description is given by Dioscorides that should be sufficient for specific identification. The purple dot in the centre of the flower is considered characteristic for wild carrot.[67] Many Renaissance authors tell us, however, that Dioscorides described three kinds of carrot – a Cretan one, one like wild celery and one like coriander. Returning to Beck's translation of Dioscorides, we find:

> Daucos [*Athamanta cretensis* L.]
> 1. Daucos: there is one kind called Cretan, having leaves like those of fennel but smaller and finer, a stem that is one span tall, an umbel like that of coriander, and white flowers; they contain seed that is white, rough, pungent when chewed, and fragrant; the root is a finger thick and one span long. It grows in rocky and sunny places. And there is another kind that nearly resembles wild celery; it is spicy and fragrant, and it tastes pungent and hot. The Cretan is superior.
> 2. The third kind resembles coriander in foliage and it has white flowers. Its top and fruit are similar to dill's, the umbel is like that of carrot it is full of longish seed like cumin and it is pungent.[68]

A note in Beck's translation, citing Liddell, Scott and Jones, identifies the three species as *Athamanta cretensis*, *Peucedanum cervaria* and *Psychotis amnis* respectively.

Matthioli is adamant that the entry on staphilinos, which he terms also pastinaca, is not wild carrot. The term 'pastinaca' adds further complexity. He maintains that no Greek or Arabic authority describes this plant as having red roots and appears familiar with Dioscorides' two kinds, both, apparently, being eaten in Italy in his time and both having white roots – hence his designation of staphilinos as not carrot, but parsnip (*Pastinaca sativa*), a designation Beck reserves for elaphoboscon and sisaron.[69]

Pliny made the question of specifying the carrot no easier, referring to daucus and pastinaca in several places. He speaks of four types of daucus distinguished by Diodotus, but 'There is no point in giving the details of these, as there are but two species.... If one really desires to add a third kind, there is one like staphylinos, called wild carrot'.[70] Andrews adds that Plutarch (45–120 CE) spoke of several kinds, while Oribasius (c. 320–400 CE) gave staphilinus as a synonym for daucus, which the Romans called pastinaca.[71] Matthioli contests the synonym idea, citing Galen who has two separate entries, 'daucus... that some call staphilinos' – Matthioli suggests here that Galen's phrasing implies that Galen does not agree with this designation – and pastinaca, both domestic pastinaca (sativa) and wild pastinaca (agrestis).[72] Hence two separate plants. Matthioli affirms Dioscorides' three kinds of daucus. William Turner (c. 1508–68), however, disagrees, arguing for staphilinos as carrot. Under the heading 'Of the garden and wild carot', he takes Matthioli to task in some detail for his error. He goes on to recruit Ruel, Fuchs and Dodoens as allies to his own opinion, citing Theophrastus' reference to coloured roots in further refutation of Matthioli's stance. Turner is more cautious, however, in dealing with Dioscorides' three kinds of daucus, 'Of wylde Carot [*Daucus carota*]'.[73] Having rehearsed the difficulties and confusions between daucus and staphilinos through various authors (omitting Matthioli here), he concludes, like others, that their close similarity would obviate problems of exchange of use:

> Wherefore although daucus and staphilinos were two sundry herbs and divers in form, yet forasmuch as they agree in virtue, the error of them cannot be great which take the one for the other, specially seeing that Aetius writeth that daucus is called staphilinos and staphilinos daucus.[74]

Turner does then venture to suggest, albeit tentatively, his own identification of the second and third plants of Dioscorides' three daucus entries. Though he has not, he says, seen the first as far as he knows, the second might be rough saxifrage and the third bisacutum.[75]

Parkinson despaired of sorting the carrots out. He says in *Theatrum botanicum*, of daucus, dauke or wilde carrots, 'Although there be many sorts of these Daukes or wilde Carrots, yet because I cannot well tell how to separate them I must packe them all into this one chapter'.[76] He describes then 16 sorts, including the true daucus of Candy, mountain fine-leaved dauke, coriander-leaved dauke and others. Compare, however, the entry for 'Pastinaca tenuifolia, Carrots', where he includes common yellow carrot, wilde carrots, wilde carrots of Naples, prickly wilde carrots of Naples and wilde carrots with hairy stalkes.[77] In another chapter, 'Pastinaca latifolia, parsnip' he says is probably the elaphoboscon of Dioscorides.[78]

Dodoens has yet a different version and seems to confound Dioscorides' two entries. He claims the Daucus of Candie and the one that resembles wild parsley are 'both yet unknown',[79] while the third he goes to some lengths to identify, drawing in the detail of the purple centre that we found under staphilinos in Dioscorides rather than under the third term of daucus:

> For this kind of Daucus there is now taken the herbe which some do call wilde Carrot... for it hath leaves like Coriander, but greater, and not much unlike the leaves of the yellow Carrot. Its flowers be white, growing upon tuffets or rundels, like to the tuffets of the yellow Carrot; in the middle whereof is found a little small flower or twain of a brown red colour turning to blacke.[80]

Gerard adds his slightly different version to the confusion, that daucus described with red roots is properly called in Greek 'staphilinos', but in the Latin 'pastinaca sativa' has the addition 'tenuifolia' to differentiate it from garden parsnip with white roots.[81] Wild carrot is differentiated:

> the wilde Carrot is called in Greek staphilinos agrios: in Latine, Pastinaca sylvestris tenuifolis: in shops Daucus: and it is used in stead of the true Daucus, and not amisse, nor unprofitably: for Galen also in his time doth testifie that it was taken for Daucus, or bastard parsley, and is without doubt Dauci sylvestris genus, or a wilde kinde of bastard Parsly, so called of Theophrastus.[82]

Parsnip he terms, for clarity, 'Pastinaca latifolia sativa':

> the herbarists of our time do call the garden Parsneps staphilinos and Pastinaca, and therefore wee have surnamed it Latifolia, or broad leafed, that it may differ from the other garden Parsnep with narrow leaves, which is truly and properly called Staphilinus, that is, the garden Carrot.[83]

Andrews throws some light on the confusion, though it is nevertheless no uncomplicated matter.[84] Daucos, apparently, was a term of generic force, applied to several plants including wild carrot and species of *Athamanta*: 'the common characteristic seems to have been a bitter, pungent root with a cathartic effect'.[85] Staphilinos, on the other hand, was a specific term for cultivated carrot as early as the fourth century BCE, with 'agrios' added to denote the wild variety. In the classical period, he continues, the distinction between staphilinos and daucus broke down and both terms applied to cultivated and wild carrot. Pastinaca was generic, like daucos, and applied to carrot, both cultivated and wild, and extended to other plants as well, including parsnip. This gave rise to many common names for both parsnip and carrot across Europe, but the one or other usually specific to a particular region, that is, referring either to carrot or parsnip depending on locality. Andrews adds further comment on the colour, that while Theophrastus referred to yellow and black-rooted forms of daukon (as wild plants), there is no mention of colour in Dioscorides, Pliny, Galen nor Oribasius (affirming Matthioli's claim), and this must be a significant omission in that had there been a colour, reference would undoubtedly have been made to it. He thus concludes that in the classical era the root of all varieties was white. Colour only emerged later, he argues, following hybridization with the Afghan carrot.[86] The reference to colour in Theophrastus, however, still leaves some doubt and allows no absolute conclusion.

Despite identification problems, however, Matthioli, Turner and others do agree that the actions of staphilinos and daucus are not dissimilar. Matthioli declares that their properties in Dioscorides and Galen accord so well that in the absence of the one the other may safely be used.[87]

Plants lacking description: Hyssop

If the fund of detail did not serve to ease interpretation of wild carrot, hyssop sets us an opposite task. 'It's a well known herb', says Dioscorides, 'which comes in two kinds; for one grows on mountains and the other in gardens; the best grows in Cilicia'.[88] There is no further description. The problems stem from reference to other plants which Dioscorides likens to hyssop. The leaf of oregano, he says, is similar to that of hyssop, 'and the flower head is not wheel-like, but as if divided, and at the end of its twigs the seed is not thickly packed'.[89] For *Aster linosiris*, Imortelle (*chrysocome* in Greek), Dioscorides writes: 'It is a little shoot having the size of a span, foliage in clusters, resembling that of hyssop'.[90] Neither description confirms our present hyssop as that of Dioscorides.

As usual, the Renaissance authors have differing opinions on the matter. While Jean D'Alechamps (1513–88) does not commit himself, expressing only that it is not clear what plant the hyssop of Dioscorides was,[91] Dodoens declares against the familiar hyssop being that of the Ancients, albeit relying on the testimony of others, 'as is sufficiently declared by certaine of the best learned writers of these daies'.[92] Gerard describes five hyssops, appending a note to the fifth, 'Hyssopus parva angustis foliis, dwarfe narrow leaved Hyssope', explaining, 'this is by most writers judged to be Hyssope used by the Arabian physitions, but not that of the Greekes, which is neerer to Origanum and Marjerome as this is to Satureia or Savorie'.[93]

The opinions of Parkinson and Matthioli, however, are strongly opposed. Parkinson, who has much to say on the subject, asserts that it is the true hyssop of the Arabians, but not that of Dioscorides or other Greek authors:

> as all doe acknowledge except Matthiolus, who doth earnestly contend, that our garden Hysope is the same of Dioscorides, whose arguments are too weake, to perswade any to be of his opinion, for the description of Dioscorides his Hysope hath no face or true resemblance with ours.[94]

Parkinson elaborates alternative suggestions from other authors, for example that:

> Lugdunensis [D'Alechamps] setteth forth a round leafed Hysope, which he taketh to be the true Hysope of Dioscorides... Lobel also propoundeth another, that is our pot Marjerome to be the right... but Fabius Columna confuteth that of Lobel and Pena, as well for that the tufted heads, are more like unto wilde Marjerome, then unto Chrysocome, or garden Marjerome, as Cratevas, Serapio, Isaak, Mesues and others doe compare them.[95]

He tells us that Fabius Columna (1567–1640) would have us believe that Polium montanum is the true Hysope, others argue for Gratiola. Referring to Jean Bauhin's (1541–1613) suggestion of Rosemary, Parkinson strays into the biblical references of vinegar offered to Christ on the cross on a stalk of hyssop. Having put all these arguments, however, he eventually rejects them all. Intriguingly, though, among the several hyssops which he describes, he includes a 'round leafed hyssop... Hyssopus foliis Origani' – that is, hyssop with leaves of oregano.[96]

Matthioli puts up a stout defence in favour of the plant being Dioscorides' hyssop. He argues firstly a wrong translation by an earlier author and consequent perpetuation of that error. Matthioli prefers Oribasius' and others' versions which read for Oregano 'Oregano heracleoticum, which some call Cunila, has leaves like hyssop; but the umbel is not circular like a wheel but is much divided'[97] – the semicolon is crucial here, it seems, clarifying that only the first part of the sentence refers to hyssop and not the rest.

Fuchs, rather more concisely, sides with Matthioli, arguing similarly:

> Those who think that this is not the true Hyssop of Dioscorides are in error. For it clearly has leaves like those of oregano but slightly narrower. Nothing more than this was noted by Dioscorides.[98]

Matthioli continues his refutation with the chrysocome comparison, here suggesting the word *coma* can refer to leaves and shoots as well as flowers and corymbs, citing examples from Pliny and Virgil in his defence. He writes further that Dioscorides compares the leaves of Symphytum petraeum to oregano, having recently observed this plant himself and its likeness to hyssop. Moreover, since Dioscorides described plants of similar genus together, its context immediately before stoechade, 'which emulates our hyssop closely in leaf and flower', adds further weight to the argument.[99] Finally, and perhaps most convincingly of all, he suggests that the familiar hyssop plants possess all the strengths and virtues that Dioscorides claims for it 'as I have tested'.[100]

Parkinson, despite his opposing stance, ends up in the same practical position, declaring, perhaps rather surprisingly:

> Now although the true Hysope of Dioscorides, and the other Greekes, is not yet certainly knowne, yet assuredly this which is knowne, and generally received, may safely be used in the stead thereof, untill the true Hysope may be knowne.[101]

Andrews draws a more modern conclusion. Having studied hyssop through a range of economic, geographical and demographic filters, he concludes that our modern hyssop is indeed the hyssop of the Ancients (though not the hyssop of the Bible).[102] Beck, however, sets Dioscorides' hyssop entry not under *Hyssopus officinalis*, but *Satureia graeca*, a kind of savoury.[103] So the debate continues...

Returning to the text of *De materia medica*, it is encouraging that there have been recent additions to scholarly work on the transmission of knowledge. There has been an illuminating and comprehensive review of 12 texts from the Hippocratic corpus to the *Spanish Pharmacopoeia* of 1865. Hyssop is given in ten texts, elecampane in nine and wild carrot in eight.[104] In addition, three papers by Leonti and his team compare ethnobotanical surveys in the Mediterranean with textual sources and argue for a significant influence of written texts on traditional usage of herbal medicines in Europe.[105]

Conclusion

We have investigated the argument that, through his travels, Dioscorides observed and described the medicinal plants of southern Europe and Asia Minor. Although we have argued that the evidence for this claim is limited, we have shown that Dioscorides was at pains to discuss the identification, quality and sources of medicinal plants. We have then suggested that studies of Pliny and other authors have been significant in explicating the text of Dioscorides. The Renaissance authors were also keen to observe and identify medicinal plants, and we have argued that modern scholarship is needed to build on the work of previous generations. This requires input from classicists and botanists but also from herbalists who have a breadth of clinical knowledge and experience of prescribing medicinal plants.

Recommended reading

Dendle, Peter, and Alain Touwaide. *Health and Healing from the Medieval Garden.* Woodbridge: Boydell and Brewer, 2008.
Nutton, Vivian. *Ancient Medicine.* London: Routledge, 2004.
Ogilvie, Brian W. *The Science of Describing: Natural History in Renaissance Europe.* Chicago: University of Chicago Press, 2006.
Tobyn, Graeme, Alison Denham, and Margaret Whitelegg. *The Western Herbal Tradition: 2000 Years of Medicinal Plant Knowledge.* Edinburgh: Churchill Livingstone/Elsevier, 2011.
Totelin, Laurence M. V. *Hippocratic Recipes: Oral and Written Transmission of Pharmacological Knowledge in Fifth- and Fourth-Century Greece.* Boston: Brill, 2009.

Notes

1. Cited in Charles G. Nauert Jr, 'Humanists, Scientists, and Pliny: Changing Approaches to a Classical Author', *American Historical Review* 84, no. 1 (1979): 83.
2. Graeme Tobyn, Alison Denham, and Margaret Whitelegg, *The Western Herbal Tradition: 2000 Years of Medicinal Plant Knowledge* (Edinburgh: Churchill Livingstone/Elsevier, 2011).
3. Ibid., ix. The most comprehensive study of the historical use of individual herbs, that of Maud Grieve, *A Modern Herbal: The Medicinal, Culinary, Cosmetic and Economic Properties, Cultivation and Folklore of Herbs, Grasses, Fungi, Shrubs and Trees with All Their Modern Scientific Uses*, ed. C. F. Leyel, repr. 1931 ed. (London: Peregrine Books, 1976), requires extensive updating to incorporate the findings of research into medicinal plants.
4. Jerry Stannard, 'Pliny and Roman Botany', *Isis* 56, no. 4 (1965): 420, 424.

5   Nauert, 'Humanists, Scientists, and Pliny', 74–6.
6   Brian W. Ogilvie, *The Science of Describing: Natural History in Renaissance Europe* (Chicago: University of Chicago Press, 2006).
7   Dioscorides, *Pedanius Dioscorides of Anazarbus: De materia medica*, translated by Lily Y. Beck (Hildesheim: Olms, 2005); John Scarborough, 'Dioscorides of Anazarbus for Moderns – an Essay Review', *Pharmacy History* 49, no. 2 (2007): 76–80.
8   John M. Riddle, 'Dioscorides', in *Catalogus translationum et commentariorum: Mediaeval and Renaissance Latin Translations and Commentaries: Annotated Lists and Guides, Vol. 4*, ed. F. Edward Cranz and Paul O. Kristeller (Washington, DC: Catholic University of America Press, 1980), 1–41.
9   Alain Touwaide, 'The Legacy of Classical Antiquity in Byzantium and the West', in *Health and Healing from the Medieval Garden*, ed. Peter Dendle and Alain Touwaide (Woodbridge: Boydell and Brewer, 2008), 15–28. For more on the Islamic contribution to Western medical texts, see also ch. 4 in this book. For more on trade between Islamic lands and the West, see ch. 6.
10 See Dimitri Gutas, *Greek Thought, Arab Culture: The Graeco-Arabic Translation Movement in Baghdad and Early 'Abbāsid Society (2nd–4th/5th–10th c.)* (London: Routledge, 1998); John Scarborough, 'Early Byzantine Pharmacology', in *Symposium on Byzantine Medicine*, ed. John Scarborough (Washington, DC: Dumbarton Oaks, 1984), 213–32.
11 John M. Riddle, *Dioscorides on Pharmacy and Medicine* (Austin: University of Texas Press, 1985).
12 The core curriculum advised for the training of Western herbal practitioners refers to 'historical antecedents', including reference to *De materia medica*. European Herbal and Traditional Medicine Practitioners Association, *The Core Curriculum for Herbal and Traditional Medicine: Producing Safe and Competent Practitioners* (Tewkesbury: EHTPA, 2007), 99.
13 John Scarborough and Vivian Nutton, 'The Preface of Dioscorides' Materia Medica: Introduction, Translation and Commentary', *Transactions and Studies of the College of Physicians of Philadelphia (5th series)* 4, no. 3 (1982): 187–227.
14 Ibid., 196.
15 For example, this claim is made by Roy Porter, *The Greatest Benefit to Mankind: A Medical History of Humanity from Antiquity to the Present* (London: Fontana Press, 1999), 79.
16 Scarborough and Nutton, 'The Preface of Dioscorides', 196.
17 Riddle, 'Dioscorides', 2.
18 Vivian Nutton, *Ancient Medicine* (London: Routledge, 2004), 175.
19 Roy W. Davies, *Service in the Roman Army*, ed. David Breeze and Valerie A. Maxfield (Edinburgh: Edinburgh University Press, 1989), 209–29.
20 Nutton, *Ancient Medicine*, 179–82.
21 David L. Kennedy, ed., *The Roman Army in the East*, Supplementary Series No. 18 (Ann Arbor, MI: Journal of Roman Archaeology, 1996), 85–6.
22 'Dioscorides of Anazarbus', *Encyclopaedia of Life Science (eLS)* (2002), http://onlinelibrary.wiley.com/doi/10.1038/npg.els.0003612/full (accessed 8 February 2013).
23 Dioscorides, *De materia medica*, II, 70. These mountains are the eastern Appenine mountains, Abruzzo province, Italy.
24 Ibid., I, 36.

25 Ibid., III, 60. For more on cumin, see also ch. 6 in this book.
26 Nicholas G. L. Hammond, ed., *Atlas of the Greek and Roman World in Antiquity* (Park Ridge, NJ: Noyes Press, 1981).
27 Marie-Hélène Marganne, 'Les références à l'Égypte dans la *matière médicale* de Dioscoride', in *Serta Leodiensia secunda: mélanges publiés par les classiques de Liège à l'occasion du 175e anniversaire de l'Université* (Liège: Université de Liège, 1992), 309–22.
28 Laurence M. Totelin, *Hippocratic Recipes: Oral and Written Transmission of Pharmacological Knowledge in Fifth- and Fourth-Century Greece* (Boston: Brill, 2009), 145–61.
29 David Magie, *Roman Rule in Asia Minor to the End of the Third Century after Christ* (Princeton, NJ: Princeton University Press and Oxford: Oxford University Press, 1950), 1582.
30 See Elisabeth Rathmayr, 'Die Skulpturenausstattung des C. Laecanius Bassus Nymphaeum in Ephesos', http://homepage.univie.ac.at/elisabeth.trinkl/forum/forum0908/48bassus.htm (accessed 7 February 2013).
31 See T. Bezeczky, 'The Laecanius Amphora in Brijuni', Institut für Kulturgeschichte der Antike, http://www.oeaw.ac.at/antike/index.php?id=230 (accessed 7 February 2013).
32 John F. Healy, *Pliny the Elder on Science and Technology* (New York: Oxford University Press, 1999), 23.
33 Pliny the Elder, *Natural History. Vol. 1, Preface and Books I–II*, trans. and ed. H. Rackham (Cambridge, MA: Harvard University Press, 1949), 109.
34 Pliny the Elder, *Natural History: In Ten Volumes. Vol. 6 Libri XX–XXIII*, trans. W. H. S. Jones (Cambridge, MA: Harvard University Press, 1969), 359.
35 Mary Beagon, *Roman Nature: The Thought of Pliny the Elder* (Oxford: Clarendon Press, 1992), 216; Barry Baldwin, 'The Career and Works of Scribonius Largus', *Rheinisches Museum für Philologie* 135 (1992): 75–82.
36 Max Wellmann, 'Sextius Niger, eine Quellenuntersuchung zu Dioscorides', *Hermes* 24, no. 4 (1889): 530–69.
37 Max Wellmann, 'Beiträge zur Quellenanalyse des älteren Plinius', *Hermes* 59, no. 2 (1924): 93–105.
38 Scarborough and Nutton, 'The Preface of Dioscorides', 202–8; Marganne, 'Les références à l'Égypte', 310–11.
39 Erotianus, *Erotiani vocum Hippocraticarum collectio: Cum fragmentis*, ed. Ernst Nachmanson (Uppsala: Appelbergs Boktryckeri, 1918), 51.
40 Scarborough, 'Early Byzantine Pharmacology', 213–32.
41 Scarborough, 'Dioscorides of Anazarbus'. The authors would like to thank John Scarborough for further information on the topic of Erotian.
42 Riddle, *Dioscorides on Pharmacy and Medicine*, 13.
43 Minta Collins, *Medieval Herbals: The Illustrative Traditions* (London: British Library, 2000).
44 Dioscorides, *De materia medica*, III, 132.
45 Pliny the Elder, *Natural History: In Ten Volumes. Vol. 7 Libri XXIV–XXVII*, trans. W. H. S. Jones, 2nd ed. (Cambridge, MA: Harvard University Press, 1956), 191.
46 Healy, *Pliny the Elder*, 5–23.
47 S. S. Renner et al., 'Dioscorides's *bruonia melaina* Is *Bryonia alba*, Not *Tamus communis*, and an Illustration Labeled *bruonia melaina* in the *Codex Vindobonensis* Is *Humulus lupulus* Not *Bryonia dioica*', in *Proceedings of the IXth EUCARPIA*

Meeting on Genetics and Breeding of Cucurbitaceae, ed. M. Pitrat (Avignon: Inra, Centre de Recherche d'Avignon, Génétique et Amélioration des Fruits et Légumes, Montfavet (France), 2008), 273–80.
48   Jerry Stannard, 'The Plant Called Moly', Osiris 14 (1962): 254–307.
49   George Keiser, 'Rosemary: Not Just for Remembrance', in Dendle and Touwaide, Health and Healing, 180–204.
50   Jacques André, Les noms de plantes dans la Rome antique (Paris: Belles Lettres, 1985).
51   Giovanni Aliotta, Le piante medicinali del corpus Hippocraticum (Milan and Naples: Guerini e Associati; Istituto Italiano per gli Studi Filosofici, 2003).
52   Peter Dendle and Alain Touwaide, 'Introduction', in Dendle and Touwaide, Health and Healing, 1–15.
53   Tobyn et al., Western Herbal Tradition, 201–10.
54   Dioscorides, De materia medica, I, 28.
55   Verbascum niveum Ten. subsp. niveum. See Flora Italiana, 'Genere/Genus: Verbascum – Famiglia/Family: Scrophulariaceae', http://luirig.altervista.org/flora/verbascum.htm (accessed 7 February 2013).
56   For example, see Peter H. Davis, James Cullen and M. J. E. Coode, Flora of Turkey and the East Aegean Islands (Edinburgh: Edinburgh University Press, 1965).
57   Pietro A. Matthioli, Commentarii, in libros sex Pedacii Dioscoridis Anazarbei, De materia medica (Venice: In Officina Erasmiana, apud Vincentium Valgrisium, 1554), vol. 3, 367.
58   Paula Findlen, 'The Formation of a Scientific Community: Natural History in Sixteenth-Century Italy', in Natural Particulars: Nature and the Disciplines in Renaissance Europe, ed. Anthony Grafton and Nancy Siraisi (Cambridge, MA: MIT Press, 1999), 369–400.
59   Frederick G. Meyer, Emily E. Trueblood and John L. Heller, eds., The Great Herbal of Leonhart Fuchs: De historia stirpium commentarii insignes, 1542, vol. 2, reprint, facsimile (Stanford: Stanford University Press, 1999), 141.
60   Rembert Dodoens, A New Herbal, or Historie of Plants, trans. Henry Lyte (London: Edward Griffin, 1619), 242.
61   Philippe J. Van Meerbeeck, Recherches historiques et critiques sur la vie et les ouvrages de Rembert Dodoens (Dodonaeus), first ed., 1841 (Utrecht: HES, 1980), 6.
62   John Gerard, The Herbal: Or, General History of Plants, the Complete 1633 Edition, ed. Thomas D. Johnson (New York: Dover Publications, 1975), 792–3.
63   John Parkinson, Theatrum botanicum: The Theater of Plants, or, an Herball of a Large Extent (London: Tho. Cotes, 1640), 654.
64   Nicholas Culpeper, Culpeper's Complete Herbal: A Book of Natural Remedies for Ancient Ills (Ware: Wordsworth Editions, 1995), 98.
65   T. J. Tutin, ed., Flora Europaea; Vol. 2. Rosaceae to Umbelliferae (Cambridge: Cambridge University Press, 1968), 374.
66   Dioscorides, De materia medica, III, 52.
67   Tobyn et al., Western Herbal Tradition, 145.
68   Dioscorides, De materia medica, III, 72.
69   Ibid., III, 69, and II, 113; Matthioli, De materia medica, vol. 3, 353.
70   Pliny, Natural History, Vol. 7, 217–19.
71   Alfred C. Andrews, 'The Carrot as a Food in the Classical Era', Classical Philology 44, no. 3 (1949): 182–96.
72   Matthioli, De materia medica, vol. 3, 374.

73 William Turner, *A New Herball, Part 1*, ed. George T. L. Chapman and Marilyn N. Tweddle, and with indexes compiled by Frank McCombie, vol. 1 (Cambridge: Cambridge University Press, 1995), 187.
74 Ibid., 187.
75 Ibid., 187.
76 Parkinson, *Theatrum botanicum*, 896.
77 Ibid., 901.
78 Ibid., 944.
79 Dodoens, *New Herbal*, 204.
80 Ibid., 204.
81 Gerard, *Herbal*, 1028.
82 Ibid., 1028.
83 Ibid., 1025.
84 Andrews, 'Carrot', 184-6.
85 Ibid., 186.
86 Ibid., 195.
87 Matthioli, *De materia medica*, vol. 3, 354.
88 Dioscorides, *De materia medica*, III, 25.
89 Ibid., 27.
90 Ibid., IV, 55.
91 Jacques D'Alechamps, *Historia generalis plantarum* (Lugdini: Apud Gulielmum Rouillium, 1586).
92 Dodoens, *New Herbal*, 162.
93 Gerard, *Herbal*, 578-80.
94 Parkinson, *Theatrum botanicum*, 3.
95 Ibid., 3.
96 Ibid., 3.
97 Matthioli, *De materia medica*, vol. 3, 332-3.
98 Leonhart Fuchs, *De historia stirpium* (Basileae: In Officina Isingriniana, 1542), 840.
99 Matthioli, *De materia medica*, vol. 3, 332-3.
100 Ibid.
101 Parkinson, *Theatrum botanicum*, 4.
102 Alfred C. Andrews, 'Hyssop in the Classical Era', *Classical Philology* 56, no. 4 (1961): 230-47.
103 Dioscorides, *De materia medica*, III, 25.
104 Paula De Vos, 'European Materia Medica in Historical Texts: Longevity of a Tradition and Implications for Future Use', *Journal of Ethnopharmacology* 132, no. 1 (2010): 32-9.
105 Marco Leonti, 'The Future Is Written: Impact of Scripts on the Cognition, Selection, Knowledge and Transmission of Medicinal Plant Use and Its Implications for Ethnobotany and Ethnopharmacology', *Journal of Ethnopharmacology* 134, no. 3 (2011): 542-55; Marco Leonti et al., 'The Causal Dependence of Present Plant Knowledge on Herbals – Contemporary Medicinal Plant Use in Campania (Italy) Compared to Matthioli (1568)', *Journal of Ethnopharmacology* 130, no. 2 (2010): 379-91; Marco Leonti et al., 'A Comparison of Medicinal Plant Use in Sardinia and Sicily – De Materia Medica Revisited?', *Journal of Ethnopharmacology* 121, no. 2 (2009): 255-67.

11

William Turner: A Milestone in Botanical Medicine

Marie Addyman

Introduction

Ten years after the death of William Turner in 1568, the writer William Harrison (1535–93) described the Northumbrian-born physician as 'the father of English physic'.[1] This praise would have gratified Turner. All his life, even when a career change in 1551 led to a ministry within the English Church, he referred to himself as a physician, both defending and exalting his calling as sanctioned by God in the Bible, and taking pride in the academic training which permitted him to use that title. But to modern eyes, Harrison's title seems odd. Is it a tribute to Turner's success rate in practice? To his theoretical knowledge? To his published work? To some as yet unknown contribution to medical science? Does either Harrison's praise of him as a physician or some modern writers' contempt for him in the same role help us at all in estimating his work?

Early- and mid-twentieth-century writers concentrated on Turner's importance for the future of botany in terms of his work on plant identification, celebrating his achievements as 'the father of English botany';[2] but they regretted the necessary basis of this in 'superstitious' or outmoded medicine. So until recent times, Harrison's assertion has been bypassed. At worst, Turner has been accused of being 'not particularly important as a physician'.[3] More usually, he is seen as irrelevant to modern medicine, stuck in a defunct Galenism and an inaccurate physiology which his writings helped to perpetuate for far too long. At best, the medical aspects of his writings have been downplayed. However, with the initiatives within modern medical herbalism to interrogate its origins and history, evidenced by a collection such as this,[4] Turner's older title merits re-examination. What emerges is a paradox. On the one hand, with regard to available theory and practice he arguably left Tudor medicine exactly where he found it; on the other, his work in establishing accurate medicaments is the unacknowledged basis of all subsequent practice.

It is the aim of this chapter to examine this paradox, and to demonstrate how and why its two opposing terms are so distinctively intertwined. So, initially Turner's context within sixteenth-century medical theory and practice will be considered, for in order to show how and where Turner did achieve something notable in its implications for the future of medical herbalism, it is necessary to examine and admit the limiting conditions within which his achievements struggled to emerge. In the second half of the chapter, his outstanding achievement in identifying medicaments within the limits of available sixteenth-century terminology will be analyzed.

To do so, a reminder of what is known of Turner's life is helpful.[5] Born in Morpeth, Northumberland, around 1508, he went up to Pembroke College, Cambridge, in 1526 and, after gaining his BA and his MA degrees, he went on to read physic. As a student, he published a short, seminal Latin work on plant names, the *Libellus de re herbaria*.[6] He went abroad in 1541, completing his medical training in Ferrara and Bologna. After travelling in Switzerland and staying around Bonn and Cologne, he became court physician to Anna of Oldenburg, Regent of East Friesland, in 1544. During this decade he wrote a Latin book on birds, made contact with the leading natural historians Konrad Gessner (1516–65) and Leonhart Fuchs (1501–66), and met leading European reformers. On the accession of Edward VI in 1547, he returned to England as physician to Protector Somerset, to whom he dedicated English works on plants, *The Names of Herbes* (1549) and Part 1 of his *Herball*. Whether from choice or compulsion, he changed career in 1551 to become Dean of Wells, an appointment curtailed by the accession of Catholic Mary as Queen of England. Abroad again, he spent some time at Weissembourg near Strasbourg, probably returning to his old profession of physician. After returning, with the accession of Elizabeth, to his previous post at Wells, over the next decade he completed his tri-part *Herball*, and wrote books on mineral baths, wines and theriacs. His long illness due to the stone induced him to seek permission to leave Wells and live in London. He was buried in St Olave's Church, Hart Street, in July 1568.

Turner in the context of sixteenth-century medicine

A concentration on sixteenth-century, male, learned medicine deals with only a minority of practitioners in the field of medical provision. There were 150 medical graduates from Oxford and Cambridge combined between 1500 and 1550;[7] even if we add in people like Turner who got his doctorate in Italy, this minority does not represent the extent and variety of medical practitioners in the England of his time. Nor did it necessarily offer the best treatment available. It is clear from his own writing that Turner never found a cure within the physic in which he believed for his own suffering from that typical Tudor affliction, 'the stone'. The best he could offer in explanation was essentially empirical guesswork within a humoral framework.

Any consideration of Turner's life and work is determined by the general uncertainties referred to above. It is not clear if his medical practice was only that of an aristocratic or royal servant, since it is unknown in what capacity he practised at Weissembourg during the mid-1550s. Overall, the influence of his foreign experiences is clear in terms of his natural history but very partially understood in terms of his medicine. In comparison, the Dutch religious refugees who thronged to England in the reigns of Edward VI and Elizabeth I are recognized as having had a real influence on English health care, moving it towards organizing poor relief and medical attention within the local parish.[8] In Wells, therefore, such a responsibility would not have devolved from the cathedral, so that Turner's involvement in physic would have been more ad hoc, within a circle of known acquaintance ranging from the highest to the middle-ranking. For instance, he wrote privately, as requested, to Cecil in 1564 about the problematical, and possibly suspicious, death of Lady Dyer; and he also prepared medicaments for a merchant's wife in Bristol.[9] The unlikelihood of him practising formally in London at least is strengthened by the fact that after 1555 the Royal College of Physicians tried to isolate the clerical providers of physic from their own licensed practitioners, at least in London, as well as sometimes actively refusing to license foreign graduates.[10]

With these limitations in mind, I want to address some of the things we do know and thereby reach out to some particular questions. The medical historian Ian Maclean has suggested that there were three phases of medical scholarship in the sixteenth century.[11] The second phase, between 1525 and 1565, when Greek editions and Latin translations proliferated in Western Europe, coincided almost identically with Turner's involvement in medicine from 1526 to his death in 1568. Over this period, Turner, who most likely had learnt Latin during his grammar school education at Morpeth, was taught Greek by Ridley at Cambridge, and used both original texts and contemporary Latin translations and commentaries as essential tools in his research. In consequence, he was able to transmit authentic classical prescriptive advice to his English readership. This familiar advice considered as potential medicaments all of God's 'creatures', as Turner and his contemporaries called them. So he recommended those 'stones' and mineral products prevalent in the medical recipes of the period: as well as *terra sigillata*, prescribed from time immemorial, Part 1 of the *Herball* alone contains references to nitre (saltpetre), litharge (lead monoxide), salgammy (rock salt) and stibium (antimony).

But while sixteenth- and seventeenth-century physicians continued to recommend the elaborate and ancient classically derived antidotes known as theriacs, to prescribe *mumia* and to use animal products such as hen's dung,[12] their medicine relied primarily on plants. However, it would be wrong to assume that learned herbal medicine was holistic in the modern sense of the word, as it emerged either in the herbals or in the *cap-à-pe* (head to foot) lists derived from Anglo-Saxon manuals.[13] In these works, symptoms are very clearly divorced from people in an abstract and structured way. There is no built-in sympathy for the patient in the sixteenth-century methodology of the herbal – that is not its task. On the other hand, herbals do reflect tacit social and psychological assumptions. Turner's terse factual entries constantly reinforce psycho-physical stereotypes, particularly in his acceptance of 'the mother' as indicating a range of both physical and emotional complaints.[14] Furthermore, while herbs accounted beneficial in moderating or curing baldness regularly occur without adverse comment, like some of his classical predecessors he condemned women's vanity in seeking to beautify themselves:

> Some weomen sprinkle the floures of Cowislip to whytre wine/ and after stil it and washe their faces with that water to driue wrinkles away/ and to make them fayre

in the eyes of the worlde rather then in the eyes of God/ whom they are not afrayd to offende with the sluttishnes/ filthines/ and foulnes of the soule.[15]

Written records of this kind do not totally represent the actual patient–doctor encounter, because they inevitably omit the patient's own record of symptoms which was the founding element in diagnosis.[16] But what is an available assumption is that the learned doctor would match individual experience of illness with the template of disease based on humoral theory.[17] Turner followed this pattern of expectation because he was 'doctus' or learned. That is, he was examined and passed not for his diagnostic skills with actual plants or actual patients, but because he was literate: he had read, could recite, answer questions and speak about, the key texts of the medical syllabus.[18] Moreover, though Turner probably would have been obliged to attend some lectures on anatomy in Italy and though it was increasingly advocated that physicians should show knowledge of anatomy, he never referred in his writings to either anatomy or physiology.[19]

The major concern in learned medicine was how to rectify the specific imbalance presented by the body, a process of medication sometimes aided by recommended diet. Late in life, when Turner gave advice on diet as part of the regimen attendant upon medicinal bathing, he followed Galenic principles, as they had been restated by Marsilio Ficino (1433–99).[20] These dictated that, for instance, vegetables were boiled twice to remove their overactive natural properties; pears were bad when raw, but were acceptable when well cooked.[21] Indeed, overall, the essential role of vegetables as part of the diet was not understood: the wealthy groups in England who could afford a physician like Turner tended to avoid eating fruit and vegetables, seeing them as the necessary portions of the more impoverished classes.[22]

While there is no evidence as to how Turner conducted a consultation, his writings show that he operated from within Galenic principles, which he explained in the opening address prefacing Part 3, in his comments on the degrees of herbs. Herbs, as products of nature, possessed the four essential qualities (hot, cold, wet, dry) in different 'degrees' from a natural mean. The dangerous herbs were the extreme ones: opium poppy (*Papaver somniferum*), cold in the fourth degree, would 'put out or quench the natural heat'.[23] The complete *Herball* was finally published in 1568, the year that Turner died, showing that all his life he remained a committed Galenist. Although it seems likely that when he was passing through Switzerland in the early 1540s he would have heard about the furore created by Paracelsus (1493–1541) in Basel, his only reference to him is in the list of authors he consulted in composing his book on medicinal baths.

As a Galenist, Turner, like his peers, would have rounded off the process of prescribing restorative medicinal herbs by prescribing procedures such as bloodletting. Since these procedures (for those who could pay for them) were undertaken by the surgeon, Part 3 is dedicated to them, in what is an unprecedented gesture in his works. Turner usually dedicated his writings to royal or aristocratic patrons, so the praise in Part 3 'To the right worshipfull Feloweship and Companye of Surgiones of the cityc of London', within the dedication of the completed *Herball* to Queen Elizabeth, is a recognition of their important role in medical practice overall.[24]

What many of the medicaments listed in Part 3 particularly indicate is that Turner, like his contemporaries, defended vigorously the need to prescribe forceful expulsives for health's sake. These purgatives were not just for physical problems but for the more ambiguous mental/emotional/spiritual ones. So, he advocated 'Sene' (senna, *Cassia acutifolia*) as something which:

> scoureth awaye and purgeth alwaye gentlye melancholye and burnt choler, from the braine, from the sensible partes, from the hart, lunges, liuer and milte, and therefore it is good for diseses that sprynge of the humores of those places as are melancholike and olde agues. And Sene maketh a man to be ioyful and merye, for it taketh away the humore and cause that maketh man sad without cause.[25]

So in spite of warnings contained in the list of the degrees of herbs, throughout his *Herball* he was active in recommending medicines which modern herbalists consider dangerous and potentially fatal: *Paris quadrifolia* (herb paris), which he declared to be entirely suitable for children according to his own judgement and that of his peers;[26] and 'hellebore' (strictly, *Veratrum album*, rather than *Helleborus niger*), which he was prescribing for women and children at the period when one of his Italian contemporaries was offering serious reservations about the widespread use of helleborism in exorcisms practised on men.[27] In these cases, as with prescribing for 'the mother', boundaries between physical and spiritual factors were not readily separated.

For the most part, in his general principles Turner and his university-trained colleagues were at one, but the stereotype needs to be tested against the actuality. As the dedication to the surgeons shows, he was reasonably democratic in his recognition of non-university providers, perhaps because he never strikes us as being an elaborate theorist, but always a practical practitioner. This may relate to his early experiences in Morpeth, but it would certainly seem to be confirmed by his experiences in Germany during his exiles there. In all his writings, Turner himself referred approvingly to the insights and experience of apothecaries from both England and the continent, while recognizing that the slack practices of some needed to be improved. The goal of recognizing a contribution within physic at the same time as improving training, which surfaced in the dedication to the surgeons, allowed him where the apothecaries were concerned to cite their useful knowledge, and to refer to *succedanea* (legitimate substitutes) when appropriate.[28] He also routinely included their terms alongside the terminology received from Greek and Latin sources, and better-known vernaculars: the Greek *Karos* (*Carum carvi*) is 'carui' in apothecary parlance; Centaurium magnum (*Centaurium erythraea*) is their 'ruponticum'.[29] This open-mindedness in Turner therefore avoids any suggestion of a rift between learned physicians and other practitioners: he strikes us, overall, as a democratic outsider rather than an elitist insider when writing and practising in England. In fact, he appears never to have joined the Royal College of Physicians, though there was a brief flurry around 1550 when it was mooted that he become their President. However, he did know, and must at times perforce have cooperated with, the established royal physicians. Drs Owen (1499–1558), Wotton (1492–1555) and Wendy (c. 1499–1560) were all referred to as having 'muche knowledge in herbes', though he also reproved them for not sharing their knowledge in print.[30]

However, Turner's democratic frame of reference to non-university colleagues did not explicitly include women. Where women received payment for services, for instance as midwives, parts of the medical establishment condemned them out of hand, though others saw them as a source of knowledge and experience, and contributed to their training. A handbook for midwives in English, giving technical terminology and diagrams, was published in 1540 and had gone through ten editions by 1604.[31] But Turner's frequent references to the herbs which could be used for 'women's diseases' show no indication of published recipes or modes of analysis. And the diffuse, but essential, provision by women of medical care within the local community, linked to gardening skills and supplied by the mistress of the great house, was never recognized by Turner. Yet, paradoxically, it would be this group who would have formed part of Turner's target audience. One known owner of his *Herball*, Lady Grace Mildmay, was daughter-in-law of Sir Walter Mildmay who was one of the mid-Tudor monarchs' most trusted financial officials – though lack of evidence of ownership does not of itself indicate lack of access to herbals within this class.[32] Meanwhile, the poorer women of the labouring classes received only the contemptuous designation of 'old wives' in the Preface to Part 1.[33] This was a term John Gerard (c. 1545–1612) would also use, but both he and John Parkinson (c. 1567–1650) referred to women as medical carers, gardeners and plant-collectors. However, while Turner did not acknowledge women explicitly, he offered such clarity in listing the practical application of his individual species that they would have been immediately useful to literate women running large households. Like Pliny and Dioscorides before him, he indicated whether plants should be prepared in water, milk, wine or honey, and how this affected their range of uses.

Who then did Turner expect to read and use his *Herball*? Written in English, and printed in the populist black-letter type, Turner's work falls somewhere in the mid-Tudor market between a technical textbook and a popular handbook.[34] The tension inherent in this statement surfaces throughout. On the one hand, there was the intention to make the use of recognizable medicaments available to any literate reader, whether lay or professional, and, implicitly, whether male or female. On the other hand, Turner was presenting the latest scholarship and his own research in plant identification, which took him well beyond the needs of someone reaching hastily for an immediate remedy. So the emphasis in *The Names of Herbes* (1549) on plants from East Friesland was not as useful as, say, knowledge of the neighbouring French flora would have been. And the 'confutations' with contemporary writers which inflated the second part of the *Herball*[35] would also have been beyond the needs of either the householder or of the average physician, who could well have been tempted to instruct his apothecary on the basis of an easier, if less accurate, herbal.

These confutations, which can protrude so uncomfortably, act as a reminder that there was no literary format available which fitted Turner's needs: a herbal did not entirely suit what he was aiming to do. The sometimes cumbersome organization of his own herbal is concomitant with him pushing out of the boundaries of a traditional genre as part of a fast-growing field of reference. Medical books of various kinds, as demonstrated by McConchie, by this time were regularly being written in English.[36] This cut authors off from a European market, but it enabled them to provide a broader service to their countrymen (a service which they defended against the accusation that they were betraying the secrets of their profession to the ignorant). Turner's writings were part of this movement to improve the knowledge and training of English practitioners, which lagged so far behind the sophisticated training and practice of medical practitioners in northern Italy or in the German lands. Adopting a familiar trope of the time, he wrote in the Preface to Part 1 of the *Herball* of physic as an enterprise sanctioned and praised in the Bible by God himself: the man who would 'take paynes to set out any herball' was as good 'unto his countre' as the soldier who took blows in its defence.[37] So he would have been gratified that McConchie offers evidence that his *Herball* did come to be used extensively by contemporary doctors, surgeons and apothecaries, giving substance to Harrison's eulogizing of the 'father of English physic'. Whereas MacLean thought his work was irrelevant, McConchie claims that 'Turner was the most widely read English writer in the medical field', a tribute to the 'prime importance' of herbals in medical practice and to the superior quality of his own.[38]

Turner would have been gratified because at the very end of his life he looked back on his career as a writer on physic with some bitterness. None of Turner's natural history writings strike us as having been written in a mood of good cheer, and all of his dedications typically requested protection by a patron from unspecified enemies or detractors, but the final dedication to Elizabeth which prefaced his complete tri-part *Herball* looked back on his authorial career with discontent and jealousy. This envy was not, as might have been expected from an English work, directed to the English royal doctors who had all made more money and gained more land and property than him,[39] but to the two great continental authorities Leonhart Fuchs and Pietro Andrea Matthioli (1501–77). Measuring himself against them, he commented bitterly that if a reader checked out the first part of his *Herball* against their writings, he would easily perceive, 'that I taught the truthe of certeyne plantes whiche these aboue named writers either knew not at al/ or ellis erred in them greatlye'.[40] According to this final self-assessment, Turner got there first but others, writing in Latin for the international market, got the credit.

Turner's contribution to medical botany

Turner's aim, reiterated over his life, produced results in his writings which make them still valuable, since he was endlessly interested in the all-healing products of nature and the help they could bring to his fellow-men. All medicaments were God's creatures; all had some beneficent purpose. Driven by this purpose, it was, arguably, the interplay between Turner's native curiosity concerning 'the creatures' and his formal training which sharpened his skills in identifying the plants forming the basis of his prescriptions. This was an effort which, as a by-product, helped further the contemporary process of extending an available vocabulary.[41] So, if he remained inevitably within an inadequate and inaccurate paradigm for describing the body and its ills; if he ignored the progress of knowledge in anatomy; if he bypassed the work on chemical preparations initiated by Paracelsus; and if his usage of available medicines was faulty and sometimes dangerous, nevertheless, his overriding concern with identifying medicaments so as to use them accurately within the constrictive paradigms of his times led not only to seminal developments in plant identification within English botany, but also provided a basis from which an ongoing tradition of herbal medicine could, eventually, rest securely.

Against this background, Turner's achievement can be more thoroughly appreciated. He was not the first writer to provide any kind of medical handbook in English. Nor was he the first writer to write about plants in English. Just before he went up to Cambridge, two English herbals were published in the 1520s. One of them, *The Grete Herball*, stayed in print continuously under differing titles throughout Turner's life, though the fact that publications slowed down suggests that his own herbal may have affected the market.[42] The other, known as *Banckes' Herbal* (1525) after its publisher, demonstrates graphically just how different Turner's productions were. This is Banckes' entry for 'Arbrotinum' (*Artemisia abrotanum*):

> this herb Arbrotinum, men call it southernwood. The virtue of this herb is thus, that if they break the seed and drink it with water, it healeth men that have been bitten by any venomous beast. Also, this herb destroyeth worms in [a] man's womb. Also, powder of this herb meddled with barley meal unbindeth and breaketh hard apostumes. Also, this herb burnt and the ashes meddled with oil, it restoreth where any man lacketh hair. This herb is hot and dry.[43]

This entry was followed later in this short book by one for 'Southernwood', but there was no suggestion as to whether 'arbrotinum' and 'southernwood' were different plants: neither one was described; although the same name occurred in the second entry, there was no back reference to the earlier one; and the recommended usages were not identical.[44] Yet Banckes' writing represented a long-standing medieval tradition which stayed in fashion over the century. Just as Turner was preparing Part 1 of his *Herball* for press, there appeared an English version of *The Book of Secrets* of Albertus Magnus (c. 1200–80). This, as well as detailing 'the marvels of the world', dealt with a selected list of plants in a way which closely resembles that in Banckes' compilation of 20 years earlier.[45]

It becomes clear that Turner was aiming for something beyond the scope of a respected – though largely useless – tradition if we compare Banckes' entry with Turner's in *Names* (1549) for 'Arbrotonum':

> Abrotonu is called in greke Abrotonum, in englishe Sothernwod, in duche Affrush, in frenche Auronne. There are two kyndes of Sothernwod, the male and the female. The male groweth plentuously in gardines in Englande, it is founde in Italy in plentie inough. Sothernwod is hote and dry in the thirde degree.[46]

– and with Part 1 of the *Herball* in 1551:

> [as in 1549, then] Dioscorides maketh two kinds of Sothernwode. The one kind is the male and it groweth in gardens and nowhere else, and this is our common Sothernwode. The other kind is the female, and divers learned men have supposed the herb, called in English lavander cotton to be this kind.[47]

Turner's entries would be seen by a modern botanist as full of errors. He perpetrated defunct and imprecise ideas about male and female plants based on size and colour rather than on structural roles in propagation, and he conflated in the second entry two completely different genera. But errors such as these are valuable because they are completely transparent and therefore open to correction, either by Turner himself or by somebody else. They are a contribution to knowledge, a certain stage at which knowledge has arrived, not a completely impenetrable and uncorrectable construct such as offered by Banckes' herbal. Moreover, the medical information which followed could be matched up by a principled apothecary to specific plant material, rather than being a matter of grabbing what was to hand in response to a garbled prescription. Hence Turner's work is seminal in setting standards of observation as well as in contributing specific data to what would later emerge as an official pharmacopoeia.

The brief comparison above is a reminder that Turner was writing in English specifically to provide and discuss reliable names and descriptions of the native and foreign plants found in the classical texts, prescribed by physicians and surgeons, supplied by apothecaries and used in home health care. To achieve this, his writings required both an unprecedented exactitude of observation as well as scrupulousness in comparing his own findings with existing verbal and written accounts of those plants. As the entries for 'Arbrotonu-Southernwood' show, this search began with ascertaining names: Turner's reforming tendencies in physic used the techniques of contemporary philology in a way which reflected the humanist training of his era. Medical herb lore in the Western tradition founded itself on Dioscorides, Pliny and Galen. Texts of these writers, although they had not been entirely lost, had to some extent been distorted and confused over centuries of copying and commentary. Consequently, it was not clear which plants people were talking and writing about. However, the humanist drive in the universities of northern Italy to recover these texts and to identify their contexts had not only spread to northern Europe by the circulation of printed texts, but had encouraged men like Turner to study there, taking their knowledge and training back to their native country in an enterprise that was European in its encyclopaedic aims, while specific in the attention paid to each country's place in a pan-European flora.[48] What Turner brought back to plant research is what gives him the right to that old title of 'father of English physic': however slow the trickle of his influence, after the completion of his *Herball* in the year of his death, herbal medicine in England would be able to identify more accurately the plant medicaments which were its mainstay.

Certainly Turner's England, at the time when he began his enterprise of providing accurate information about plant medicaments, had its problems. For one thing, the Mediterranean flora listed by Dioscorides was obviously not always identical to that of a cooler, northern Europe country. For another, in England the names differed from county to county, from district to district. A daisy (*Bellis perennis*) was a banewort or a ewe-gollan in his native Northumberland, but twelve disciples, twelve frills, or a baby's pet in Somerset.[49] Turner had difficulty ascertaining something as obvious to us as a daffodil.[50] Nobody had collated regional differences in England or established them within a European flora, yet this is what he set out to do: a huge task, conducted within a life which was disrupted by politics, made stressful by 'the stone', and aided to only a very small degree by his peers in England.

So, inter alia, Turner's work transmitted to his peers and successors the importance of obtaining knowledge of local flora. Beginning as a boy in Northumberland, wherever he went in England (or Europe) he studied plants and named their habitats. His herbals are full of specific references not just to regions but to the variety of habitats he had experienced: woods, marshes, coasts, fields, roadsides or mountains. In this, he reflected the traditional practice of folk botany in its pursuit of the 'generic-specieme' designated by Scott Atran: the concept of a plant as known in its local form, and therefore neither exclusively a genus or a species, but combining the qualities of both by being a 'sort of/kind of'.[51] But in another sense he was ahead of his time, and fairly isolated in his task. Gerard would refer spasmodically to his friends and colleagues finding different plants across the country in the 1590s, but it would be the seventeenth century before men like Thomas Johnson (c. 1600–44) and John Goodyer (c. 1592–1664) regularly organized themselves into English plant-hunting expeditions.[52] So, when, a century after the first part of Turner's *Herball*, Nicholas Culpeper (1616–54) reversed the trend for ever larger and fatter tomes by declaring that only English herbs were needed for English ailments, he could do so partly at least because by then he was secure in the knowledge that they could be identified accurately.

Turner never shared Culpeper's insular brief. Whether by inclination, experience or training, or, most likely, by a combination of all three, his work on native species was always emphatically contextualized within European medical theory. He praised his Italian master, Antonio Musa Brasavola (1500–55), and the medical tradition in Ferrara which had brought such learning to physic;[53] he corresponded with major figures in Germany and Switzerland, including Gessner and Fuchs; and his publisher secured the use of Fuchs' woodcuts, the best of their day, for his own herbal.[54] But the masters he revered were not just the living ones of his own times. To his own empirical observations, to the comments and writings of his contemporaries, he brought his ability to work directly from Greek and Latin, so that he could study the available textbooks in which learned physic was rooted. David Gardner-Medwin, in a lecture given to celebrate the 500th anniversary of Turner's birth, demonstrated in detail that his herbal contains the earliest extant English translation of Dioscorides – something normally attributed to Goodyer's unpublished work of a century later.[55] Likewise, in the last years of his life, as new plants, and potentially new remedies, infiltrated Europe from the Americas, he extended his range further by offering as Part 3 of his *Herball* a description of plants which were not in Dioscorides' master work of the first century, but which men of the sixteenth century were beginning to use regularly. At the same time, in extending his brief beyond the classical masters, he found himself relying on 'the Arabianes', the medieval masters rejected by the purists of his generation, for information about plants they had known and recommended. Hence Guaiacum (*Guaiacum officinale*) 'oute of Calcutte/Java' [sic], the plant then being used for syphilis, was described alongside the precious medieval spices, nutmeg and mace, discussed by the Arabians.[56]

Turner set about his task constrained by the intrinsic problems affecting any writer on plants in his era with no knowledge of genus and species. The 'kindes', 'formes', 'manneres' and 'sortes' which he and his peers automatically referred to were all insecurely understood variants of Atran's monotypical generic-specieme.

There was confusion, as the 'Arbrotonu–Southernwood' entries show, between male and female plants, a terminology based on colour or size rather than on the microscopic knowledge of pollination, which only began to be generally understood in the late seventeenth century.[57] Likewise, there was a general hesitancy going back for centuries in differentiating between wild and horticultural forms. And Turner had only a very thin vocabulary available to describe the different species he listed. His frequent references to 'black' flowers or plants indicate the paucity of his colour vocabulary, and the treatment of flowers as variegated forms of foliage demonstrate that neither the words 'petal' nor 'sepal' were available to him. Consequently, he overused very simple forms of analogy as a descriptive mechanism. His conflation of two entirely different genera under one word 'selendine' in Part 2 of the *Herball* (1562) includes the following description of the greater celandine (*Chelidonium majus*):

> the leaues are lyke crowfote leaues, but softer and blewish gray in color. The flowre is lyke the flowre of wall gelauore, otherwise called hartes ease.... The iuice that is in it is lyke saffrone, bitinge sharps.... It hath a small codde lyke unto homed popye and long, but it is euer smaller.[58]

Yet at the same time he was capable of other analogies, so sharp and striking that, while they would not help the seeker to identify a species, they would certainly help to fix it afterwards in the memory. Random selections from any pages of the *Herball* throw up vivid descriptions: for example, Aristolochia longa (*Aristolochia clematitis*) 'bryngeth furth fruite lyke blacke peares and sede lyke mennes hertes', and dodder (*Cuscuta europaea*) is 'lyke a great red harpe strynge'.[59]

In these descriptions, Turner was assuming – or hoping – that a physician, a surgeon or an apothecary would be a natural historian, with some of his own direct knowledge of plants, and further enabled by this *Herball* to refuse to use dangerous or shoddy substitutes. So if the modern botanist is dismayed that he demonstrated the Tudor physician's lack of interest in the flower in preference for the medically useful parts (seeds, leaves, shoots and roots), for his contemporaries he provided tools whereby the physician could identify accurately the plants he described. He demonstrated the possibility of checking textual accuracy from field work and back again, and insisted on the necessity of this procedure. His books performed this task for his fellow practitioners by comparing texts in the classical languages, and encouraging by his example a cluster of related skills. So, for instance, he replaced generalized hearsay with context and specificity: Turner's use of 'they say' – common in early texts – is far less frequent than Gerard's would be later, and much more cautious. These tactics helped him to define clearly his field of enquiry: namely, how a plant could be recognized and as a result how it could be used according to best medical practice. To achieve this, he admitted and included what he did not know and pointed to the need for such knowledge as was not yet available, by making corrections all the time in research that was envisaged as ongoing and part of a cooperative field. Admittedly, this cooperation frequently exhibited itself in fierce contempt for what he believed somebody had got wrong! All too often the target was his Italian contemporary Matthioli, whose annotations on Dioscorides on more than one occasion were declared to be 'nothyng worth',[60] and whose quarrelsome nature, like that of Fuchs, Turner could on such occasions easily match.[61]

In order to bring this methodology strictly and clearly within the province of English medical plants and English medical needs, he adopted a series of procedures for dealing with those native species he believed to be useful. Wherever he could, he usually recorded and adopted the existing native use of names, retaining regional variants, sorting them, comparing them and, crucially, identifying the same plant under different names. As with some of his other procedures, this impacted on botany as well as physic: the first recorded use of the word 'daffodil' to typify the yellow-trumpeted, poisonously bulbous plant of English woods and meadows came from Turner. Likewise, when he invented a new name when no vernacular one was available, the results penetrated horticulture and botany as well as medicine. Spindle tree (for *Euonymus europaeus*) and monk's hood (for *Aconitum napellus*) came from contemporary German; 'loosestrife' was a literal translation of the classical Greek *lysimachia*.[62] The result of this activity is that Turner provided the first reliable descriptions for future botanists of about 300 native plants.[63] But for his contemporaries, whose reliance on plants to provide both day-to-day relief and aid in the treatment of major disease, injury or trauma was unstinting (whether misplaced or not), the benefits of identifying the same plant under its different names, and accepting a name for something which previously had no proper name, were incalculable.

This is not to say Turner could provide all the answers. Sometimes, as we saw, he asserted an alarming belief in the acceptable uses of dangerous plants, not always or entirely protecting his readers by simply indicating their degrees of lethal heat or coldness. At the time that he published an innovative analysis of wines, he was also defending the mystique of theriac; *mumia* and animal products appeared in his works just as they did in those of his contemporaries; and he had intended, he said, to write about the useful medicinal properties not only of minerals but of birds. Yet while it is realistic to acknowledge how limited our knowledge is of him as a practising physician, and realistic to examine the paradigms and cultural conditions in which he worked, it is unrealistic to insist that, as well as describing every plant as accurately as possible, he should have been able to overhaul both their medical application and the general medical paradigms of his time. The compromise is to accept that traditionally accepted best practice was his guide, reinforced by rigorous and scrupulous scholarship. And he knew at least some of the tradition's limitations, in his realization that some plants should be incorporated within the medical flora even though they were unknown within the classical medical line running from Dioscorides.

Indeed, this stubborn curiosity and eclecticism is what makes him so instructive and so influential. Sometimes, reading the different parts of his *Herball*, it seems all too apparent that Turner was attempting to use a non-existent vocabulary to perform a task which had not been invented. But he had a heroic stab at the task, and medicine in the future could establish its practice on the secure identification he provided of its basic constituents, just as scholarly method could adapt his rigorous analytical practices.

Recommended reading

Addyman, Marie. *William Turner: Father of English Botany*. Morpeth: Castle Morpeth Borough Council, 2008.
Arber, Agnes. *Herbals, Their Origin and Evolution: A Chapter in the History of Botany, 1470–1670*. 3rd ed. Cambridge: Cambridge University Press, 1986.
Jones, Whitney R. D. *William Turner: Tudor Naturalist, Physician and Divine*. London: Routledge, 1988.
Raven, Charles E. *Early Naturalists from Neckam to Ray: A Study of the Making of the Modern World*. Cambridge: Cambridge University Press, 1947.
Webster, Charles, ed. *Health, Medicine and Mortality in the Sixteenth Century*. Cambridge: Cambridge University Press, 1979.

Notes

1 See William Harrison, *The Description of England: The Classic Contemporary Account of Tudor Life*, ed. Georges Edelen, new ed. (Washington: Folger Shakespeare Library and Dover Publications, 1994), 289.

2 Charles E. Raven, *Early Naturalists from Neckam to Ray: A Study of the Making of the Modern World* (Cambridge: Cambridge University Press, 1947). See also Agnes Arber, *Herbals, Their Origin and Evolution: A Chapter in the History of Botany, 1470–1670*, 3rd ed. (Cambridge: Cambridge University Press, 1986), and, more recently, Anna Pavord, *The Naming of Names: The Search for Order in the World of Plants* (London: Bloomsbury, 2005).

3 Antonia McLean, *Humanism and the Rise of Science in Tudor England* (London: Heinemann Educational, 1972), 195.

4 Work initiated by Barbara Griggs, in her different editions of *Green Pharmacy*. See Barbara Griggs, *New Green Pharmacy* (London: Vermillion, 1997).

5 A biographical summary is given in Raven, *Early Naturalists*, chs IV–VI, and in Whitney R. D. Jones, *William Turner: Tudor Naturalist, Physician and Divine* (London: Routledge, 1988).

6 Turner's natural history writing can be accessed as follows:
(i) *Libellus de re herbaria, 1538: [and] the Names of Herbes, 1548*, facsimiles with introductory matter by James Britten, B. Daydon Jackson and W. T. Stearn (London: The Ray Society, 1965). The date 1548 is 'old-style' and should be 1549.
(ii) *A New Herball, Part 1*, Vol. 1, ed. George T. L. Chapman and Marilyn N. Weddle (Ashington: Mid Northumberland Arts Group and Carcanet Press, 1989). This is based on the 1551 text.
(iii) *A New Herball, Parts II and III*, ed. George T. L. Chapman, Frank McCombie and Anne U. Wesencraft (Cambridge: Cambridge University Press, 1995). This is based on the 1568 text.
(iv) *The First and Seconde Partes of the Herbal of William Turner Doctor in Phisick Lately Oversene, Corrected, and Enlarged* (Cologne: By [the heirs of] Arnold Birckman, 1568).
(v) Arthur H. Evans, ed., *Turner on Birds*, Kessinger reprint ed. (Cambridge: Cambridge University Press, 1903).

(vi) *A Book of Wines... [a Facsimile of the Edition of 1568.]*, ed. Sanford V. Larkey and Philip M. Wagner (New York: Scholars' Facsimiles and Reprints, 1941).
(vii) *A Booke of the Natures and Properties... of... Bathes* (Cologne, 1562/1568).
(viii) The letter to Gessner on fishes is translated and annotated in A. Wheeler, P. Davis and E. Lazenby, 'William Turner's (c. 1508-1568) Notes on Fishes in His Letter to Conrad Gessner', *Archives of Natural History* 13, no. 3 (1968): 291-305.

7   Mary Lindemann, *Medicine and Society in Early Modern Europe* (Cambridge: Cambridge University Press, 1999), 105, Table 4.1.

8   See Andrew Pettegree, *Foreign Protestant Communities in Sixteenth-Century London* (Oxford: Clarendon Press, 1986); Deborah E. Harkness, *The Jewel House: Elizabethan London and the Scientific Revolution* (New Haven, CT: Yale University Press, 2007), especially chs 1 and 2.

9   Lansdowne MS. VIII, no. 78; a version is provided by George T. L. Chapman, 'William Turner of Morpeth, Northumberland (1508-68)', *The Scottish Naturalist* (1986): 11-27. The information concerning the merchant's wife comes by courtesy of Frances Neale, former archivist of Wells Cathedral, who is preparing extracts of the commonplace book for publication.

10 The standard account of the College's achievements is that by George Clark, *A History of the Royal College of Physicians of London*, vol. 1 (Oxford: Clarendon Press for the Royal College of Physicians, 1964). A more recent defence is in Elizabeth L. Furdell, *The Royal Doctors: Medical Personnel at the Tudor and Stuart Courts* (Rochester, NY: Rochester University Press, 2001). Meanwhile, R. S. Roberts had offered a much more clinical assessment of the College's ongoing attempts to establish a monopoly, in 'The Personnel and Practice of Medicine in Tudor and Stuart England. Part II: London', *Medical History* 8, no. 3 (1964): 217-33. See also Margaret Pelling, *The Common Lot: Sickness, Medical Occupations and the Urban Poor in Early Modern England* (London: Longman, 1998); Margaret Pelling and Charles Webster, 'Medical Practitioners', in *Health, Medicine and Mortality in the Sixteenth Century*, ed. Charles Webster (Cambridge: Cambridge University Press, 1979), 165-235.

11 Ian MacLean, *Logic, Signs and Nature in the Renaissance: The Case of Learned Medicine* (Cambridge: Cambridge University Press, 2002).

12 Turner refers more than once to *mumia*. For a general history of the use of mumia, see Richard Sugg, *Mummies, Cannibals and Vampires: A History of Corpse Medicine from the Renaissance to the Victorians* (London: Routledge, 2011). On theriacs, see Gilbert Watson, *Theriac and Mithridatum: A Study in Therapeutics* (London: Welcome Historical Medical Library, 1966).

13 See, for example, Bald's *Leechbook* in Stephen Pollington, *Leechcraft: Early English Charms, Plant Lore, and Healing* (Norfolk: Anglo-Saxon Books, 2000).

14 This will be discussed in detail in Marie Addyman, *Physic and Philosophy: William Turner's Botanical Medicine* (forthcoming).

15 Turner, *A New Herball, Parts II and III*, 716.

16 For an overview of these practices, see Peter Elmer, ed., *The Healing Arts: Health, Disease, and Society in Europe, 1500-1800: A Source Book* (Manchester: Manchester University Press in association with the Open University, 2004), chs 1-3; Nancy G. Siraisi, *Medieval and Early Renaissance Medicine: An Introduction to Knowledge and Practice* (Chicago: University of Chicago Press, 1990); Andrew Wear, Roger K. French and Iain M. Lonie, eds., *The Medical Renaissance of the Sixteenth Century* (Cambridge: Cambridge University Press, 1985). English medicine immediately

prior to Turner's times is discussed in Carole Rawcliffe, *Medicine and Society in Later Medieval England* (Stroud: Sutton, 1995).

17   For more on classical approaches and the humoral framework, see chs 2 and 9 in this volume.

18   Pliny the Elder, *Natural History: In Ten Volumes. Vol. 6 Libri XX–XXIII* and *Vol. 7 Libri XXIV–XXVII*, trans. W. H. S. Jones (Cambridge, MA: Harvard University Press, 1969 and 1956 respectively). Turner wrote that he studied 'physik and philosophy' in his dedication to Part 2 of the *Herball*. See Turner, *A New Herball, Parts II and III*, 23. For the general background for these terms, see Edward Grant, *A History of Natural Philosophy: From the Ancient World to the Nineteenth Century* (Cambridge: Cambridge University Press, 2007).

19   See Jonathan Sawday, *The Body Emblazoned: Dissection and the Human Body in Renaissance Culture* (London: Routledge, 1995).

20   Noga Arikha, *Passions and Tempers: A History of the Humours* (New York: Harper Perennial, 2007), 126, quotes Ficino's list of foods which should be avoided to combat melancholy: both in principle, and in detail, the recommendations of the fifteenth-century Italian and the sixteenth-century Englishman are similar. For an early overview of balneological writing, see Arnold C. Klebs, 'Balneology in the Middle Ages', *Transactions of the American Climatological and Clinical Association* 32 (1916): 15–37, and for a modern one, Roy Porter, ed., *The Medical History of Waters and Spas*, Medical History Supplement No. 10 (London: Wellcome Institute for the History of Medicine, 1990), which includes Roy Palmer's essay on Italian baths in the Renaissance, taking its title from Turner, 'In our Lyghte and Learned Tyme', ibid., 14–22.

21   Mark Grant, ed., *Galen: On Food and Diet* (London: Routledge, 2002), 141, for an example on cabbage. For contemporaries, see F. J. Furnivall, ed., *The Fyrst Boke of the Introduction of Knowledge Made by Andrew Borde, of Physycke Doctor: A Compendyous Regyment; or, a Dyetary of Helth Made in Mountpyllier* (London: Published for the Early English Text Society by N. T. Trübner and Co., 1870), and Thomas Vicary, *The Anatomie of the Bodie of Man*, ed. F. J. Furnivall and P. Furnivall (London: Early English Text Society, 1888), ch. 1.

22   The Italian writer Giacomo Castelvetro, exiled in England under James I, wrote his own account of his native land's use of these to try and improve the diet of his host country. Giacomo Castelvetro, *The Fruit, Herbs and Vegetables of Italy: An Offering to Lucy, Countess of Bedford*, trans. Gillian Riley (London: Viking, 1989). For an account of the food of the rich in the early modern world, see Alison Sim, *Food and Feast in Tudor England* (Stroud: Sutton, 1997); or more generally, Kate Colquhoun, *Taste: The Story of Britain through Its Cooking* (London: Bloomsbury, 2007), chs 7–9; J. C. Drummond and Anne Wilbraham, *The Englishman's Food: A History of Five Centuries of English Diet*, revised by Dorothy Hollingsworth (London: Pimlico, 1991). For a graphic account of the food of the poor in early modern Europe, see Piero Camporesi, *Bread of Dreams: Food and Fantasy in Early Modern Europe*, trans. David Gentilcore (Cambridge: Polity Press in association with B. Blackwell, 1989).

23   Turner, *A New Herball, Parts II and III*, 632 et seq.

24   Ibid., 631.

25   Ibid., 707.

26   Turner refers to herb paris (*Paris quadrifolia*, which he termed 'one berrye') on different occasions. The clearest reference to it being harmless is in Turner, *A New Herball, Parts II and III*, 44.

27 For exorcisms using dangerous herbs, see Piero Camporesi, *The Incorruptible Flesh: Bodily Mutation and Mortification in Religion and Folklore*, trans. Tania Croft-Murray (Cambridge: Cambridge University Press, 1988).
28 Pamela Smith and Paula Findlen, *Merchants and Marvels: Commerce, Science and Art in Early Modern Europe* (London: Routledge, 2002), 122, includes tables of *succedanea* from Lobelius' herbal of 1581. See also Leslie G. Matthews, 'Royal Apothecaries of the Tudor Period', *Medical History* 8, no. 2 (1964): 170–80.
29 Turner, *A New Herball, Part 1*, 118, 123.
30 Ibid., 26.
31 See Elaine Hobby's ch. 4 in this book.
32 For Grace Mildmay, see Elizabeth L. Furdell, *Publishing and Medicine in Early Modern England* (Rochester, NY: Rochester University Press, 2002), 96; also Rachel Weigall, 'An Elizabethan Gentlewoman: The Journal of Lady Mildmay, Circa 1570-1617', *Quarterly Review* 215 (1911): 119–38. For a list of female owners of herbals, see Rebecca Laroche, *Medical Authority and Englishwomen's Herbal Texts, 1550-1650* (Farnham: Ashgate, 2009), Appendix B.
33 Turner, *A New Herball, Part 1*, 25 et seq.
34 Furdell, *Publishing and Medicine*; MacLean, *Logic, Signs and Nature*; Henry S. Bennett, *English Books and Readers, 1475 to 1557: Being a Study in the History of the Book Trade from Caxton to the Incorporation of the Stationers' Company* (Cambridge: Cambridge University Press, 1952).
35 Turner, *A New Herball, Parts II and III*. As an example, see his long discussion of *Pinus sylvestris*, 197 et seq.
36 R. W. McConchie, *Lexicography and Physicke: The Record of Sixteenth-Century English Medical Terminology* (Oxford: Clarendon Press, 1997). McConchie lists some, though not all, of the medical works published in Tudor England and discusses the issue of writing in English in ch. 2 in particular.
37 Turner, *A New Herball, Part 1*, 26–7.
38 McConchie, *Lexicography and Physicke*, 91 et seq.
39 It is not clear if Turner owned any permanent property at all during his life, and certainly not deriving from the practice of physic. Turner's will is discussed in Jones, *William Turner*, 47. Regarding the gains made by the royal doctors, Dr Owen for instance had acquired property in nearby Bristol in the reign of Henry VIII. See John Latimer, *Sixteenth-Century Bristol*, reprint of 1908 ed. (Charleston, SC: Bibliolife LLC, 2009), 33.
40 Turner, *The First and Seconde Partes*, iii, preface to the complete *Herball* of 1568.
41 Turner's vocabulary penetrated English usage through his share in the debate over coining new plant-names, though he and those of his contemporaries who wrote herbals did not extend medical vocabulary in general. See McConchie, *Lexicography and Physicke*, especially ch. 7 and appendices, 125, for his comment on herbalists. See also Leah Knight, *Of Books and Botany in Early Modern England: Sixteenth-Century Plants and Print Culture* (Farnham: Ashgate, 2009).
42 Eleanour S. Rohde, *The Old English Herbals*, reprint of the 1922 ed. (New York: Dover Publications, 1971), gives a bibliography of English herbals.
43 Sanford V. Larkey and Thomas Piles, eds., *An Herbal [1525] Edited and Transcribed into Modern English* (New York: Scholars Facsimiles and Reprints, 1941), 7.
44 Ibid., 75.
45 Michael R. Best and Frank H. Brightman, eds., *The Book of Secrets of Albertus*

Magnus of the Virtues of Herbs, Stones, and Certain Beasts, revised ed. (Boston: Samuel Weiser, 1999).
46 Names of Herbes in Turner, Libellus de re herbaria, 149.
47 Turner, A New Herball, Part 1, 219.
48 See Scott Atran, The Cognitive Foundations of Natural History (Cambridge: Cambridge University Press, 1990); Brian W. Ogilvie, The Science of Describing: Natural History in Renaissance Europe (Chicago: University of Chicago Press, 2006).
49 Geoffrey Grigson, The Englishman's Flora, facsimile of 1955 ed. (London: Phoenix House, 1987), 374.
50 Turner, Libellus de re herbaria, 197.
51 Atran, Cognitive Foundations, ch. 2.
52 Raven, Early Naturalists, section D, 227 et seq.
53 Vivian Nutton, 'The Rise of Medical Humanism: Ferrara, 1464–1555', Renaissance Studies 11, no. 1 (1997): 2–19.
54 On the publishing tradition associated with Fuchs' illustrations, see Arber, Herbals, ch. VII; Wilfrid Blunt and William T. Stearn, The Art of Botanical Illustration, revised 1994 ed. (Woodbridge: Antique Collectors' Club in association with Royal Botanic Gardens, 1950), 64 et seq.
55 David Gardner-Medwin, 'William Turner and Medicine' (paper presented at Turner 500 and Hancock 200: Naturalists in North-East England Conference, Newcastle University, 6–8 September 2008). See also David Gardner-Medwin's 'Down the Long Series of Eventful Time', in Medicine in Northumbria: Essays in the History of Medicine in the North East of England, ed. David Gardner-Medwin, Anne Hargreaves and Elizabeth Lazenby (Newcastle-upon-Tyne: The Pybus Society for the History and Bibliography of Medicine, 1993), 1–23, written while he was Honorary Secretary for The Pybus Society. The biographical details of Turner's life are subsequently being updated by the author, but Gardner-Medwin's analysis remains insightful.
56 Turner, A New Herball, Parts II and III, 670, 676. For a review of the contribution of the Islamic medical writers, see Peter Pormann and Emilie Savage-Smith, Medieval Islamic Medicine (Edinburgh: Edinburgh University Press, 2007). For a different slant on Islamic–Western indebtedness, see Bernard Lewis, The Muslim Discovery of Europe (London: Weidenfeld and Nicolson, 1982).
57 Some pioneering, exploratory work was done by Turner's near-contemporary Cesalpino. See Pavord, Naming of Names, 228 et seq.
58 Turner, A New Herball, Parts II and III, 395.
59 Turner, A New Herball, Part I, 72, 120.
60 Turner, A New Herball, Parts II and III, 70.
61 For arguments between Fuchs and Matthioli, and of each with other writers, see Pavord, Naming of Names, chs XII and XV. Only Gessner refrained from such quarrels, valuing all his correspondents including Turner (ch. XVIII).
62 For a discussion of Turner's naming strategies, see Knight, Of Books and Botany, ch. 3, and Addyman, Physic and Philosophy (forthcoming).
63 A list of these is provided by George A. Nelson, 'William Turner's Contribution to the First Records of British Plants', in Proceedings of the Leeds Philosophical and Literary Society, Scientific Section (Leeds: Leeds Philosophical and Literary Society, 1959), 109–38.

12

John Parkinson: Gardener and Apothecary of London

Jill Francis

Introduction

'I will endeavour to set downe and declare so much, as I hope may by reason perswade many in the truth'.[1]

Thus writes John Parkinson, who stands as an important figure in the history of the early modern period as a gardener, apothecary and writer who lived and worked in the city of London from the late sixteenth century until his death in 1650. Throughout his long working life, Parkinson earned his living and reputation as an apothecary, preparing and dispensing plant-based and other medicines from his shop on Ludgate Hill, as well as growing and cultivating the plants that were the essential tools of his trade on a substantial plot in Long Acre near Covent Garden, further outside the City walls to the west.[2] He is now best known as the author of two major publications: *Paradisi in sole paradisus terrestris: or, A Garden of all Sorts of Pleasant Flowers*, a remarkable gardening book published in 1629, on which his reputation as a gardener and writer still rests, and *Theatrum botanicum: The Theater of Plants*, a comprehensive new herbal which represented the culmination of his life's work as an apothecary, published in 1640.[3] Rarely however, are these two important aspects of his life – gardener and apothecary – considered together. This chapter aims to do just that, in order to demonstrate how each of these areas informed and enhanced his own work and also to deepen our own understanding of Parkinson the gardener, the apothecary and the world in which he lived.

Theatrum botanicum was a monumental work of over 1,700 pages, drawing on Parkinson's 50 years of experience of growing and working with plants. Its form was that of a conventional herbal, describing 'those Plants that are frequently used to helpe the diseases of our bodies', but updated to include, in Parkinson's own words, 'many hundreds of new, rare and strange plants from all parts of the world' as well as to amend, he goes on, 'all the many errors, differences and oversights of sundry Authors that have formerly written of them'.[4] As this chapter will show, this is no false modesty: although working within a traditional genre, Parkinson's great herbal was firmly rooted in the new empirical methods of scientific observation and experiment.

On the other hand, *Paradisi in sole* does not fit neatly into any recognized genre, but represents, as will be demonstrated, a radical departure in contemporary horticultural writing, recommending plants and flowers not only for their uses and virtues but also, and for the first time, 'those that are beautiful flower plants, fit to store a garden of delight and pleasure'.[5] A cursory glance reveals that it is set out in a similar way to the traditional herbal, with descriptions of the place, the time, the names, and so on, of hundreds of plants. However, in addition to its emphasis on ornamental plants, what also makes this book different are the closely written chapters at the beginning of each section (viz. the Garden of Pleasure, the Kitchen Garden and the Orchard) which contain detailed and intensely practical advice on gardening and growing plants. This in itself was a new departure from the herbal, but these chapters also include, for instance, Parkinson's views on current trends – what people 'nowadays' are doing in their gardens – some of which he approves of and some of which he does not. He grapples with moral issues such as gardeners playing God and trying to control nature, and despairs over idle and ignorant gardeners who don't know how to deal with the new 'outlandish' plants.[6] In particular, he is at pains to dispel 'false tales and reports', striving instead, as noted at the head of one chapter, to present the 'truth' and, more particularly, a truth that he has discovered through his own observation and experience.[7]

It would seem that once freed from the constraints of working within a particular genre, Parkinson was able to produce a book that was innovative and original: a book that reveals much about the man, his work and his attitudes to the plants that he grew in his garden and used in his apothecary shop. It is for this reason that it is appropriate to examine his great work on gardening alongside the more obvious source of his herbal in order to extend our knowledge of the practice of herbal medicine in the early modern period.

Methodology

In modern-day terms, John Parkinson could well be described as an interdisciplinary man, an approach which can be helpfully emulated by present-day historians of the period. As a historian of early modern gardening practices, I would specifically identify three aspects of appropriate methodologies which can be brought to bear on this current discussion.

The first, as already alluded to, concerns the interdisciplinary nature of the study. One of the editors of this volume, Anne Stobart, has articulated her 'vision of a shared multiplicity of histories for medical herbalists to identify with'[8] and it would seem that the overlaps between the work of the apothecary and the work of the gardener, as epitomized in the person of John Parkinson, offer a perfect opportunity to demonstrate how one area of expertise can usefully inform the other to the benefit of both. However, despite potential cross-overs between the history of gardening and the history of herbal medicine – the work of practitioners in both areas being firmly rooted in the study of plants – it appears that whilst no study of gardening of this period would be complete without some mention of John Parkinson as the gardener and garden writer, Parkinson as the apothecary has apparently attracted less attention. One reason for this rests in the enduring quality of *Paradisi in sole*: his herbal has not stood the test of time in the same way. Perhaps because this is how Parkinson is now remembered – for his gardening book – it is inevitable that he has been claimed by, and 'pigeon-holed' into, garden history with the result that he is simply less visible to medical historians.

A brief overview of recent studies would seem to support this. For instance, Deborah Harkness' *The Jewel House*, an otherwise excellent overview of the community of scientists, botanists, medical practitioners and gardeners living and working in Elizabethan London, or Lauren Kassell's *Medicine and Magic in Elizabethan London* contain no mention at all of John Parkinson.[9] Andrew Wear's *Health and Healing in Early Modern England* does contain one reference to Parkinson's *Paradisi in sole*, but only to make a passing comparison with the Garden of Eden.[10] There is no mention of Parkinson's medical knowledge, his medicinal herbal or that he was a practising apothecary, despite all of these topics being covered in this book. Rebecca Laroche's work on Englishwomen's herbal texts does include a discussion of Parkinson's two books, to illustrate her analysis of the role of women in the ownership and use of herbals. Although Laroche considers the possibility that Parkinson may have oriented his texts in a gendered way towards women and men, this does little to further our knowledge of Parkinson and the relationship between his roles as the apothecary and the gardener.[11] On the other hand, any book covering the history of gardening during this period will almost always mention John Parkinson, referring to him as the author of *Paradisi in sole*, generally regarded as the 'first great English gardening book', noting the pun on his name in the title,[12] and with some references to his various comments on particular plants.[13] Other writers note Parkinson's originality, although there is little attempt to offer any kind of analysis as to the significance of his work in gardening history.[14] This omission has begun to be addressed in recent studies such as Rebecca Bushnell's *Green Desire: Imagining Early Modern English Gardens*, which explores extensively what was original about Parkinson's *Paradisi in sole*, identifying a new emphasis on cultivating plants for beauty and pleasure; and Anna Parkinson's biography of Parkinson, *Nature's Alchemist*, which reconstructs his life and times from his books and the few known facts about him.[15]

Detailed consideration of Parkinson's contribution to both the history of medicine and the history of gardening is still found wanting, and the disciplinary constraints outlined above can seriously impede our understanding. This chapter will attempt to address this issue, demonstrating that for the garden historian an analysis of the work of the apothecary can greatly enhance an understanding of the work of the gardener at this time, and vice versa: the student of the history of herbal medicine can gain a broader understanding of their subject through an increased appreciation of the work of the gardener.

Second, it is important to stress the necessity of returning to original resources in order to get past the 'idle tales and fancies', as Parkinson called them, to try and uncover something nearer 'the truth'.[16] As academic disciplines, the history of both gardening and herbal medicine are still relatively new and although (or maybe because?) there is great general interest in both subjects, any serious scholarly study in either field tends to be hampered by popular myths and traditions which appear to go unchallenged. For example, in the case of early modern gardens, despite a conspicuous absence of concrete evidence (there are, for instance, no extant gardens from this period, and relevant documentary archives are at best scant), a picture of Elizabethan and early Stuart gardens appears firmly fixed in the modern mind, being perpetuated through numerous historical garden recreations which serve to give substance to traditional and sometimes fanciful notions which do not necessarily stand up to scrutiny.[17] In living up to received, if inaccurate, expectations, the pursuit of 'truth', in the sense of presenting actual evidence and considered interpretation, can unfortunately be lost. In order to gain an enhanced understanding of the contemporary viewpoint, therefore, it is of critical importance that original sources are approached anew, unhampered by later editorial decisions or popular misconceptions which have established themselves during the intervening years. In this chapter, a detailed study of John Parkinson's gardening book and his herbal will repay dividends in this regard: the words that Parkinson actually wrote reveal a great deal about the practicalities of working as a gardener and as an apothecary in early modern London, and offer a contemporary, but uniquely personal, view of the world in which he lived and worked. At the same time, the inherent difficulties in matching the prescription offered by contemporary literature to actual practice will also be addressed.

Third, and finally, with regard to specific methodologies, it is crucial to our understanding of the evidence that we are able to set these works firmly within the social, cultural and intellectual context of the times in which they were written. Gardening, like medicine, is an activity that crosses many social boundaries, and how it was viewed and carried out by various members of society would have been informed by the prevailing notions and environments in which they lived.[18] Examination of these contexts not only offers fresh occasion for beneficial interdisciplinary insight, but also furthers our knowledge and understanding of the early modern world.

This chapter therefore provides a necessarily brief overview of the somewhat scanty biographical evidence we have for John Parkinson, before moving on to comment on the context of the times within which he was living and working, and within which his published books have to be set. The remainder of the chapter looks in closer detail at the two books for which Parkinson has become so well known, exploring what they reveal to us of his original approach to both the art of the apothecary and the art of gardening.

Biographical details

Opposite the first page of the opening chapter of *Paradisi in sole* is depicted a portrait of its author, John Parkinson (see Figure 12.1). The surrounding text declares him as 'John Parkinson, Apothecary of London' and it shows a woodcut illustration of him aged 62.[19] The family coat of arms in the bottom left-hand corner, the Latin text, his mode of dress and the shield of the Worshipful Society of Apothecaries in the bottom

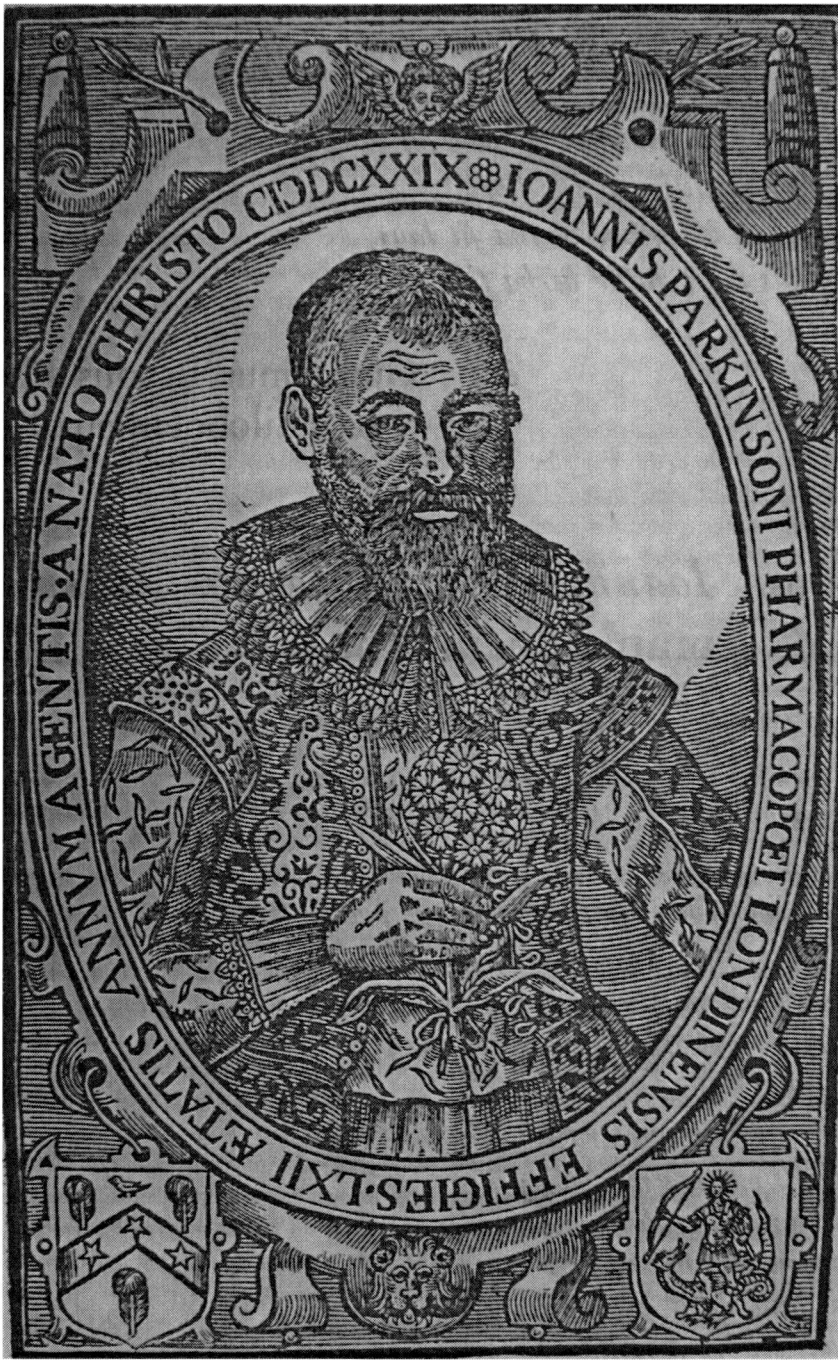

Figure 12.1 Portrait of John Parkinson. Illustration from *Paradisi in sole, paradisus terrestris* (1629; repr. 1904). Courtesy: Special Collections, Cadbury Research Library, University of Birmingham.

right-hand corner all reveal him as a man of learning and some substance, defining his status as a gentleman and as a respected member of his profession.[20] This is John Parkinson, the apothecary who devoted most of his long life to the research, writing and publication of *Theatrum botanicum*, probably the most detailed and accurate medicinal herbal ever printed in English, which would be used as a standard text by medical students for well over a hundred years after his death in 1650.[21]

However, at the same time the portrait also reveals John Parkinson, the gardener. In his hand he is holding a single flower stem, a Sweet William (*Dianthus barbatus*) or 'Sweet John' as it was sometimes known.[22] Apart from the thinly disguised play on his name, what is interesting about this particular plant is that, by his own definition, it has no medicinal uses. In his description of this plant, under the heading 'The vertues', Parkinson simply states: 'We have not knowne any of these used in Physicke'.[23] This book, the portrait is telling us, is offering something new to the reader: not only are plants to be valued for their uses and virtues, the subject of most books about plants and flowers up to this point, but they can also be recommended solely as ornaments and delights for the garden. This portrait encapsulates perfectly the person of John Parkinson: the apothecary, concerned with the medicinal properties of plants, and the gardener, concerned with beauty and ornament.

There is little extant documentary evidence regarding the young John Parkinson, but as we know from the portrait that he was 62 years old in 1629, then it follows that he must have been born around 1567–8. Recent research has traced the coat of arms depicted at the bottom of the portrait to one carved over the doorway of a farmhouse near Whalley in Lancashire, linking him to the family of Parkinsons living there at the time, and it is likely therefore that this is where he spent his formative years.[24] How or why he came to London is unknown, but by 1584 Parkinson was living in the city where he was to spend the rest of his adult life. He signed up as an apprentice apothecary to Francis Slater, a freeman of the Company of Grocers (the Worshipful Society of Apothecaries was not yet in existence), gained his freedom from the Company in 1593, and by 1594 had established his own shop in Ludgate.[25] He was instrumental in the setting up of the Society of Apothecaries, which was eventually incorporated by royal charter on 6 December 1617, recognized at last as a distinct and separate body from the Grocers' Company.[26] John Parkinson's name is recorded as one of the founding members both on the Grant of Arms to the new Society and as one of the assistants who appeared at the first meeting of the Society to take their oaths at Grey's Inn Court before the Attorney General and the king's physicians, Dr Atkins and Dr Mayhern.[27] Parkinson was elected as a warden of the Society in 1620.[28] These early years were not easy ones for the Society, many problems continuing as a result of the split from the powerful Grocers' Company. The legal wranglings eventually reached the Star Chamber, but the session, presided over by Sir Francis Bacon (1561–1626), found heavily in favour of the Apothecaries, reiterating the provisions and ruling of the 1617 charter that from now on only members of the Society were allowed to make and sell medicines, the Grocers' Company losing their rights to do so.[29] The result of this judgement was that it gave apothecaries a legitimate basis on which to build their businesses and opened the way for men such as John Parkinson to practise a trade that was at last becoming respected. The Society of Apothecaries had the personal backing of the king and reflected the spirit of the times, representing an essential step forward in the foundation of a scientific medical system, the mixing and dispensing of medicines now being properly regulated by the new Society.[30]

However, despite that fact that assistants were appointed for life, and although Parkinson was to remain a member of the Society, he resigned from office in 1621. No reason was given for his resignation, so we can only speculate that now that the essential task of establishing the apothecaries as a recognized body was completed, he preferred to withdraw from the complicated affairs of people and politics and return to his work of tending his plants, mixing his medicines and writing his books. Nevertheless, his reputation as an apothecary continued to grow over the years: he was a major contributor to two manuals for the correct identification and dispensing of medicines, the new *Pharmacopoeia* commissioned by the College of Physicians (1618), and the Society of Apothecaries' own *Schedule of Medycines* (1619);[31] he published his two major books; and by 1640 his expertise had been officially recognized in his appointment as Botanicus Regius, Herbalist to King Charles I.[32] Unfortunately for Parkinson, this appointment did not come at a particularly auspicious time to enhance his career, the king's political difficulties causing him to move his court to Oxford just two years later. John Parkinson remained in London, and having lived long enough to witness the execution of his royal patron, died in 1650 at the age of 82, with little except his reputation: his record in the burial register reads, 'John Parkinson: A Famous Botanist'.[33] His name has lived on, however, through his two published works: *Theatrum botanicum*, written by Parkinson the apothecary; and *Paradisi in sole*, written by Parkinson the gardener.

Parkinson's books and their context

In order to fully appreciate the originality of Parkinson's work – and before embarking on the promised consideration of the social and cultural context within which it was produced – it might first be helpful to offer some background to the genre of English gardening and botanical literature within which it needs to be set.

The first books of horticultural interest began to appear in England in the sixteenth century, their distribution and popularity aided simultaneously by the spread of Renaissance humanist scholarship and the advent of the new print culture which enabled books to be produced and sold relatively cheaply. Books on husbandry, herbals and, later, books concerned specifically with gardening, were all being produced and distributed, at first in Latin, but increasingly in the vernacular. The end of the century saw the publication of John Gerard's (c. 1545–1612) immensely popular *The Herball, or Generall Historie of Plantes* (1597), which was reprinted, substantially updated and improved by Thomas Johnson (c. 1600–44) in 1633, proving so popular that it was again reprinted in 1636. Four years later, John Parkinson's *Theatrum botanicum* was published which, it has been argued, was probably the last in the genre of the great herbals.[34] Alongside these publications were gardening books, the first book in English solely dedicated to the art of gardening being Thomas Hill's *Brief and Pleasaunt Treatise How to Dresse, Sowe and Set a Garden*, published in 1558.[35] Between this and the publication of Parkinson's *Paradisi in sole*, a number of new gardening manuals were written and published, including two revised editions of Hill's book with new titles, *The Proffitable Arte of Gardening* (1568) and *The Gardeners' Labyrinth* (1577),[36] Gervase Markham's *The English Husbandman* (1613) and William Lawson's *New Orchard and Garden* (1618), which ran to 13 editions as well as being reproduced numerous times within other publications.[37]

However, one particular problem which faces the historian when attempting to judge the distance between representation and actual practice is that much of this early gardening literature was, in one way or another, derivative.[38] The classical texts of the Greeks and Romans, as noted above, formed the basis of the intellectual humanist legacy of the period, and to compile works from known sources was perfectly acceptable, so perhaps it is not surprising to find that the first English gardening books relied heavily on both the received wisdom of the ancients as well as contemporary Dutch and French Renaissance writers.[39] In 1572, Leonard Mascall declared, 'I have taken out of diverse authors this simple work into our Englishe tongue'[40] (and the greater part of Mascall's book is a translation of an extremely popular French publication), and Thomas Hill states with no apology that 'I have not given thee any labour of mine owne, but rather have collected the sayinges and writings of many aunciente authours'.[41] Although little is known about Thomas Hill, it is apparent that he earned his living as a compiler and translator of books and pamphlets on a wide range of subjects, so the likelihood is that he was no gardener himself, and indeed he never claims to be.[42] The point here is that he bases his authority for what he is writing in the classics, and for him – and his readers – that was authority enough.

Other books were simply direct translations. Richard Surflet's translation of *Maison rustique, or the Countrie Farme* (1600), for instance, was originally published in French in 1564 by Charles Estienne as *L'agriculture et maison rustique*, a very popular work which was reprinted numerous times between 1564 and 1598; Surflet's version was a direct translation into English of the 1598 edition.[43] And many of these gardening books were reprinted and republished over many years, sometimes under the same author, albeit often after his death, or sometimes with a changed name and title. On other occasions, texts were simply reprinted under a different author's name.

However, although the general practice of translating works from Italian and French sources was both acceptable and desirable, it unfortunately leaves us with the difficulty of not really knowing to what extent these earliest books reflected actual contemporary practice in England. And in the particular case of gardening literature, the problem is even more pronounced because advice and practices could not simply be transplanted from Mediterranean climates to England. The sunnier, warmer and drier conditions in the countries where the books were first written would have been very different to those found in England at the same time, and the directions contained therein would not necessarily apply.

As we move into the seventeenth century, however, there is a discernible change in the way that gardening writers were approaching their work. Unlike Thomas Hill, who ensures that his readers are aware of his authoritative sources and that their work is not diminished by any advice of his own, authors such as Gervase Markham and William Lawson were beginning to change the emphasis. Markham, for instance, in his edited edition of Surflet's 1600 translation of *Maison rustique, or the Countrie Farme*, published in 1616, claims that he has 'Now newly Reviewed, Corrected and Augmented... the Husbandrie of France, Italie and Spain, reconciled and made to agree with ours here in England'.[44] Unfortunately, despite these claims, Markham does not actually change any of the original text, but simply adds to it, with the result that the reader is often faced with contradictory information. On the other hand, just two years later, William Lawson published his *New Orchard and Garden*, saying that, although he admires the work of the ancients, he will leave them to 'their times, manner and several countries', recognizing that their advice does not appertain to the English garden. Instead, his advice is based on his long experience of working in his 'Northern Orchard and country Garden'.[45] His book appears then to live up to its title, representing a new approach to gardening and gardening advice. However, it was for John Parkinson to make this change explicit: not by adding to ancient writings as Markham had done, or setting them aside as Lawson had done, but by actively rejecting them as a valid source of authority.[46] This was a new and radical departure and it means that we can view what Parkinson has to say in a different light to that of his predecessors. As previously noted, his aim is to 'perswade many in the truth'[47] by setting down what he has learned through his own observation and experience. What we see is a man moving with the times, reflecting the changes he sees around him in his own work.

So what then were these changes? And why were they happening? Whilst we must always beware of making arbitrary chronological divisions to define historical periods, it is inevitable that as the long reign of Elizabeth I came to a close, the new century and the reign of a new monarch would bring with it new aspirations and possibilities for the future. The spread of printed material, increased opportunities for foreign travel, the opening up of new trade routes all had the effect of both making available, and creating a demand for, luxury and exotic goods.[48] Curious and extraordinary plants were arriving on English shores from all over the world. In 1597, John Gerard describes many plants in his *Herball* that he had obtained from 'forren places', including ginger 'digged up' from 'Domingo in the Indies'; tulips, that 'strange and forrein floure', from the Middle East; crocuses from Spain and Italy; potatoes and tobacco from the Americas.[49]

But just three decades later, John Parkinson writes of Gerard that 'since his dates we have had many more varieties than he ever heard of... as may be perceived by the store I have here produced'.[50] Already, the choice of plants available to the apothecary and to the gardener was far greater than it had been at the end of the previous century, and Parkinson saw it as an obligation to pass on his new-found knowledge through his books: 'For I have always held it a thing unfit, to conceale or bury that knowledge God hath given, and not to impart it'.[51]

At the same time, ideas and attitudes towards other humanist concepts such as the commonwealth, individual prosperity and social mobility were also shifting. In the sixteenth century, ideas of pleasure, luxury and recreation were strongly associated with idleness and self-indulgence, and as such were frowned upon as they were non-productive and contributed nothing to the common good. However, by the early decades of the seventeenth century, this was changing: the pursuit of individual profit and prosperity was now recognized as a factor in maintaining social stability; the opening up of international markets made trade in luxury goods both possible and desirable; and the rise in conspicuous consumption was by now unstoppable. The acquisition of goods that were not strictly necessary – satisfying wants rather than needs – became acceptable.[52] And, as already mentioned, during the early years of the seventeenth century there was an increasing acceptance of the emerging concept of observation and experiment, a view which slowly displaced the unchallenged wisdom of ancient authorities which had underpinned the humanist ideals of the previous century, as well as the magic, witchcraft and 'idle fables', as John Parkinson dismissed them, popularly employed to help explain the inexplicable in everyday life.[53]

Ancient truths and errors

Although this latter view was not entirely new,[54] it was first popularised in print by Francis Bacon who disparagingly regarded the current state of natural history, particularly within the court circles in which he moved, as entertaining but untrustworthy knowledge. His aim was to elevate the study of natural history, the utility of which was becoming more apparent as Englishmen travelled further and further away from familiar shores, to a publicly useful form of science. In his *Novum organum* of 1620, Bacon proposed a new framework for the study of natural history, 'the foundation of all', based on empirical knowledge, openly criticizing the classical approach of writers such as Aristotle and Pliny. The problem here was that knowledge was gathered indiscriminately, without any verification on the part of the author, but then presented – and accepted – as authoritative. In Bacon's view, however, knowledge was born of experience not authority.[55]

Already, we have seen how Parkinson was articulating similar ideas in his own work, and what set his writing apart from his predecessors was the fact that, rather than relying on the classical texts of ancient Greece and Rome, he firmly bases the information in his books on his own experience of growing plants in his garden. For him, the serious study of the apothecary's art required the serious study of plants, and he considered it of crucial importance to observe and understand the plants that were the essential tools of his trade. He did not write about a plant until he had seen how it would grow and had observed its properties for himself: he notes, for instance, of a variety of Spignall that 'when it is better grown up with me… I shall the better judge of it.'[56] He does not yet feel that he is in a position to make authoritative comment. He reiterates over and again that his authority is based purely on his own knowledge, gained through experience, observation and practice, and he is confident in the new scientific method as the key to knowledge. He states, for instance, in his chapter in *Paradisi in sole* on 'outlandish flowers', or flowers from overseas:

> This I doe affirm upon good knowledge and certaine experience, and not as many others doe, tell of wonders of another world, which themselves never saw nor ever heard of, except some superficiall relation, which they themselves have augmented according to their owne fansie and conceit.[57]

Parkinson's comments here are directed both at earlier authors of herbals, such as Turner and Dodonaeus, who, as he explains in his Epistle to the Reader, were writing about different places or times when many of the plants now available were unheard of, and towards more recent writers for whom he reserves his more scathing criticism. According to Parkinson, these writers presumed a knowledge of the new plants arriving from overseas – often as little more than seeds, roots or dried specimens – but they cannot possibly have understood or seen for themselves the nature of the plant. As he writes elsewhere, 'some of these errors are ancient, and continued by long tradition, and others are of later invention, and therefore more to be condemned'.[58] Parkinson, on the other hand, actually took the seeds, bulbs and roots and planted them in his own garden in Long Acre to observe how they grew and what they looked like. Some he received via fellow gardeners: for instance, his friend John Tradescant sent him a root of Indian Moly to plant in his garden.[59] On another occasion, in 1608, Parkinson commissioned the plant hunter William Boel to seek out for him new species of plants while travelling in Spain and he returned with over 200 different kinds of seeds. Parkinson wrote that 'by sowing them [I] saw the faces of a great many excellent plants'.[60] It was in this way, by careful scientific method, that he built up his extensive knowledge of plants and flowers which he then applied to both his work as an apothecary and to his gardening.

In *Paradisi in sole*, Parkinson sweeps away the long-held beliefs, ancient reports, tales and fables repeated ad infinitum by writers of the early English gardening manuals: he viewed practices such as soaking seeds in coloured dyes to make the blooms a particular colour or applying 'sents' such as cinnamon or cloves under the bark of trees to make the fruits take on those flavours as nonsensical. If anyone had actually tried these techniques, as he had done, they would know that they did not work: once they are put to the test, he says, 'they all vanish away like smoake'.[61] And put them to the test he did: he made many trials with many different types of plants of the various methods that are reported to change their natures, but he reports: 'I could never see the effect desired, but rather in many of them the losse of my plants'.[62] And elsewhere, he categorically asserts that 'there is not any art whereby any flower may be made to grow double, that was naturally single, nor of any other scent or colour than it first had by nature'.[63] This is in stark contrast to the view, for instance, of the Elizabethan commentator William Harrison (1535–93), who was marvelling over 50 years earlier that gardeners nowadays were so 'curious and cunning' that 'in the daily colouring, doubling, and enlarging the proportion of our flowers' they do 'what they like with Nature', and Parkinson grapples at length with this problem.[64] Once again, the importance of practical experimentation and observation as a basis for knowledge is emphasized: he hopes 'by reason' to 'perswade many in the truth', and one of the truths he is so anxious to convey is that nothing exists that was not found in nature first, and if men say they have created 'by art' plants that are not as they are found in nature, then they are liars, 'feigning and boasting often of what they would have, as if they had it'.[65] He asserts that all these 'rules and directions set down in bookes, so confidently, as if the matters were without all doubt or question… they are all but meere idle tales and fancies'.[66] He is absolutely confident of his own observations and experience and equally confident, if modest, in his conclusions: 'although they have not been amplified with such Philosophical arguments and reasons, as one of greater learning might have done, yet they are truely and sincerely set down'.[67]

What is demonstrated here is that Parkinson was employing a new and innovative approach to writing about plants – whether herbs for medicinal use, as in *Theatrum botanicum*; or flowers for the garden, as in *Paradisi in sole*. It was an approach which reflected changing times and attitudes, aligning itself as it did alongside the century's new ideals of advancement and knowledge, which lent an intellectual respectability to practical experiment and gave him the confidence to communicate his own experiences in this way. Of course, although Parkinson could not have known it, it was only to be another 30 years or so before the establishment of the Royal Society[68] which formally embraced scientific method and practical experiment as a legitimate source of knowledge.

The garden of pleasure

There is one further aspect of Parkinson's *Paradisi in sole* which cannot pass without mention, and a short exploration will reveal more of John Parkinson the man and how he was prepared to adapt to the changing times and attitudes around him. What made *Paradisi in sole* unique is that for the first time it placed ornamental plants and flowers firmly at both the centre of the book and at the centre of the garden. The title of the first and by far the longest part of this book is at once revealing: 'The Garden of Pleasant Flowers'. Not only is this the first book to take the beauty of plants and flowers as its principal subject, but it also describes for the first time the creation of a garden in which the beauty of the plants and flowers were to be its primary purpose. Parkinson himself declares that this is a new kind of book: 'having perused many herbals... none of them have particularly severed those that are beautifull flower plants, fit to store a garden of delight and pleasure, from the wilde and unfit',[69] and this is what he sets out to remedy, recommending plants and flowers as ornaments, delights, objects of beauty or curiosity. He feels no obligation, as for instance John Gerard did, to first and foremost attribute plants with 'uses' or 'virtues'. Gerard says of plants that 'whilst the delight is great, the use is greater, and joyned often with necessitie'.[70] Parkinson, on the other hand, relegates the description of uses and virtues of plants to the bottom of his list of reasons for writing this book: 'Fourthly [and lastly], I have also set down the Vertues and Properties of them in a briefe manner' he writes in the preface.[71]

Pragmatists may reasonably wonder how much the fact that he already had another book on herbal plants in progress actually influenced this editorial decision, but the fact remains that here was a different book, almost exclusively concerned with plants and flowers for the garden of pleasure. The first plant Parkinson describes is the Crowne Imperiall (*Fritillaria imperialis*), which he clearly admires greatly: 'for his stately beautifulness deserveth the first place in this our Garden of delight'. He devotes a full folio page to how it looks and includes a fabulous woodcut drawing of the flower, but dismisses the virtues with 'I know of none' (see Figure 12.2).[72]

As already mentioned, for the previous 30 years, plants had been arriving in London from all over the world and, although no plant hunter himself, Parkinson's

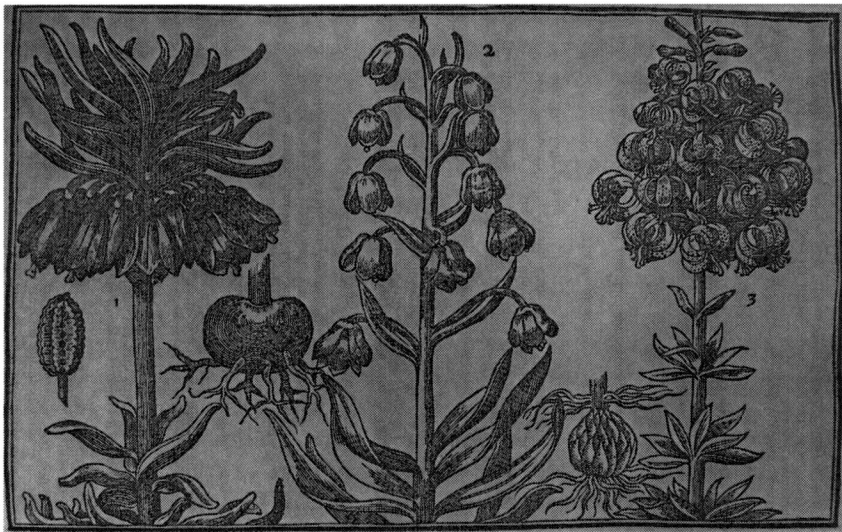

Figure 12.2 Crowne Imperiall (*Fritillaria imperialis*). [Plant numbered 1.] Illustration from *Paradisi in sole, paradisus terrestris* (1629; repr. 1904). Courtesy: Special Collections, Cadbury Research Library, University of Birmingham.

interest, both as an apothecary and as a gardener, made him a passionate collector and cultivator of these exotic plants. Although he briefly mentions English flowers, he devotes far more attention to his descriptions and instructions on cultivation for these 'outlandish' flowers recently brought from across the seas, many of which were bulbs such as crocus, tulips, iris, anemones, and so on. He admires these fine flowers for many reasons but, for him, their outstanding quality is that they help to provide colour and interest in the garden throughout the year.[73] Although native plants such as primroses and violets showed their faces in the spring, most flowers that traditionally adorned the English garden only had a brief flowering season during the summer, leaving the garden bereft of colour for much of the year. So, of the new outlandish plants, Parkinson enthuses that they 'shew forth their beauty and colours so early in the yeare, that they seeme to make a Garden of delight even in the Winter time'.[74] What these exotic introductions were doing then was more than just providing new varieties of flowers, but also introducing a whole new way of furnishing a garden, because plants could now be selected in order to provide flowers in the garden for every month of the year.

Having said all this, of course, at the same time Parkinson fully acknowledges the utilitarian nature of most people's gardens. 'Many men,' he says, 'must be content with any plat of ground',[75] and he is not for one moment suggesting replacing kitchen herbs and vegetables with ornamental flowers. What he is doing is recommending them as a desirable addition for those who are in a position to be able to indulge in this luxury – for luxury it is: unlike vegetables and herbs, ornamental flowers produce no 'profit'. He includes a section on the kitchen or herb garden and a section on the orchard, mentioning that he still has to write the fourth part, the garden of 'simples'.[76] This eventually evolved, of course, into his *Theatricum botanicum*.

Conclusion

So what in the end are we to make of John Parkinson's contribution to the history of herbal medicine and to gardening? Although the main subject of this chapter has been Parkinson the apothecary, we have found ourselves again and again having to consult his gardening book, *Paradisi in sole*, because it is within the pages of this book, rather than his herbal, that he reveals so much about his methods of working and his attitudes and reactions to the world in which he lives. Thus Parkinson looks both forwards and backwards in the history of writing about plants: the culmination of his life's work, *Theatrum botanicum*, although engaging with modern empirical methods, was one of the last in the genre of the great herbals and as such represents the end of an era. On the other hand, *Paradisi in sole* was revolutionary in its approach, looking forward to a time when the ornamental garden would reign supreme and gardening for pleasure would become widely accepted. In conclusion, I would suggest that in our search for some 'truth' regarding both the history of gardening and of herbal medicine in the early modern period, John Parkinson has proved an invaluable guide, and exploring extant texts as written by contemporaries is a worthwhile method of investigation. In applying the same keen observation and experiment to both areas of his work, John Parkinson provides an early modern example of the benefits of interdisciplinary study; perhaps the reason he was such a skilful and meticulous apothecary was because he was also a passionate and knowledgeable gardener.

Recommended reading

Harkness, Deborah E. *The Jewel House: Elizabethan London and the Scientific Revolution*. New Haven, CT: Yale University Press, 2007.

Henderson, Paula. *The Tudor House and Garden: Architecture and Landscape in the Sixteenth and Early Seventeenth Centuries*. London: Yale University Press, 2005.

Parkinson, Anna. *Nature's Alchemist: John Parkinson, Herbalist to Charles I*. London: Frances Lincoln, 2007.

Willes, Margaret. *The Making of the English Gardener: Plants, Books and Inspiration, 1560–1660*. New Haven, CT: Yale University Press, 2011.

Notes

1. John Parkinson, *Paradisi in sole paradisus terrestris* (London: H. Lownes and R. Young, 1629), 22.
2. Anna Parkinson, *Nature's Alchemist: John Parkinson, Herbalist to Charles I* (London: Frances Lincoln, 2007), 92; John N. D. Riddell, 'John Parkinson's Long Acre Garden 1600-1650', *Journal of Garden History* 6, no. 2 (1986): 112-24. Parkinson himself refers to 'my garden in Long acre' in John Parkinson, *Theatrum botanicum: The Theater of Plants, or, an Herball of a Large Extent* (London: Tho. Cotes, 1640), 609.
3. These two texts will be referred to as Parkinson, *Paradisi in sole*, and Parkinson, *Theatrum botanicum*.
4. Parkinson, *Theatrum botanicum*, 1, title page.
5. Parkinson, *Paradisi in sole*, Epistle to the Reader.
6. Ibid., 13, 463.
7. Ibid., 22-3.
8. Anne Stobart, 'Challenging Research for the History of Herbal Medicine' (paper presented at Herbal History Research Network conference on 'Researching the History of Western Herbal Medicine: Appraising Methods and Sources: Branching Out in Early Modern Medicine', 16 July 2010, London), 1.
9. Deborah E. Harkness, *The Jewel House: Elizabethan London and the Scientific Revolution* (New Haven, CT: Yale University Press, 2007); Lauren Kassell, *Medicine and Magic in Elizabethan London: Simon Forman; Astrologer, Alchemist, and Physician* (Oxford: Clarendon Press, 2005).
10. Andrew Wear, *Health and Healing in Early Modern England* (Aldershot: Ashgate, 1998), 139.
11. Rebecca Laroche, *Medical Authority and Englishwomen's Herbal Texts, 1550-1650* (Farnham: Ashgate, 2009), 28-42.
12. *Paradisi in sole paradisus terrestris*, to be rendered 'Park in Sun's [= Parkinson's] Earthly Paradise': Parkinson, *Paradisi in sole*, publisher's note on the first page.
13. See, for instance, Paula Henderson, *The Tudor House and Garden: Architecture and Landscape in the Sixteenth and Early Seventeenth Centuries* (London: Yale University Press, 2005); Edward Hyams, *A History of Gardens and Gardening* (London: Dent, 1971); Roy Strong, *The Renaissance Garden in England* (London: Thames and Hudson, 1979); Roy Strong, *The Artist and the Garden* (London: Published for the Paul Mellon Centre for Studies in British Art by Yale University Press, 2000).
14. See, for instance, Miles Hadfield, *A History of British Gardening* (London: Spring Books, 1960), 78-9; Ann Leighton, *Early English Gardens in New England* (London: Cassell, 1970), 146-54.
15. Rebecca Bushnell, *Green Desire: Imagining Early Modern English Gardens* (New York: Cornell University Press, 2003); Parkinson, *Nature's Alchemist*.
16. Parkinson, *Paradisi in sole*, 22, 24.
17. This problem has recently been identified and explored by a number of garden historians, including Henderson, *Tudor House and Garden*, esp. 3; Alexander Sampson, '*Locus amoenus*: Gardens and Horticulture in the Renaissance', *Renaissance Studies* 25, no. 1 (2011): 1-23, esp. 22; and Jill Francis, '"A Ffitt Place for any Gentleman"? Gardens, Gardeners and Gardening in England and Wales, c. 1560-1660' (unpublished PhD thesis, University of Birmingham, 2011), esp. 385-412.
18. The author here defines gardening as any activity relating to the cultivation of plants and trees within an enclosed space specifically set aside for this purpose.

19 Parkinson, *Paradisi in sole*; the publisher's notes give the full translation as 'Portrait of John Parkinson, London apothecary, at 62 years of age, 1629 A.D.'.
20 There is evidence to indicate that one way of attaining 'professional' status was through membership of a company, and that to be admitted as a member of a company was a sign that one had achieved gentry status: see, for instance, Steven Rappaport, *Worlds within Worlds: Structures of Life in Sixteenth-Century London* (Cambridge: Cambridge University Press, 1989), 258–9. Also see Steve Rea and Richard Cust, 'The Courts of Chivalry 1634–1640', http://www.court-of-chivalry.bham.ac.uk (accessed 17 June 2013), Case 367, Leming v. Clopton: On 28 January 1637, Leming petitioned against Clopton for challenging his gentility. One piece of evidence presented which successfully proved Leming's entitlement to call himself a gentleman was the fact that he had been a warden of the Company of Ironmongers.
21 Parkinson, *Nature's Alchemist*, 288.
22 Although it is not labelled by Parkinson in the portrait, he does discuss the various varieties of this plant and includes illustrations from which it is possible to identify the flower in the portrait. See Parkinson, *Paradisi in sole*, 319–21.
23 Parkinson, *Paradisi in sole*, 320.
24 Parkinson, *Nature's Alchemist*, 16.
25 Ibid., 53, 92.
26 This was the culmination of a long-running dispute between the grocers and the apothecaries. Until this time, the importers, keepers and retailers of drugs, spices and perfumes were all united under the auspices of the Company of Grocers, and although the art or 'mistery' of the apothecary, legally requiring seven years' apprenticeship, had been officially recognized by Act of Parliament since 1540, they still had no part in the governing body of the company and therefore no control over their own craft. See Juanita Burnby, *A Study of the English Apothecary from 1660–1760*, Medical History Supplement, Vol. 3 (London: Wellcome Institute for the History of Medicine, 1983), 8–22.
27 Wall, *Worshipful Society of Apothecaries*, Plate XXIV and Plate V.
28 See Juanita Burnby, 'Parkinson, John (1566/7–1650)', in *Oxford Dictionary of National Biography* (Oxford: Oxford University Press, 2004), http://www.oxforddnb.com/view/article/21372 (accessed 27 June 2013).
29 Wall, *Worshipful Society of Apothecaries*, 8–22.
30 Ibid.
31 Royal College of Physicians of London, *Pharmacopœia Londinensis* (London: Printed [by E. Griffin] for Iohn Marriot and are to be sould at his shop in Fleetstreete in St Dunstons Churchyarde, 1618). This work was translated into English in 1649. See Nicholas Culpeper, *A Physical Directory or a Translation of the London Dispensatory, Made by the College of Physicians in London* (London: Peter Cole, 1649). The *Schedule of Medycines*, referred to by Anna Parkinson, *Nature's Alchemist*, 176, was apparently never actually published.
32 Burnby, 'Parkinson'; Parkinson, *Theatrum botanicum*, To the Reader. Parkinson signs himself with this title.
33 Parkinson, *Nature's Alchemist*, 284.
34 See, for instance, ibid., 288–91.
35 Thomas Hill, *A Most Briefe and Pleasaunte Treatise, Teachyng How to Dresse, Sowe, and Set a Garden* (London: John Day, 1558).
36 Thomas Hill, *The Proffitable Art of Gardening* (London: Thomas Marshe, 1568) and *The Gardeners Labyrinth* (London: Henry Bynneman, 1577).

37 Gervase Markham, *The English Husbandman* (London: T. S. for John Browne, 1613); William Lawson, *A New Orchard and Garden: With, the Country-Houswifes Garden*, London: Alsop for Roger Jackson, 1618; repr., facsimile ed., with an introduction by Malcolm Thick (Totnes: Prospect Books, 2003). For more on the growth of printed agricultural and horticultural literature, see Joan Thirsk, 'Making a Fresh Start: Sixteenth-Century Agriculture and the Classical Inspiration', in *Culture and Cultivation in Early Modern England*, ed. Michael Leslie and Timothy Raylor (Leicester: Leicester University Press, 1992), 15–34; also Bushnell, *Green Desire*.
38 This idea, and its implications, is explored at length in Francis, 'A Ffitt Place', 29–51.
39 For more on ancient Greek texts, see also chs 2, 9 and 10 in this book.
40 Leonard Mascall, *A Booke of the Arte and Maner, Howe to Plant and Graffe All Sortes of Trees* (London: Henrie Denham for John Wight, 1572), sig. Aiiii^v.
41 Blanche Henrey, *British Botanical and Horticultural Literature before 1800: Comprising a History and Bibliography of Botanical and Horticultural Books Printed in England, Scotland, and Ireland from the Earliest Times until 1800. Volume 1: The Sixteenth and Seventeenth Centuries* (Oxford: Oxford University Press, 1975), 63–4; Thomas Hill, *The Proffitable Art of Gardening: Now the Third Tyme Set Fourth* (London: Henry Bynneman, 1579), sig. Aaiii.
42 Thirty-eight titles, including reprints and editions, are listed on the *English Short Title Catalogue* at the British Library as 'gathered' and 'englished' by Hill. See also Francis R. Johnson, 'Thomas Hill: An Elizabethan Huxley', *Huntington Library Quarterly* 7, no. 4 (1944): 329–51.
43 Charles Estienne, *Maison rustique, or the Countrie Farme* (London: Edm. Bollifant for Bonham Norton, 1600); Charles Estienne, *L'agriculture et maison rustique* (Paris: For Iaques Du-Puys, 1564).
44 Gervase Markham, *Maison rustique, or, the Countrey Farme* (London: Adam Islip for John Bill, 1616), title page.
45 Lawson, *New Orchard and Garden*, sigs. A^3, A^{3v}, title page, sig. A^2.
46 Parkinson, *Paradisi in sole*, Epistle to the Reader.
47 Ibid., 23.
48 For more on this, see Linda L. Peck, *Consuming Splendor: Society and Culture in Seventeenth-Century England* (Cambridge: Cambridge University Press, 2005); Keith Thomas, *The Ends of Life: Roads to Fulfilment in Early Modern England* (Oxford: Oxford University Press, 2009).
49 John Gerard, *The Herball or, Generall Historie of Plantes* (London: Edm. Bollifont for John Norton, 1597), sig. A1^v, 55, 116, 123, 285, 780. For the medieval trade in medicinal plants and spices, see ch. 6 in this volume.
50 Parkinson, *Paradisi in sole*, Epistle to the Reader.
51 Ibid.
52 David Pennington, 'Beyond the Moral Economy: Economic Change, Ideology and the 1621 House of Commons', *Parliamentary History* 25, no. 2 (2006): 214–31; Peck, *Consuming Splendor*, 2; Thomas, *Ends of Life*, 139.
53 Parkinson, *Paradisi in sole*, 24.
54 Deborah Harkness has identified a thriving community of natural scientists working in London in the sixteenth century, concerned with the study of the natural world in an active and practical way, already laying the foundations of a new empirical culture based on scientific experiment: Harkness, *Jewel House*, 15–56.
55 Paula Findlen, 'Francis Bacon and the Reform of Natural History in the Seventeenth Century', in *History and the Disciplines: The Reclassification of Knowledge in Early*

Modern Europe, ed. Donald R. Kelley (Woodbridge: University of Rochester Press, 1997), 239-60.
56 Parkinson, *Theatricum botanicum*, 889.
57 Parkinson, *Paradisi in sole*, 8.
58 Ibid., 22. It is difficult not to see his specific target here as John Gerard, whose *Herball* of 1597 was by now widely condemned as being plagiarized and inaccurate. For more on this, see Marcus Woodward, ed., *Gerard's Herball: The Essence Thereof Distilled by Marcus Woodward from the Edition of Th. Johnson, 1636* (London: Minerva, 1971), Introduction, xv-xvii. Also, Harkness, *Jewel House*, 15-18.
59 Parkinson, *Paradisi in sole*,141.
60 Parkinson, *Theatrum botanicum*, 1108.
61 Parkinson, *Paradisi in sole*, 23.
62 Ibid.
63 Ibid., 22.
64 William Harrison, *The Description of England: The Classic Contemporary Account of Tudor Life*, ed. Georges Edelen, new ed. (Washington: Folger Shakespeare Library and Dover Publications, 1994), 265; Parkinson, *Paradisi in sole*, 22-5.
65 Parkinson, *Paradisi in sole*, 22, 23. Parkinson acknowledges that it is possible that flowers can be made 'somewhat fairer or larger' by the intervention of man, but he offers an alternative explanation. Whilst maintaining that nature cannot be changed or altered – that is in God's hands – what the gardener can do, by careful selection of the better flowers, nurturing and 'good ordering', is to improve what can be found in nature. The role of the gardener was not to try and control nature, but to work in harmony with it in order to bring it to perfection.
66 Ibid., 24.
67 Ibid., 25.
68 For more on the Royal Society, founded in 1660, see Michael Hunter, *Establishing the New Science: The Experience of the Early Royal Society* (Woodbridge: Boydell Press, 1989).
69 Parkinson, *Paradisi in sole*, Epistle to the Reader.
70 Gerard, *Herball*, The Epistle Dedicatorie.
71 Parkinson, *Paradisi in sole*, Epistle to the Reader.
72 Ibid., 27-8.
73 Ibid., 8-10. In these pages, Parkinson describes the 'pride, beauty and earlinesse' of many spring-flowering bulbs, including the 'stately and delightfulle forme' of the tulip of which he claims 'there is no Lady or Gentlewoman of any worth that is… not delighted with these flowers'.
74 Ibid., 8.
75 Ibid., 3.
76 Ibid., [5ᵛ].

Part Four

The Multi-disciplinary Nature of the History of Herbal Medicine, and Contributions from Archaeology and Ethnobotany

Introduction

Susan Francia and Anne Stobart

As we have pointed out elsewhere in this book, the history of herbal medicine has not hitherto been widely considered as a subject for rigorous academic study, and pertinent research that has been carried out is scattered among a range of academic disciplines. A researcher interested in investigating the history of the use of plants as medicines has therefore to search far and wide to discover, and be able to draw on, past written and other sources. These may be found in such obvious areas as garden history, pharmaceutical history and medical history; but there are other academic disciplines which not only offer sources but also have a great deal to contribute to future research through providing appropriate methods and techniques, as well as ways in which to understand how people in the past both thought about and used plants.

Art history offers a perspective on the way people in the past visualized and depicted medicinal plants, and how they made a record of their descriptions and attributions. Studies of artistic works and botanical illustrations have included some aspects of herbal medicines.[1] Literary studies contribute further analysis of printed texts, their provenance and attribution, and the attitudes of their writers, centred in the world-view of the times in which they lived. There have been studies of plants in specific works such as in the Bible[2] and in the works of Shakespeare.[3] Health concerns and treatments have also been explored in the context of the theatre.[4] Language studies provide not only translations of key sources but also further analysis of the words used to depict medicinal plants, including lists of synonyms, which may help to trace the introduction of, and the trade in, medicinal plants.[5] Food history is uniquely intertwined with the history of herbal medicine as, in the world-view of the past, food was not considered as distinct from medicine; the two were both integral parts of the philosophy of health.[6] For example, in the 1390s, instructions to a young wife in the art of housewifery contained many recipes, including some specifically for the sick, such as a drink made of barley, liquorice and figs; and another of honey, yeast, ginger, long pepper, grains of paradise, and cloves.[7]

There are many more areas of academic study which may reveal information pertinent to herbal history. Archaeology gives us a window into the lives of people of past cultures, including their use of plants for both food and medicine, and also uncovers the distribution of plants in historic time. Anthropology can provide another window on people and their cultures, together with an exposition of different philosophies and practices of medicine. Ethnobotany, the study of the relationship between people and plants, can provide a particularly valuable contribution to the history of herbal medicine. And the hitherto little studied field of oral history has a great deal to give to the study of how plants were used in history.[8]

Once again, the advent of the Internet has provided significantly more resources which are freely available. Images relating to the history of herbal medicine, including medieval art, botanical illustrations and many others are available through the British Library and the National Library of Medicine.[9] The University of Michigan hosts a database which lists plants used by native peoples of North America.[10] Compilations of oral remembrances about herbal remedies are still being made, through the Ethnomedica project coordinated through the Royal Botanic Gardens at Kew.[11] Such examples are just an indication of the range of resources being made available in electronic form.

In this section we have two chapters which explore the contributions of archaeology and ethnobotany in relation to selected aspects of the history of herbal medicine. Brian Moffat and co-researchers at the Soutra Hospital Archaeo-ethnopharmacological Research Project have been studying human and plant remains since 1986. The medieval Soutra Hospital provides an ideal site for an archaeo-medical investigation which explores medical practice through the survival of remains of distinctive waste produced. This chapter discusses two plants found in combination at the site: St John's wort (*Hypericum perforatum*) and valerian (*Valeriana officinalis*), identifying their possible geographical sources and analyzing the texts known to be available to the Augustinian Order to infer possible preparations and uses of this combination of medicaments. Scottish oral tradition is also accessed to further illuminate a window into the past history of herbal medicine.

Anna Waldstein discusses the contribution which ethnobotany, itself a highly interdisciplinary field, can make to the history of herbal medicine. Her focus in this chapter is on Aztec medicine and in particular the work of Bernard Ortiz de Montellano, who looks at both the Aztec world-view and that of colonial officials, and concludes that there was an empirical logic in Aztec use of medicinal plants. Anna offers an overview of ethnobotanical considerations and a wider perspective on the global movement of medical knowledge and practices throughout time. Ethnobotanical approaches to the interpretation and critical analysis of historical documents offer a very interesting way of researching historical texts. They also provide new types of analytical methods which could be of use to the evaluation of herbal therapeutic practices in the future.

Notes

1   Jean A. Givens, Karen M. Reeds and Alain Touwaide, eds., *Visualizing Medieval Medicine and Natural History, 1200–1500* (Aldershot: Ashgate, 2006).
2   Lytton J. Musselman, *A Dictionary of Bible Plants* (Cambridge: Cambridge University Press, 2011); James A. Duke, *Herbs of the Bible: 2000 Years of Plant Medicine*, ed. Mary A. Telatnik (Loveland, CO: Interweave Press, 1999).
3   Eleanour S. Rohde, *Shakespeare's Wild Flowers, Fairy Lore, Gardens, Herbs, Gatherers of Simples and Bee Lore* (London: Medici Society, 1935); Frederick G. Savage, *Shakespeare's Flora and Folk-Lore* (Stratford-upon-Avon: Shakespeare Press, 1923).

4   Tanya Pollard, *Drugs and Theater in Early Modern England* (Oxford: Oxford University Press, 2005).
5   See, for example, Tony Hunt and Michael Benskin, eds., *Three Receptaria from Medieval England: The Languages of Medicine in the Fourteenth Century* (Oxford: The Society for the Study of Medieval Languages and Literature, 2001); Irma Taavitsainen and Päivi Pahta, *Medical Writing in Early Modern English* (Cambridge: Cambridge University Press, 2011).
6   For overviews of food history, see J. C. Drummond and Anne Wilbraham, *The Englishman's Food: A History of Five Centuries of English Diet*, revised by Dorothy Hollingsworth (London: Pimlico, 1991); Reay Tannahill, *Food in History*, revised ed. (Harmondsworth: Penguin, 1988). For the medieval era, see Melitta W. Adamson, *Food in Medieval Times* (Westport, CT: Greenwood Press, 2004); Terence Scully, *The Art of Cookery in the Middle Ages* (Woodbridge: Boydell Press, 1995).
7   Eileen Power, ed., *The Goodman of Paris (Le ménagier de Paris): A Treatise on Moral and Domestic Economy by a Citizen of Paris c. 1393* (London: The Folio Society, 1992), 192–3.
8   Daniel R. Woolf, 'The "Common Voice": History, Folklore and Oral Tradition in Early Modern England', *Past and Present* 120, no. 1 (1988): 26–52.
9   See British Library, 'Images Online', https://imagesonline.bl.uk/; and National Library of Medicine, 'Images from the History of Medicine', http://ihm.nlm.nih.gov/luna/servlet/view/all (both accessed 15 June 2013).
10 'Native American Ethnobotany: A Database of Foods, Drugs, Dyes and Fibers of Native American Peoples', http://herb.umd.umich.edu/ (accessed 15 June 2013).
11 'Ethnomedica. Remembered Remedies: Researching the Herbal Traditions of Britain', http://www.kew.org/ethnomedica/ (accessed 15 June 2013).

Archaeological Sources for the History of Herbal Medicine Practice: The Case Study of St John's Wort with Valerian at Soutra Medieval Hospital

Brian Moffat

Introduction and methodology

The history of herbal medicine is a field which lends itself readily to cross-disciplinary study, and archaeology is one of the most obvious academic disciplines which intersects with the history of plants. Archaeological investigations often recover plant remains, which have been studied to ascertain what our ancestors ate, but rarely investigate how plants were used as medicines. The ongoing investigations of the Soutra Hospital Archaeo-ethnopharmacological Research Project (SHARP) provide a potentially very fertile source of data on plants used during the medieval period in a medicinal context. This is a clear area in which the history of herbal medicine and another academic discipline can support each other on an ongoing basis. This chapter examines how the field of archaeology can contribute to the history of herbal medicine, by focusing on the investigations carried out at a medieval monastic site at Soutra, in south-east Scotland. The project was set up to investigate all aspects of pharmacological and medical practice at this medieval monastery, founded by the Augustinian Order. This order specialized in caring for the sick and infirm, as well as the aged and poor. Travellers and pilgrims were also offered hospitality.[1] The monastery at Soutra formed part of a pan-European Augustinian network, across which medical and pharmacological information, books, seeds and plants would have been shared and circulated.

A further academic discipline which has the potential to intersect usefully with the history of herbal medicine is that of literary analysis. At Soutra this discipline has been used to help investigators understand the uses to which plants would have been put during the lifetime of the monastery, and this collaboration between archaeology and historical literary studies is another example of the potential benefits of cross-disciplinary research. The investigations at Soutra use both archaeo-botanical analysis and also literary analysis of the extant library catalogues of all Augustinian houses in Britain, to determine the medieval medical practices being carried out at Soutra. This type of investigation, combining archaeological findings and historical literary analysis, is believed to be unique.

Apart from archaeological and literary analysis, a third strand of analysis at Soutra uses oral tradition, which can provide information which is either not readily seen or not present in the extant literature from medieval times. Oral tradition forms another potentially rich area which intersects with the history of herbal medicine, and the SHARP investigations have been able to benefit from the rich oral tradition in Scotland. The fourth strand of analysis used at Soutra is collaboration and discussion with the discipline of modern medical herbalism, which is able both to provide suggestions for the possible uses of plants in the past and also to reveal, via modern scientific analysis, the plant chemicals responsible for their mode of action.

Our investigations at Soutra, therefore, utilize all four types of analyses in parallel: archaeological, literary, oral tradition and modern herbal practice, to attempt to reconstruct a picture of how certain plants, found in quantity in the archaeological investigations, might have been used in the medical practice of the medieval monastery. This chapter provides one case study of how different disciplines may usefully interact to underpin the field of the history of herbal medicine.

Soutra medieval hospital, site and situation

Information in this chapter is digested from a number of SHARP publications since the project began.[2] The house of the Holy Trinity at Soutra, or Soltre, stood on top of Soutra Hill, where only a tiny burial vault, Soutra Aisle, now stands. The Aisle serves as a monument to the 'once powerful monastery', as a plaque records.[3] Based on the Soutra cartulary or charter-collection, it is certain that the hospital was founded before 1164 CE and was still operating, in a depleted state, in 1650 CE.[4] This cartulary indicates that it was the best-endowed hospital in Britain north of York, with extensive and ever-accumulating estates. Charters or deeds to lands were the normal means by which medieval monasteries of all kinds acquired and retained lands within the contemporary legal world.

Run by the Master and Brethren of the Augustinian Order, Soutra stood, as the highest hospital and monastery in the British Isles, upon the principal highway, Via Regia or Royal Road, between Edinburgh and London.[5] It is one day's gentle ride south of Edinburgh (see Figure 13.1). At the hospital's North Gate, the Via Regia joined the Via Publica north-eastwards to Haddington. These were the only highways in medieval east-central Scotland. The Via Regia formed the shortest crossing of the Southern Uplands, some four or five miles, which contrasted with distances of over 40 miles to the west and east.[6] At the head of the pass, Soutra has been called the 'St Bernard's of Scotland', after the renowned Augustinian hospital in the High Alps. Although St Bernard's Hospice stands today at 2,472 m in the High Alps,[7] this is not as fantastical as it may sound; we have experienced snow-drifts here at Soutra in excess of 45 ft/14 m deep.

Archaeological Sources for the History of Herbal Medicine Practice   255

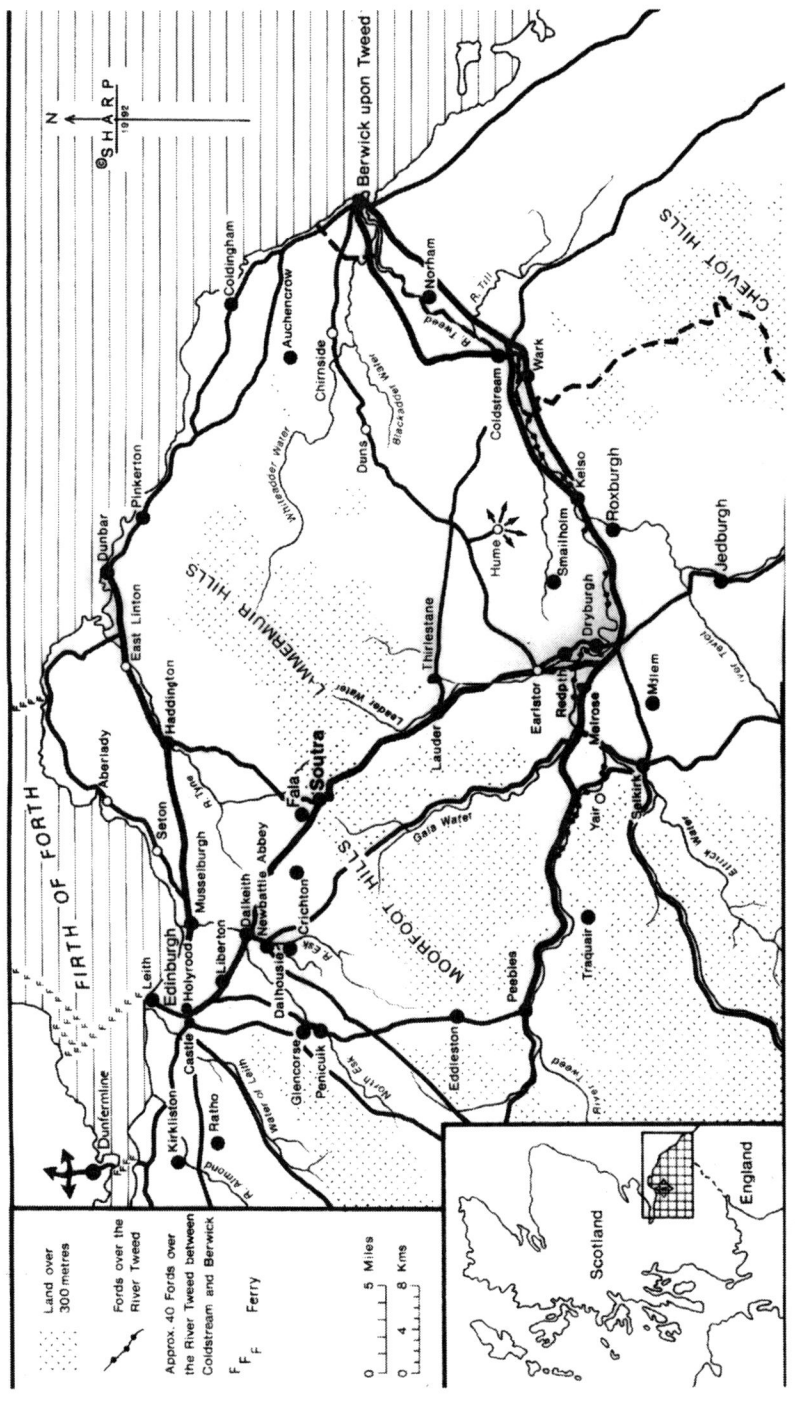

Figure 13.1 Map of medieval South-east Scotland. Illustration courtesy of Soutra Hospital Archaeo-ethnopharmacological Research Project.

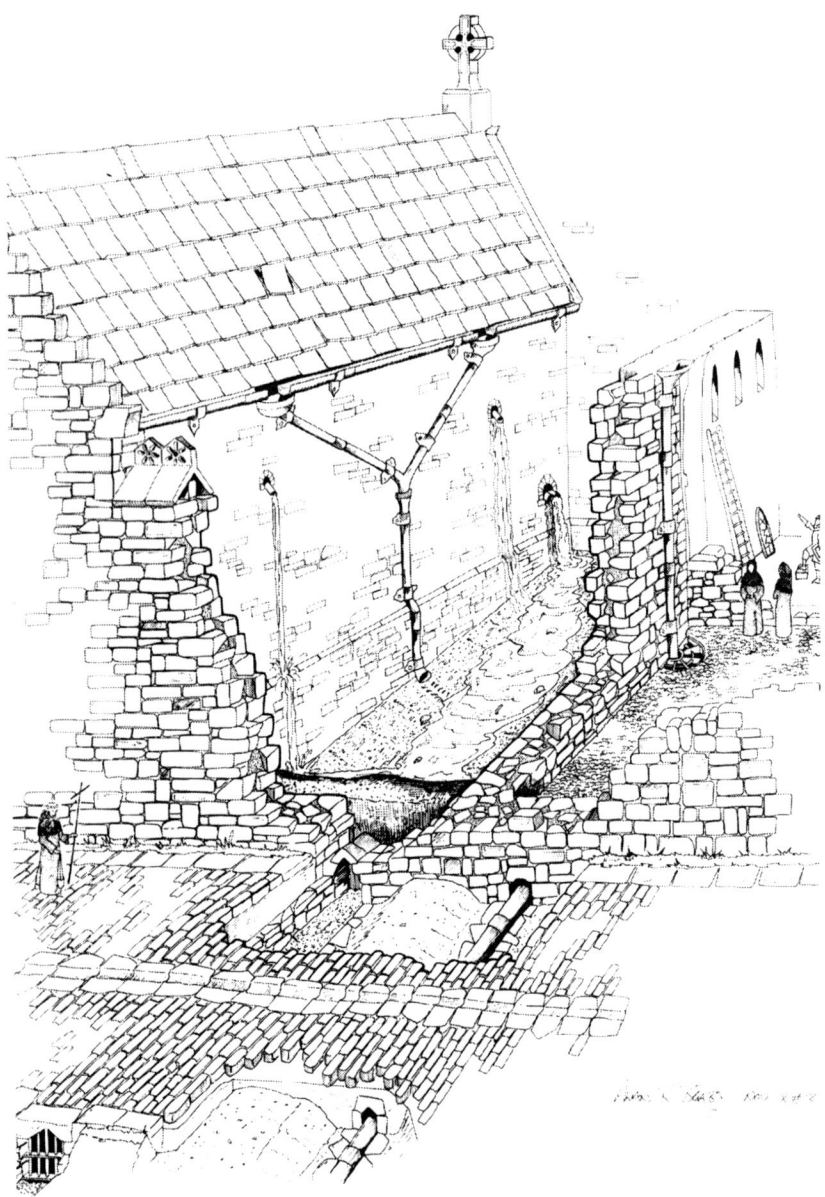

Figure 13.2 Reconstruction of the drain blocked with 'medical waste' at Soutra. Blockage dates to 1300–1320 CE. Illustration courtesy of Soutra Hospital Archaeo-ethnopharmacological Research Project.

The reasons for selecting Soutra for this type of investigation were fourfold:

1. The site is precisely located at and around the hilltop. It always has been isolated, and remains so. This isolation allows for the specific identification of medical waste belonging to the hospital.[8]
2. The hospital was well documented and generally well funded, so that the extensive medieval Soutra estates may be carefully delimited.[9]
3. The absence of buildings at Soutra (except Soutra Aisle), whilst disappointing for traditional archaeological investigation, allows access to the hospital drains. The preparatory geophysical surveys allowed us to produce a subterranean ground-plan of the entire built area. At that time, in 1986, this was the most extensive such survey in Europe.[10]
4. SHARP investigators sought advice from forensic scientists in order to ascertain what ground conditions led to optimized preservation of organic remains. These specific and specified clay minerals underlie the entire Soutra site.

Coupled with this, we needed to know how to routinely and rapidly identify medical waste. Over six years, SHARP investigators read through medical manuals and related records, asking what the practices described would produce in the form of waste. Three criteria for the distinctiveness of medical waste emerged: (a) human blood from many sources (here it is sufficient to mention that routine bloodletting was a monastic speciality and voluminous); (b) lead (Pb) – which taints all waste passing along plumbed pipes; and (c) key drug plants, particularly those exotic to the site. SHARP investigators set out to systematically search for all three in drains (notably the main drain or *cloaca magna*), pits and ditches, and to intensify study once they were established to exist (see Figure 13.2).[11]

Library catalogues of the Augustinian monasteries

The Soutra investigation could not rationally proceed without the Corpus of British Medieval Library Catalogues (CBMLC). The first volume was issued in 1990; it has reached 16 volumes that deal with the catalogues of monastic orders.[12] If physical residues from making and using medieval medicines are not interpreted through contemporary key medical and allied works, then any 'findings' would necessarily remain speculation and surmise. The twin volumes of the CBMLC ascribed to the Augustinian Canons and the Augustinian (or Austin) Friars were the SHARP investigators' focus.[13] They form an enthralling guided tour around the libraries, with priming from the editors' footnotes together with careful interpretation. All extant Augustinian library catalogues with substantial medical sections were examined.[14] These Augustinian monastic houses were: Lanthony (Monmouthshire/Gwent); Leicester (Leicestershire); Thurgarton (Nottinghamshire); Waltham (formerly Essex, now in the London Borough of Waltham Forest); as well as the York Friars. These are, of course, chance survivals. No analogous Augustinian catalogues survive for Scotland or Ireland.

Two types of works were sought within the CBMLC. First, *Sinonomiae*, or compilations of synonyms of plant-names combining, it was hoped, names in Latin, French and English. Ambiguous plant names form a crucial obstacle to study across the centuries. Second, practical everyday herbal manuals or herbals were sought. Of the *Sinonomiae*, the titles which emerged were *Alphita* (named after barley-meal, a preparation used in poultices and much else) and *Sinonomia Bartholomei*. The editor of *Sinonomia Bartholomei* links this with the great Augustinian hospital, St Bartholomew's, at Smithfield in London. It survives and thrives as a great modern hospital under the same name. The title of only one herbal emerged, *De viribus herbarum* (Concerning the powers of herbs), variously attributed to Macer, Macer Floridus or Odo Magdunensis. In the five Augustinian houses there were, in their library catalogues, respectively 0, 1, 2, 0 and 1 copies of the *Sinonomiae*. Copies of Macer were, respectively, 1, 3, 1, 0, 2.[15] Two points arise here: first, the fourth catalogue for Waltham Abbey logs nil and nil. This is due to its early date: late twelfth century or early thirteenth century. Mowat dates the *Sinonomiae* to post-1387 and c. 1465. And Macer is conventionally agreed to date to around 1100 CE. Second, there are numerous imprecise titles in all catalogues and the CBMLC editors can make little of them.[16] It is possible that there is some under-recording of these three key titles.

Waltham Abbey excepted, these three texts of *Alphita*, *De viribus herbarum* and *Sinonomia Bartholomei* are standard to Augustinian houses and have no real, identifiable rivals.

Archaeological data on St John's wort (*Hypericum perforatum*) and valerian (*Valeriana officinalis*) from the Soutra drain

Much of the work at SHARP has considered plants and medical approaches, but in this chapter the focus is on identification and interpretation of St John's wort and valerian.[17] Five independent teams of archaeobotanists have agreed on the identification of seeds in one sample from the Soutra drain (see Table 13.1) and all were struck by the excellent state of preservation.[18]

No other seeds or identifiable plant detritus were logged from this sample. Batches of modern and medieval seed were counted and measured on the basis of volume; the ratio of *Hypericum* spp. to valerian was agreed to be four to one.[19] The seed cache (a deposit of seeds together which has been recovered for study) is being further screened for mineral or chemical additives.

Table 13.1 Seed count of sample (Soutra Aisle (SA) 735; 1996/7).

Common name	Latin name	Number of seeds
St John's wort	*Hypericum perforatum*	1,420
Slender St John's wort	*Hypericum pulchrum*	310
St John's wort undifferentiated	*Hypericum* spp.	64
Total St John's wort spp.		1,794
Common valerian	*Valeriana officinalis*	560

The sources of the St John's wort

It is useful to try to analyze the possible sources of the plant remains, to determine how the monastery was sourcing its material. The Soutra seeds are confidently and precisely dated – from pottery, glass and ironwork all found in a continuously sealed deposit – to the period 1300 to 1320 CE.[20] The plants may have been cultivated in gardens, or may have been indigenous wild plants. Could the species be of local origin? This is likely, since both are to be found today in the Scottish Wildlife Trust's Linn Dean Nature Reserve, 1 km east of Soutra Aisle. This spectacular gorge is tiny (2 ha) and may be pinpointed because Linn Dean Head is the traditional southward limit of Midlothian or Edinburghshire. First, the west side and then the east side became the property of the monastery, so that all of it was owned by the brethren by about 1250 CE. SHARP investigators estimate that it holds in excess of 360 species of plant, an astonishingly high total, including many of the species recovered from the hospital drains.[21] Several species of St John's wort are to be found today on the drier, sunnier gorge sides, while valerian thrives only on a distinct area of valley bog. In addition, perforate St John's wort grows within 0.5 m of the edge of the excavated drain today.

But it is possible that either, or both, plants were also cultivated in the monastic gardens. In John Harvey's *Mediaeval Gardens*, he tabulates the plants that are recommended in 22 gardeners' manuals:[22] St John's wort first appears in 1305, and valerian in 1375, and both intermittently afterwards. This might suggest some pressures on the plants in the wild, or that additional supplies were needed on site. Harvey pointed out that four to five million medicinal recipes survive from the Middle Ages in Europe, and noted the challenge of finding out which were selected for use. The way of doing this is to use archaeological investigations to uncover methodically what types of plants were in use in large quantities in medieval monastic hospital sites.

Preparation and uses of St John's wort with valerian at Soutra, with reference to Macer's herbal, *De viribus herbarum*

The significant textual source of the period is Macer's herbal, which is organized into 77 chapters, each given over to one species and headed by synonyms for it. Although a modern edition of Macer in Middle English has existed since 1949, this is primarily a linguistic exercise.[23] Studies of Macer in French, German and Dutch are far more advanced;[24] from Latin it reached almost all European vernacular languages, and editions were printed up to 1700 and beyond. However, SHARP investigators sense that 1700 is a watershed between Macer as a practical manual and Macer as an historical study.

The basic 77 chapters of Macer's herbal have two telling properties. First, they centre, unlike previous texts, on the flora of northern Europe.[25] Herbal manuals prior to this had a broadly Mediterranean flora. John Riddle, author of *Dioscorides in Pharmacy and Medicine*, emphasizes this to us – specifying his subject's *De materia medica* as probably the most renowned herbal of the ancient world.[26] Second, they are organized *ab capite ad calcem* (literally from head to shoe, or from top to toe) – and this certainly facilitates consultation. SHARP investigators have analyzed Frisk's edition of Macer's herbal – the 614 single, simple recipes and 861 composite ones, typically strung together – totalling 1,475 recipes. In *SHARP Practice 6*, the recipes are broken down into those (good) for named parts of the body of all people, for women, for complaints that are localized, and those that have a generalized locus or are non-specific.[27]

Macer routinely advocates the steeping of seeds, technically called maceration, as the main everyday means of preparing a medicine. Once the maceration is complete as per the recipe, the seeds are spent, redundant and, as waste, are only fit to be discarded. Once recovered by the SHARP researchers working in the hospital drains, centuries afterwards, the physical remains of identifiable seeds are matched with a documented recipe in Macer's herbal. The significant finding of seeds suggests which precise recipe was selected for use, and Macer's herbal manual tells what it was to be used for. Retrospectively, we learn the diagnosis of the medieval physician, and what measures he took to deal with it. This is the essence of the SHARP investigation at Soutra.[28] Here we are concerned with a single recipe – a combination of St John's wort and valerian. Table 13.2 gives *Sinonomiae* entries for both St John's wort and valerian.[29]

In modern herbal practice, according to authoritative sources, a combination of St John's wort and valerian would be used as a preparation for depression combined with a mild soporific.[30] SHARP investigators studied both current knowledge on these herbs, and the possibility of their use for what was, in medieval times, termed 'melancholy'.[31] Macer had no chapter devoted to St John's wort, and valerian only figures in the supplement (ch. 104). Furthermore, he had very little stress on any matter that might be termed mental illness, let alone melancholy. Other herbals cited St John's wort only for use in treating wounds – as a vulnerary – in a great variety of forms and procedures.[32] Melancholy is rarely a theme in medieval herbals, although it must be added that, from a modern-day perspective, it is only in the sphere of 'nervous illness' that St John's wort and valerian are compatible and combinable.

Table 13.2 Medieval names for St John's wort and valerian according to the *Sinonomiae*.

Plant	Text	Names
St John's wort	*Alphita*	Herba Sancti Johannis, ypericon, scopa regea, triscalamus, herba perforata, fuga demonum idem, g[allic]e herbe Johan, anglice, Seynt Jones uurt
Valerian	*Alphita*	Valeriana, amantilla, martura uel marturella, benedicta, seu idem, g[allice], et angl[ice], ualeriane
St John's wort	*Sinonomia Bartholomei*	Ypericon, herba Sancti Johannis

Sources: J. L. G. Mowat, ed., *Sinonoma Bartholomei: A Glossary from a Fourteenth-Century Manuscript in the Library of Pembroke College, Oxford*, Anecdota Oxoniensia, Medieval and Modern Series, Vol. 1, Part 1 (Oxford: Clarendon Press, 1882), 25; —, ed., *Alphita: A Medico-Botanical Glossary from the Bodleian Manuscript, Selden B.35*, Anecdota Oxoniensia, Medieval and Modern Series, Vol. 1, Part 2 (Oxford: Clarendon Press, 1887), 78, 189.

Melancholy and its descriptions in medical literature

There are many modern social histories of melancholy, including Stanley W. Jackson's (1986) *Melancholy and Depression from Hippocratic times to Modern Times*. His treatment of Greco-Arabic writings on the matter of melancholy is unusually detailed, thoughtful and fully referenced. He cites, in particular, Averroes (1126–98 CE), Constantinus Africanus (c. 1015–87 CE), and the Paris-based encyclopaedist, Bartholomaeus Anglicus (fl. 1250 CE). All writers emphasize 'purgation'.[33] How do these figure in the catalogued Augustinian libraries? If we do not consider translations, the extant library catalogues reveal that there were four copies of Averroes, 23 copies of Constantinus Africanus, and six copies of Bartholomaeus Anglicus in those libraries. None of these works could be considered as practical manuals.

We are obliged to pick up a working definition of melancholy: in Juhani Norri's *Names of Sicknesses in English, 1400–1550*, where he offers: 'Excess of melancholy (black choler) and emotional disturbance resulting therefrom (characterised by gloomy thoughts, extreme depression, and… insane imaginings)'.[34]

More recent historical studies of melancholy by Jennifer Radden and Clark Lawlor[35] provide a combination of sociology, aetiology and taxonomy with, in Lawlor's case, a strong literary and autobiographical emphasis. Radden provides, for the Middle Ages, editions and commentaries on the writings of Avicenna (980–1037 CE) and Hildegard of Bingen (1098–1179 CE).[36] What these medieval writers do not provide are measures or procedures for the alleviation or mitigation of melancholy or melancholia. They are emphatically not practical manuals.

Neither does melancholy figure in Kenneth Kiple's monumental *Cambridge World History of Human Disease* – either in the 158 contributed chapters on named diseases or in an introductory section, by Pressman, entitled 'Concepts of Mental Illness in the West'.[37] An early and fleeting mention is made of the foundation of the hospital of St Mary of Bethlehem, in 1450 CE – to become the notorious Bedlam in London. In passing, the sole Bethlehemite foundation in Scotland was at St Germains, near Tranent in East Lothian. Founded 'possibly c. 1170', it is visible from Soutra. Its internal life is unknown. Pressman outlines the categories of insanity in the Renaissance derived from the classical system of mania, melancholy and dementia, and notes that melancholy 'held powers similar to those of the saints'.[38] It would seem that matters of melancholy were not recognized as, prima facie, medical.

Scottish and continental sources

John Higgit's *Scottish Libraries*, in the CBMLC series, has no catalogues with a substantial medical section.[39] The disappearance of such library catalogues in Scotland, and in Ireland, cries out for serious study. But, folklore of the Gaelic-speaking area, the *Gaeltacht*, has St John's wort among its most prominent and potent plants. According to the ultimate authority, the *Carmina Gadelica* (Song of the Gael), it is 'Achlasan Chaluim Chille', literally, 'Armpit package of [St.] Columba'.[40] St John's wort, as a plant once picked and crushed, is placed (and bound) within the armpit or oxter. McLean's edition of Gaelic poems expands: 'Neath my arm for ever bound… for thy power'; 'for beneath my arm'; 'arm-wort plant'; my little arm-wort'; and 'arm-wort of Columcill' – excerpted from five poems.[41] SHARP investigators have a policy of continuing to consult experts in the medicinal use of medieval patches, and have confirmation that St John's wort used in the above manner is indeed a rudimentary 'patch'. According to a recent memoir of a Highland boyhood, it was in use in the recent past:

> There was a great domestic quarrel when Herself (his guardian) found a piece of achlasan Chaluimchille on the left armpit of my vest. I had the St John's wort – the armpit package of St. Columba – on recovering from measles. Alec (the shepherd) taught me an old poem to recite on picking the powerful flower [three-stanza poem as from *Carmina Gadelica*].[42]

In addition, we asked the late Mary Beith (1938–2012), author of *Healing Threads: Traditional Medicines of the Highlands and Islands*, and long-term columnist on the subject for the *West Highland Free Press*: 'In the traditional tales she knew of, precisely what state of mind was reported as prompting the search for, and use of, St John's wort?'. She replied, 'lonely; frightened; fearful; gloomy; saturnine; melancholic – and often with a wintry Hebridean backdrop'.[43]

We may draw this influence closer to Soutra with the island of Inchcolm (literally: island of Columba) in the Firth of Forth, opposite Burntisland, Fife, and visible from Edinburgh. It was the site of an Augustinian priory and then an abbey, and remains the best preserved one in Scotland. It will be as well to set a context for St Columba (c. 521–97 CE) and his influence, and his biographer and fellow Bishop of Iona, Adamnan (627/8–704 CE). The *Oxford Dictionary of National Biography* entry is worth citing: 'Modern folklore indicates that down to recent decades [sic] he featured in traditional tales and religious sayings as hero-figure, protector or divine intermediary'.[44] The earliest recorder of the folkloric properties of St John's wort in Scotland was the Welsh polymath and originator of the notion of Celticism, Edward Lhuyd (1660–1709). In 1699–1700, he noted only that it was believed to have protective powers against witchcraft.[45] This seems broadly comparable with the entry in *Agnus castus*, a fourteenth-century herbal. Herba Iohannis is described, after a preamble on its synonyms, and what it may be confused with, then, 'The vertu of this herbe is yef [if] it be in an hows [house] it wele suffer non wykked gost a-bydyn in the hows ne entryn [entrance]'.[46]

One last point has to be confronted: an anomalous and striking name for St John's wort, in *Alphita*, is 'Fuga Demonum' – that which causes a demon to flee.[47] In a less than systematic survey, we have gathered 40 or so medieval illustrations of St John's wort with a demon 'in the frame' – clawed, horned, tailed, bat-winged, blackened. The demon is depicted at a distance and this seems to accord with the repellent properties claimed for St John's wort in common superstitious sayings. Iona Opie's *Dictionary of Superstitions* cites a fifteenth-century manuscript: 'If anyone carries hypericon or St John's wort, the devil cannot approach within the space of nine paces'.[48] Is the demon imaginably a metaphor for melancholy, or is that too far-fetched? A recent, excellently reviewed biography of Paracelsus indicates otherwise. Lured into Paracelsus' biography by an unusual statement by Mark Blumenthal in *Herbal Medicine: Expanded*

Commission E Monographs, we read: 'Since the time of Swiss physician Paracelsus (c. 1493–1541 CE) it [St John's wort] has been used to treat psychiatric disorders'.[49] Elsewhere, this continuous tradition in the use of St John's wort is routinely declared but is rarely detailed with precision and never documented.

Paracelsus' biographer, Philip Ball, provides further information.[50] In Paracelsus' impoverished childhood in the Swiss–German borderlands, the flora of his homeland – the Sihl Valley and Etzel Mountains – was to become a crucial resource for its medicinal properties, and this – once detailed – includes St John's wort.[51] Much later on, Ball adds circumspectively,

> Madness, they [Paracelsus' contemporaries and rivals] argued, was the result of an excess of melancholy or black bile. But, traditional medicine and demonology were by no means incompatible, for it was commonly thought that it was through the agency of black bile that the devil gripped the mind and soul; Luther [a final Augustinian] called this humour 'the devil's bath'.[52]

A study of the literature for the medical treatment of depression plainly yielded a very incomplete picture compounded of science and superstition, melancholy and madness, depression and demons. The SHARP investigators concluded that it is extremely difficult to extricate any literary evidence for practical uses for St John's wort and valerian in the treatment of depression in the medieval era. And yet it is obvious that the key seed cache is artificial or man-made, as no single habitat could yield and concentrate these species in this way. And its context (see Figure 13.2) is one of mass, deliberate purgation – a blood-dump of 50 m^3 – as well as powerful herbal and chemical 'dual purgatives'.[53] This fits with the theory of purgation being an essential part of the medieval treatment of depression, so St John's wort and valerian seeds are not out of place in such a context. Further research may be able to shed light on this. Or it may be that extant medieval recipe collections or receptaria simply fail to document the precise use of these herbs for this condition. The evidence, as investigated by SHARP researchers, appears in this case to be found in folk medicine rather than book medicine. But, if we move away from the study of depression, and look at what medieval manuals do tell us about the medical uses of St John's wort and valerian, we find other possible uses of these plants in combination.

Other uses of St John's wort and valerian in combination

If we forget modern-day models of how these two plants may be used in combination, and look instead at the medieval recipes for St John's wort, we are provided with an alternative picture of how medieval medical practitioners used this plant.[54] It was used in ways for which it is no longer utilized in modern practice, as is true of many medicinal plants. For example, the medieval manuals highlight the use of St John's wort as a vulnerary in the healing of wounds and fractures. Guy de Chauliac (c. 1300–68 CE), a French physician and surgeon, who wrote a lengthy and influential treatise on surgery in Latin, *Chirurgia magna*, which was translated into many other languages including Middle English c. 1425,[55] cites St John's wort as *incarnatif* (promoting the growth of new tissue in a wound or sore; promoting the closing of the lips of a wound), *mundicatif* (an ointment, powder, plaster or liquid used for cleansing a wound or ulcer) and *consolidatif* (promoting cicatrization or closing of a wound).

St John's wort is also known to have been used in fevers. Anne Van Arsdall details its use for quartan fever as described in *The Old English Herbarium*, an Anglo-Saxon medical text from about 1000 CE, which is a translation of a fifth-century Latin work.[56] The medical practitioner would have wanted to include restful sleep and it is possible that a herb that helped the patient with relaxation and sleep, such as valerian, would have benefited the healing process.[57] It is, therefore, also possible that a combination of St John's wort and valerian was used in fevers and wound healing, where both conditions would benefit from the calming and soporific effects of valerian. Finally, the *Compendium medicinae*, compiled by Gilbertus Anglicus, an English physician of the medieval era, probably written between 1230 and 1250, cites the use of St John's wort for cathalempsie (fainting fits). Once again, we have to calibrate these medical writers against the CBMLC: the *Old English Herbarium* and Guy de Chauliac (whose *Chirurgia* postdates the Soutra evidence) are both, by name, absent. A single copy of Gilbertus Anglicus is recorded at the monastic house in Leicester.[58]

Conclusions: General and particular

This chapter has indicated the possibilities of a collaboration among different academic disciplines. The investigations at Soutra provide a forum in which these academic disciplines can work together and cross-fertilize one another. Archaeological findings, historical literary analysis, oral traditional sources and modern medical herbal practice were all utilized to research the feasible historical uses for St John's wort and valerian, found in large concentrated quantities on the site of the medieval hospital. In this case, the postulation that the modern-day use of St John's wort for depression, in combination with valerian, was also valid in the medieval era could not be verified by a close analysis of the extant medieval literature available to us from the monastic community. However, this highlights some of the problems of doing medieval research, where extant literature is fragmentary and where the researcher should not expect to find information presented in a way that is comparable with modern-day literature. Or it might simply show that the uses of these two plants were so well understood that no written instructions were necessary. The oral tradition, however, provided verification for the use of St John's wort in depression and other nervous states, and this highlights the possibilities for future uses of this field to underpin studies in the history of herbal medicine. But, there are various recorded uses for which St John's wort could have been usefully employed in combination with valerian at Soutra. These are uses for which it is not usually employed in practice today.

The analysis of the archaeological findings at Soutra, in combination with an analysis of the literary works available to the Augustinian brethren at that time, and of the oral tradition handed down through the centuries, is a very interesting and fruitful addition to the range of methodologies available to the researcher. Further work which brings together archaeologists, historians and herbalists is likely to yield much more data on what was actually used in medieval herbal medicine, as opposed to what was written in the books of the time. This kind of collaborative enterprise has the potential to be used for all kinds of plant remains found on archaeological sites where hospitals or infirmaries once existed. Each type of plant investigated is likely to yield different observations in the different academic disciplines. Ongoing research of this type could eventually provide a useful and fascinating data source for researchers interested in studying the history of herbal medicine.

Cross-disciplinary investigations such as at Soutra plainly have strengths and weaknesses, consistencies and inconsistencies, verifications (of practice) and voids. On balance, insiders at SHARP favour the interpretation of St John's wort with valerian as an anti-melancholic because of: the overall context of the blood-dump – indicating the likelihood of mass (albeit unrecorded) purgation; the convincing contribution from the oral tradition; the abundant though hardly utilitarian medieval literature which centred on melancholy; the absence of any detritus in this precise location indicating wound-treatment, notably dressings and narcotic plants recovered elsewhere at Soutra; and the 'fit' with modern herbalist practice.

Recommended reading

Bryce, Derek, ed. *The Herbal Remedies of the Physicians of Myddfai*. Felinfach, Wales: Llanerch Enterprises, 1988.
Greene, J. Patrick. *Medieval Monasteries*. Leicester: Leicester University Press, 1992.
Moffat, Brian. 'The Seeds of Narcosis in Medieval Medicine: The Prehistory of Anaesthesia in Practice?'. *History of Anaesthesia Society Proceedings* 22 (1999): 7–12.
Moffat, Brian. '"A Marvellous Plant": The Place of the Heath Pea in the Scottish Ethnobotanical Tradition'. *Folio (National Library of Scotland)* 1 (Autumn 2000): 13–15.

Notes

1 Technical terms for the classes of eligible people are peppered throughout the charters. David Laing, ed., *Registrum Domus de Soltre necnon Ecclesie Collegiate S. Trinitatis prope Edinburgh... Charters of the Hospital of Soltre, of Trinity College, Edinburgh, and Other Collegiate Churches in Mid-Lothian*, vol. 109 (Edinburgh: Bannatyne Club, 1861). See also discussion in the appendices to Brian Moffat, ed., *SHARP Practice 1. First Report on Researches into the Medieval Hospital at Soutra, Lothian* (Fala: SHARP, 1986).
2 Digested from the introductory sections of the six published *SHARP Practice* reports, as well as the seventh, now in preparation. Only specific sources will be cited.
3 It is located at altitude 1200 ft/371 m; Ordnance Survey Explorer Series, No. 345

(2001): Map Reference: NGR NT 453584. Introductory pamphlets are available free from SHARP, 5 Fala Village, Midlothian, EH37 5SY. These outline 'highlights' in the medical specialisms that have been discerned and investigated through the SHARP investigations at Soutra, including: anaesthesia; blood-letting; childbirth management; dentistry; deficiency diseases and dietary supplements; disinfection and the containment of diseases; epidemic management; famine management; food and water poisoning; parasitology and purgatives; psychiatric illnesses; surgical amputation.

4   Laing, *Charters*, Charters 1 to 55. Note that this is an incomplete cartulary. When Trinity College Hospital (TCH), Edinburgh, annexed the larger part of the Soutra estates in the 1460s, the TCH charters mention Soutra as the previous owner, but perhaps a dozen such estates are absent from the original Soutra charters.

5   Ian B. Cowan and David E. Easson, *Medieval Religious Houses, Scotland*, 2nd ed. (London: Longman, 1976). This book provides an overview of the medieval hospitals of Scotland. It is not the intention of this chapter to discuss the history of the hospital as an institution, which is set out in other literature, e.g. Lindsay Granshaw and Roy Porter, eds., *The Hospital in History* (London: Routledge, 1990); Carole Rawcliffe, *The Hospitals of Medieval Norwich*, vol. 2, Studies in East Anglian History (Norwich: Centre of East Anglian Studies, University of East Anglia, 1995); Sheila Sweetinburgh, *The Role of the Hospital in Medieval England: Gift-Giving and the Spiritual Economy* (Dublin: Four Courts Press, 2004); Sethina Watson, 'The Origins of the English Hospital', *Transactions of the Royal Historical Society, Sixth Series* 16 (2006): 75–94.

6   Brian Moffat, ed., *SHARP Practice 6. The Sixth Report on Researches into the Medieval Hospital at Soutra, Scottish Borders/Lothian, Scotland* (Fala: SHARP, 1998), figs 13h, 13i.

7   Ibid., fig. 13c.

8   The succession of local maps demonstrates this. See the cover on Brian Moffat, ed., *SHARP Practice 2: The Second Report on Researches into the Medieval Hospital at Soutra, Lothian Region* (Edinburgh: SHARP, 1988) for the synopsis on this matter.

9   Based on 20 years of fieldwork. The base-maps of the main Soutra estates, clustered on Soutra Aisle, appear as figs 12a, 12b and 12c in Brian Moffat, ed., *SHARP Practice 5: The Fifth Report on Researches into the Medieval Hospital at Soutra, Lothian/ Borders Region, Scotland* (Edinburgh: SHARP, 1995). The most distant estates underline Soutra's great wealth. Furthest north was Strathmartine parish, 88 km/54 miles distant, on Tayside; furthest south was Liddel Moat/Motte estate, 93 km/57 miles distant, near Carlisle; furthest west were Wiston watermills on the River Clyde, 70 km/43 miles; furthest east were warehouses on the waterfront at Berwick-on-Tweed, 56 km/34 miles distant. As the most southerly and easterly estates lay in England, Soutra was certainly a multinational entity.

10 The Resistivity Survey is reported in Moffat, *SHARP Practice 1*, Section III, and enhanced in Moffat, *SHARP Practice 6*, fig. XA. The magnetometry survey is in Moffat, *SHARP Practice 2*, Section VI, also Moffat, *SHARP Practice 3*, 14–18. The ground-penetrating radar survey of the Soutra wells has yet to be published.

11 For the x-ray diffraction clay analysis, see Brian Moffat, ed., *SHARP Practice 3: The Third Report on Researches into the Medieval Hospital at Soutra, Lothian/ Borders Region, Scotland* (Edinburgh: SHARP, 1989), Section I. Once again, the investigations are developed through Moffat, *SHARP Practice 1*, et seq.

12 It is vital that the entire CBMLC series is together on open shelves, as it is at the

National Library of Scotland. Only then may the necessary and complex cross-referencing be accomplished.

13 Teresa Webber and Andrew G. Watson, eds., *The Libraries of the Augustinian Canons*, vol. 6, CBMLC (London: British Library in association with the British Academy, 1998); Keith W. Humphreys, ed., *The Friars' Libraries*, vol. 1, CBMLC (London: British Library in association with the British Academy, 1990).

14 All indexes were scrutinized: for named works; for named and un-named authors; for subject areas, broad and narrow. As the identification of medical material was crucial, these indexes were double-checked.

15 Webber and Watson, *Libraries*, 428; J. L. G. Mowat, ed., *Sinonoma Bartholomei: A Glossary from a Fourteenth-Century Manuscript in the Library of Pembroke College, Oxford*, Anecdota Oxoniensia, Medieval and Modern Series, vol. 1, part 1 (Oxford: Clarendon Press, 1882), 1–2; J. L .G. Mowat, ed., *Alphita: A Medico-Botanical Glossary from the Bodleian Manuscript, Selden B.35*, Anecdota Oxoniensia, Medieval and Modern Series, vol. 1, part 2 (Oxford: Clarendon Press, 1887), v. The index entry to Odo Magdunensis, otherwise Macer, in Webber and Watson, *Libraries*, 523, was found to be incomplete. The entry ought to read, in full, 'A16.467b, A20.305f (anon.), A20.1235a, A20.1238, A36.19b'. Three copies of Macer were omitted.

16 SHARP investigators estimate that perhaps 15 per cent of the titles in the medical sections above have not been able to be identified with reasonable certainty.

17 Other publications that deal with specific research topics are: (i) Brian Moffat, 'A Curious Assemblage of Seeds from a Pit at Waltham Abbey, Essex: A Study of Medieval Medication', *Essex Archaeology and History* 18 (1987): 121–3. Waltham Abbey was Augustinian. The seeds were narcotic and anaesthetic (?); (ii) Brian Moffat, 'Investigations into Medieval Medical Practice: The Remnants of Some Herbal Treatments, on Archaeological Sites and in Archives', in *Medicine in Early Medieval England: Four Papers*, ed. Marilyn Deegan and D. G. Scragg (Manchester: University of Manchester Centre for Anglo-Saxon Studies, 1989), 33–40. This centres on worm (helminth) treatments at Jedburgh Abbey (Augustinian, Borders); (iii) Brian Moffat, 'The Seeds of Narcosis in Medieval Medicine: The Prehistory of Anaesthesia in Practice?', *History of Anaesthesia Society Proceedings* 22 (1999): 7–12. This centres on narcotic and anaesthetic seeds from Soutra; (iv) Brian Moffat, '"A Marvellous Plant": The Place of the Heath Pea in the Scottish Ethnobotanical Tradition', *Folio (National Library of Scotland)* 1, Autumn (2000): 13–15. This deals with an appetite suppressant from Soutra. The scientific names for the central plant species in the above papers are, respectively: *Hyoscyamus niger*, *Conium maculatum*; *Potentilla erecta*; *Hyoscyamus niger*, *Papaver somniferum*, *Conium maculatum*; *Lathyrus linifolius*.

18 The raw data follows standard methods and manuals of identification: five teams of archaeobotanists were involved, coordinated by the late Dr John H. Harvey. Nomenclature follows Clive A. Stace, *New Flora of the British Isles*, 3rd ed. (Cambridge: Cambridge University Press, 2010).

19 Five batches of seed from each species were obtained both from cultivated (plant nurseries) and wild sources. This will form a separate study.

20 No contaminant material from subsequent periods whatever was identified. Experiments using tracer-dye, fluorescein, failed to transpose this lurid green dyestuff through the stratigraphy of the blocked drain (unpublished data).

21 A provisional species list for the Linn Dean Nature Reserve, compiled by a dozen

botanists, appears in Moffat, *SHARP Practice 6*, Section VIII. Linn Dean is routinely called Soutra's 'natural pharmacy'.
22 John H. Harvey, *Mediaeval Gardens* (London: B. T. Batsford, 1981).
23 Gösta Frisk, ed., *A Middle English Translation of Macer Floridus' De viribus herbarum*, vol. 3, Essays and Studies on English Language and Literature (Uppsala: Lundequist, 1949).
24 The acme of Franco-German study of Macer is Laurence Moulinier, 'Abbesse et agronome: Hildegarde et le savoir botanique de son temps', in *Hildegard of Bingen: The Context of Her Thought and Art*, ed. Charles Burnett and Peter Dronke (London: Warburg Institute, University of London, 1998), 139-43, 149, 151. Bingen is, of course, in the Rhineland.
25 The precise origins of Macer's flora have yet to be established. SHARP investigators have assembled some 15 passing comments on the matter. For example, a distinction he makes regarding two types of myrtle: 'Ours' that thrives on swampy or moorish ground in the north (*Myrica gale*; the bog myrtle or sweet gale), and the bush or tree that originates to the south, the Mediterranean (probably *Myrtus communis*) by implication was 'theirs'.
26 John Riddle, pers. comm.; John M. Riddle, *Dioscorides on Pharmacy and Medicine* (Austin: University of Texas Press, 1985). See also Paul T. Keyser and Georgia Irby-Massie, eds., *The Encyclopaedia of Ancient Natural Scientists: The Greek Tradition and Its Many Heirs* (London: Routledge, 2008), 1053, where only four informants on St John's wort from the ancient world are cited. Contrast this with over 200 for saffron, on the same page.
27 Macer's stock-cupboard of recipes or receipts is analyzed in Moffat, *SHARP Practice 6*, 36-41.
28 This is the twenty-third clump of seeds that SHARP has referred to Macer's herbal, *De viribus herbarum*.
29 The majority are variants of the standard medieval Latin, French and English names. Mowat, *Alphita*, 78, 189; Mowat, *Sinonoma Bartholomei*, 25.
30 Simon Mills and Kerry Bone, *The Essential Guide to Herbal Safety* (St Louis, MO: Elsevier/Churchill Livingstone, 2005), 585, 616.
31 We have found a range of scientific works on St John's wort invaluable, namely: P. A. G. M. De Smet and W. A. Nolen, 'St John's Wort as an Anti-Depressant', *British Medical Journal* 313, no. 7052 (1996): 241-42; Michael Heinrich et al., *Fundamentals of Pharmacognosy and Phytotherapy* (Edinburgh: Churchill Livingstone, 2004); Wolfgang Hensel, *Medicinal Plants of Britain and Europe*, Black's Nature Guides (London: A. and C. Black, 2008); Klaus Linde et al., 'St John's Wort for Depression – an Overview and Meta-Analysis of Randomised Clinical Trials', *British Medical Journal* 313, no. 7052 (1996): 253-58; Carol A. Newall, Linda A. Anderson, and J. David Phillipson, *Herbal Medicines: A Guide for Healthcare Professionals*, 2nd ed. (London: Pharmaceutical Press, 2002); M. Wichtl, 'Quality Control and Efficacy Evaluation in Phytochemicals', in *Plants for Food and Medicine: Proceedings of the Joint Conference of the Society for Economic Botany and the International Society for Ethnopharmacology, London, 1-6 July 1996*, ed. Hew D. V. Prendergast et al. (Kew: Royal Botanic Gardens, 1998), 309-16. In addition, we referred to the standard toxicological text for the plants: only the matter of photosensitivity arose for those taking St John's wort. See Marion R. Cooper and Anthony W. Johnson, *Poisonous Plants and Fungi in Britain: Animal and Human Poisoning* (London: Stationery Office, 1998). Even though there was no suggestion that the plants were foodstuffs,

the confirmatory texts used to ascertain this were: Miles Irving, *The Forager Handbook: A Guide to the Edible Plants of Britain* (London: Ebury Press, 2008); Andrew Jotischky, *A Hermit's Cookbook: Monks, Food and Fasting in the Middle Ages* (London: Continuum, 2011); Joan Thirsk, *Alternative Agriculture: A History from the Black Death to the Present Day* (Oxford: Oxford University Press, 1997); Wichtl, *Quality Control*; John Wilkins, David Harvey and Mike Dobson, *Food in Antiquity* (Exeter: University of Exeter Press, 1995).

32 Warren R. Dawson, ed., *A Leechbook or Collection of Medical Recipes of the Fifteenth Century: The Text of MS No. 136 of the Medical Society of London, Together with a Transcript into Modern Spelling* (London: Macmillan, 1934), 654, 686, 872; George Henslow, *Medical Works of the Fourteenth Century: Together with a List of Plants Recorded in Contemporary Writings, with Their Identifications* (London: Chapman and Hall, 1899), A27, 55, 61; B78, 117; C126, 128; Tony Hunt, *Popular Medicine in Thirteenth-Century England: Introduction and Texts* (Cambridge: D. S. Brewer, 1990), 15, 29, 39, 89. There was an anonymous *Tractatus de valeriana* at York (Humphries, *Friars' Libraries*, A8.362u), but it now seems lost.

33 Stanley W. Jackson, *Melancholia and Depression: From Hippocratic Times to Modern Times* (New Haven, CT: Yale University Press, 1986), ch. 3 and notes, 408–9.

34 Juhani Norri, *Names of Sicknesses in English, 1400–1550: An Exploration of the Lexical Field* (Helsinki: Suomalainen Tiedeakatemia, 1992), 349.

35 Jennifer Radden, ed., *The Nature of Melancholy: From Aristotle to Kristeva* (Oxford: Oxford University Press, 2000); Clark Lawlor, *From Melancholia to Prozac: A History of Depression* (Oxford: Oxford University Press, 2012).

36 Radden, *Nature of Melancholy*, sections 4 and 5.

37 Jack D. Pressman, 'Concepts of Mental Illness in the West', in *The Cambridge World History of Human Disease*, ed. Kenneth F. Kiple (Cambridge: Cambridge University Press, 1993), 59–85.

38 Cowan and Easson, *Medieval Religious Houses*, 61.

39 John Higgit, ed., *Scottish Libraries*, vol. 12, CBMLC (London: British Library in association with the British Academy, 2006).

40 Alexander Carmichael, ed., *Carmina Gadelica: Hymns and Incantations with Illustrative Notes on Words, Rites and Customs, Dying and Obsolete: Orally Collected in the Highlands and Islands of Scotland and Translated into English*, 2nd ed., vol. II (Edinburgh: Oliver and Boyd, 1928), 96.

41 G. R. D. McLean, *Poems of the Western Highlanders: From the Gaelic* (London: S. P. C. K., 1961), no. 232, 238, 249/50, 495.

42 Donald Cameron, *The Field of Sighing: A Highland Boyhood* (Edinburgh: Birlinn, 2003), 97.

43 Mary Beith, *Healing Threads: Traditional Medicines of the Highlands and Islands*, repr. 1995 ed. (Edinburgh: Polygon, 2004), 40 (her published traditional tale), 238, and personal communication.

44 See Máire Herbert, 'Columba (c. 521–597)', *Oxford Dictionary of National Biography* (Oxford: Oxford University Press, 2004), http://www.oxforddnb.com/view/article/6001 (accessed 27 June 2013).

45 John L. Campbell, *Edward Lhuyd in the Scottish Highlands, 1699–1700* (Oxford: Clarendon Press, 1963), 58.

46 Gösta Brodin, ed., *Agnus Castus: A Middle English Herbal Reconstructed from Various Manuscripts*, vol. 6, Essays and Studies on English Language and Literature (Uppsala: Lundequist, 1950), 163.

47 Mowat, *Alphita*, 78.
48 Ionie Opie and Moira Tatem, *A Dictionary of Superstitions* (Oxford: Oxford University Press, 1989), 336–7.
49 Mark Blumenthal, Alicia Goldberg and Josef Brinkman, eds., *Herbal Medicine: Expanded Commission E Monographs* (Austin, TX: American Botanical Council, 2000), 359.
50 Philip Ball, *The Devil's Doctor: Paracelsus and the World of Renaissance Magic and Science* (London: W. Heinemann, 2006).
51 Ibid., 25.
52 Ibid., 325–6.
53 A dual purgative combining Glauber's Salts and Epsom Salts, which, though named as such only in the nineteenth century, could be obtained as a by-product from coastal salt-making at salt pans. Soutra owned several salt pans around the Firth of Forth, and transported the products including 'bittern', the chemical purgative, via a Salter's Road (still named as such and still open) to Soutra. It was combined with an emetic, seeds of dog's mercury (*Mercurialis perennis*) – the species your pet dog is likely to feed on voraciously in order to make itself sick. This study will appear in SHARP Practice 7 (forthcoming).
54 See also the discussion of St John's wort by Karen Reeds, 'Saint John's Wort (*Hypericum perforatum* L.) in the Age of Paracelsus and the Great Herbals: Assessing the Historical Claims for a Traditional Remedy', in *Herbs and Healers from the Ancient Mediterranean through the Medieval West: Essays in Honour of John M. Riddle*, ed. Anne Van Arsdall and Timothy Graham (Farnham: Ashgate, 2012), 265–305.
55 Printed editions are Margaret S. Ogden, ed., *The Cyrurgie of Guy De Chauliac. [Volume I Text]*, vol. 265, Early English Text Society Series (London: Published for the Early English Text Society by the Oxford University Press, 1971); Björn Wallner, ed., *The Middle English Translation of Guy de Chauliac's Treatise on 'Apostemes': Book II of the Great Surgery/Edited from MS. New York Academy of Medicine 12 and Related MSS* (Lund: Lund University Press, 1988–9). The Middle English Dictionary Online lists extant manuscript versions of *Chirurgia magna* such as http://www.manuscriptsonline.org/resources/md/ (accessed 17 June 2013).
56 Anne Van Arsdall, *Medieval Herbal Remedies: The Old English Herbarium and Anglo-Saxon Medicine* (New York: Routledge, 2002), 216.
57 Bone and Mills, *Essential Guide*, 616.
58 Webber and Watson, *Libraries*, A20.1169.

How Can Ethnobotany Contribute to the History of Western Herbal Medicine? A Mesoamerican Answer

Anna Waldstein

Introduction

Ethnobotany, the study of relationships between plants and people, became a formal discipline in the early twentieth century. Though originally distinguished from economic botany by its focus on non-industrialized peoples, ethnobotanical research is being carried out all over the world and in all types of societies. The field is highly interdisciplinary, with contributions from botany, anthropology, archaeology, phytochemistry, ecology, pharmacology, medicine, history, religion and geography.[1] While many ethnobotanists are involved in the identification of new plant chemicals, genes and products for industrial development, they have also made great contributions to biodiversity conservation. However, the most significant aim of ethnobotany is to understand how people interpret and use plants. Medical ethnobotany focuses specifically on the ways people use plants to effect healing and has much to contribute to the study of the history of herbal medicine. Typically the work of a medical ethnobotanist involves the documentation of (1) medicinal species and their uses; (2) techniques involved in using plants as medicines (e.g. recipes, preparation and administration methods); and (3) the role of plants in shaping theories and experiences of illness and healing.

While most ethnobotanical research has been done with contemporary populations, a variety of medicinal plant scientists have started looking at historical relationships between plants and people. Heinrich et al.[2] provide a concise but rich overview of three effective approaches: 'botanico-historical' research that traces the use of particular species back through time; the application of historical linguistic data; and the use of documentary evidence from early ethnobotanical investigations. Historians interested in herbal medicine may also find merit in ethnobotanical approaches to the interpretation and critical analysis of older historical documents, such as a recent look at an early nineteenth-century Brazilian prescription book[3] and a review of malaria remedies from sixteenth- and seventeenth-century European herbals.[4] The work of Bernard Ortiz de Montellano on Aztec medicine provides a particularly robust method for applying ethnobotanical insights to the interpretation of historical documents that concern medicinal plants. By considering both an Aztec worldview and that of colonial officials (who trained Aztec scribes to develop a Nahuatl orthography), Ortiz de Montellano is able to show that Aztec use of medicinal plants had an empirical logic to it in his innovative *Aztec Medicine, Health, and Nutrition*, which was published in 1990.

This chapter shows how to apply ethnobotanical concepts to contextualize the use of medicinal plants, to achieve finer resolution in historical studies of herbal medicine and to gain a more panoramic perspective on the global movement of medical knowledge and practices throughout time. Using Ortiz de Montellano's work as a guide, it addresses the importance of socio-ecological context; political motivations of the authors of historical texts; cosmology, culture and worldview; and local concepts of efficacy as applied to herbal (and other) medicines. The chapter then explores how this ethnobotanically-informed Mesoamerican case study fits into, and helps to create, a more complete picture of global historical processes that have led to a widely shared body of medical knowledge and materials which extends throughout Central Asia, North Africa, Europe and the Americas. The main conclusion to be drawn is that ethnobotany can help answer questions about how past populations used herbal medicines, as well as how medical knowledge and materials have been shared with, adopted by, stolen from and/or forced upon, others. Combining ethnobotany and history thus increases the chances of adapting medical texts from the past to benefit people in the present.

The Mesoamerican environment and culture area

Ortiz de Montellano situates his work in historical ethnobotany on the Aztec people, a Postclassic Mesoamerican civilization. The term 'Mesoamerica' refers to a culture area, defined by common characteristics that were present during pre-Columbian times. The northern border of Mesoamerica is a bit nebulous. It is sometimes difficult to distinguish between the regions controlled by Mesoamerican civilizations and territories that were left to more nomadic and less centralized warrior-based societies, but it is somewhere in the vicinity of what is currently known as the Chihuahuan desert. For example, Kirchoff equates the Pánuco River in Sinaloa, Mexico, with the northern border of Mesoamerica.[5] While most scholars agree that Mesoamerica extends southward through Mexico, Guatemala and Belize, and ends in the eastern regions of El Salvador and Honduras, Creamer has argued that the southern border of Mesoamerica is also debatable.[6] Suffice to say that Mesoamerica overlaps extensively with contemporary Mexico.

The nation of Mexico is one of the richest in biological diversity on earth and is also home to tremendous ecological and cultural diversity. The topographic and climatic variations of Mexico create a mosaic of environmental conditions, including mountain ranges, desert regions, rainforests and coastal zones. This diversity of environments and wealth of natural resources explain why Mexico was the birthplace of the major early civilizations of Mesoamerica.[7] In addition to Mexico's majority, Spanish-speaking *mestizo* population, there are currently around 10 million people who belong to some 56 ethno-linguistic groups[8] and live in nearly all of the major ecosystems of the country. The multi-use land management strategies of these indigenous peasants tend to maintain and even increase biodiversity.[9] Mexico's robust heritage of indigenous cultures has also made it a nation with a complex cultural wealth of traditional medical systems. In Mexico, cultural and biological diversity form the basis of traditional medicine that helps support the health of the nation, largely through the use of over 5,000 species of medicinal plants.[10]

Ortiz de Montellano, alongside others, argues that 'early Mesoamerica was a cultural unit sharing a common worldview, religion, and ideas of human physiology and health'.[11] The common cultural characteristics of pre-Columbian Mesoamerica include intensive agriculture, religion manifested in monumental architecture, developed art styles expressed in several media, urban centres, expansionist politics, social stratification, specialization, markets and extensive trade, elaborate calendars, and hieroglyphic writing. In the Valley of Mexico, where the Aztec once built their capital Tenochtitlan and present-day Mexico City still stands, Tula and the Toltecs ascended to political dominance by 950 CE, the beginning of the Mesoamerican Postclassic period. This was about 200 years after the collapse of Teotihuacan, the first great metropolitan centre in Mesoamerica, which was located in the northern part of the Valley of Mexico. Although Tula never reached the scale or architectural grandeur of Teotihuacan, the city did have ties with, and influence on, other areas. Tula fell by 1200 CE, marking the beginning of the Aztec phases. Early in Aztec times, conditions appear to be similar to those around the collapse of Teotihuacan, but later Tenochtitlan-Tlatelolco became a dominant centre.[12] The Aztec, or Mexica, were a group of 'chichimec' warlords who came from the north, and claimed Toltec descent to legitimize their rule.[13] The formation of the Triple Alliance Empire (Tenochtitlan, Texcoco and Tlacopan) is generally recognized as a major turning point in the political and economic history of central Mexico. The Triple Alliance expanded and conquered neighbouring areas. As the Triple Alliance tribute was imposed on top of prior local tributes, it led to greater economic hardship and a lowered standard of living in provincial areas. Presumably this would have affected the lower classes more intensely, as they were not receiving tribute goods and services like the provincial nobility.[14]

Aztec ethnohistorical sources

The Aztec state has been one of the most intensively studied civilizations in Mesoamerica. Aztec agricultural development and standard of living,[15] trade,[16] architecture,[17] women's production[18] and even attitudes toward homosexuality[19] have all been the subject of research. During the sixteenth and seventeenth centuries, a number of ethnohistorical works about Mesoamerican cultures were produced. Bernal Diaz (b. 1492 to 1498, d. 1585)[20] wrote an account of the conquest of New Spain in 1568. He provides a fairly detailed description of the Aztec emperor Montezuma

(c. 1466–1520), and how he lived, as well as the battle/fall of Tenochtitlan. However, much of the book focuses on the exploits of Hernan Cortes. The most important ethnohistorical work on the Aztec is the *Florentine Codex*. The translators, Anderson and Dibble, consider its author, Bernardino de Sahagún (1499–1590), to be one of the best 'ethnographic missionaries' of his time. They note that he used trained Aztec informants, as well as other 'anthropological techniques'. Altogether there are 12 volumes: I. The Gods; II. The Ceremonies; III. The Origin of the Gods; IV. The Soothsayers; V. The Omens; VI. Rhetoric and Moral Philosophy; VII. The Sun, Moon and Stars, and the Binding of the Years; VIII. Kings and Lords; IX. The Merchants; X. The People; XI. Earthly Things; and XII. The Conquest. Sahagún was a remarkable scholar with an apparently insatiable appetite for information. The work is thorough and ethnographically sophisticated.

More information is available about Aztec religion and medicine than for any other American culture, as this is the best documented state-level society in the New World. Sahagún's work, for example, reveals a preoccupation with the health of both the body and the soul. Like other anthropologists,[21] Ortiz de Montellano treats these historical works ethnographically, using them as a source of ethnobotanical data. However, it is important to distinguish historical documents that were written by explorers, missionaries and conquerors from the work of trained ethnographers. For example, Diaz freely admits that he was a soldier, and was more concerned with following orders than closely observing the cultures and peoples he was conquering. The *Florentine Codex* was written with the intent of teaching missionaries to understand the Aztecs in order to convert them to Christianity.[22] The information that Sahagún collected when he specifically asked about Aztec medical knowledge focuses on illnesses and medicinal plants. Thus, Sahagún's work gives an impression of less supernatural involvement in Aztec medicine than there actually was. *Historia natural de la Nueva España* was written by the Spanish doctor Francisco Hernández and published posthumously in 1648. It is the most comprehensive work on Aztec medicinal plants, listing over 3,000, and Hernández attempted to test plants on himself and on hospital patients. However, the work is limited by his inability to let go of his own medical (humoral) models in order to understand Aztec concepts of disease (for example, he classified plants according to ascribed Galenic qualities rather than documenting Aztec medicinal plant categories).[23]

Primary sources about Aztec medicine are also influenced by the Spanish to a certain extent, as it was the Spanish who trained Aztec scribes to render Nahuatl as a written language. In 1552, Martín de la Cruz, an Aztec doctor, wrote a herbal in Nahuatl that was translated into Latin by Juan Badiano (the *Codex Badianus*). The herbal was intended to be a tool for convincing Charles V (1500–58) that Indians were capable of being educated. Thus, it was heavily influenced by European medical concepts.[24] Nevertheless, the Badianus manuscript is the oldest known medical text from the Americas that was written by indigenous physicians. The work discusses 251 plants and their uses. Only 15 plants overlap with the 255 listed by Sahagún. These include sacred intoxicants and stimulants, such as datura (*Datura stramonium*), morning glory (*Ipomoea* spp.), tobacco (*Nicotiana tabacum*) and cacao (*Theobroma cacao*).[25] In 1629, Hernando Ruiz de Alarcón published a *Treatise on Superstitions* in order to cast out paganism and syncretism in Aztec practices by recording pagan beliefs and activities to help clerics identify them. The work mentions fewer than 30 medicinal plants and gives the impression that Aztec medicine was primarily magical, that is, based on ritual.[26] As a consequence of the strong European influences on authors of Aztec medical (and other) texts, it is important to read them with a broader understanding of Aztec cosmology, worldview and culture.

Aztec society, cosmology and medicine

Some anthropologists have argued that the Aztec population was excessive and that ritual cannibalism was carried out to obtain adequate protein. However, studies of the carrying capacity of the Valley of Mexico and Aztec agricultural techniques show that it was possible to have a balanced, nutritious diet without recourse to human flesh. The *chinampa* system was key to the Aztec economy and, by extension, to the health of the population. *Chinampas* are floating agricultural plots that were constructed in lakebeds around the Aztec capital. The technology dates back to earlier phases in Mesoamerican pre-history, beginning with early piecemeal pioneering efforts at *chinampa* construction. However, large-scale *chinampa* development of later Aztec phases was planned, as evidenced by hydrological complexity and uniform *chinampa* size. At its peak, surplus production of the entire system could have been as much as 20 million kilograms per annum. It has been estimated that between one-half and two-thirds of Tenochtitlan's food needs were probably supplied by local *chinampas* alone.[27]

During early small-scale *chinampa* construction, land tenure was communal. Tenants produced tribute to a local ruler and there was little stratification among commoners. The Aztec intensification of the *chinampa* system gave rise to a distinction between 'free' commoners (*macehualtin*) and serfs (*mayeques*), but there is evidence that the two social classes enjoyed roughly the same standard of living and had a similar range of production activities.[28] Water transport was critical to the success of the system and all *chinampas* were connected to Tenochtitlan by canals. The state provided hydrological coordination and planning in exchange for rent and tribute.[29] Postclassic trends in all parts of Mesoamerica were toward the decentralization of ritual and decision-making, but with increasing economic integration. Toward the end of the period, rulers appeared to rely more on promoting economic stability (rather than religion) to retain power and there appeared to be development of a more trade-based power structure in which religion was commercialized and trading centres lacked religious architecture. Among the Aztec, more labour was going into agricultural development and craft specialization than into temple building, or even the military.[30]

Nevertheless, spiritual practice was important in Aztec society, especially as it related to healing, even if the state authorities did not invest so much power in religion. According to Aztec cosmology, there is a link between astronomical events and bodily function. Thus, from the Aztec point of view, the stability of the universe had to be maintained by feeding human flesh to the Sun. This is what the practice of human sacrifice stemmed from, rather than a cultural predisposition to excess and exoticism, that is, strange or bizarre behaviour. In fact, the Aztec worldview supported an ethic of moderation and balance, while disequilibrium was seen as a major cause of illness and disease. Throughout contemporary Mexico (and most other Latin American nations), the 'hot-cold' system of balancing bodily 'humours', foods and elements is a predominant ethnomedical theory. Evidence for the historical continuity of this theoretical system extends back to Aztec times.[31] In general, foods, illnesses, medicines and even people are classified as 'hot' or 'cold', though 'hot' and 'cold' do not necessarily refer to the actual thermal temperatures of substances, but rather to innate characteristics.[32] Browner also reminds us that there may be more to Mesoamerican equilibrium models of health than a balance of hot and cold alone. Extremes of all type (heat, cold, moisture, dryness) can cause disequilibrium, as can displaced or 'wandering' organs and clogged orifices.[33] To help regulate equilibrium and balance, the Aztec had a range of healing options, from supernatural to mundane, to choose from, and plants played key roles in most, if not all, of them.

In 1976, George Foster (1913-2006), a medical anthropologist, first defined the difference between personalistic (e.g. supernatural, wilful) and naturalistic (e.g. empirical) aspects of traditional medical systems.[34] This theoretical distinction helped to acknowledge and elucidate the coexistence of empirical and magical models of health and healing in many medical systems. Personalistic aetiologies are based on the idea that the volition or intervention of a natural or extra-natural force causes misfortune, including illness. The treatment of personalistic illnesses is the speciality of shamans, who conduct healing ceremonies aimed at appeasing angered gods or spirits, or counteracting the influence of witches or other shamans, and so on. Naturalistic causes of ill health are the product of natural events or properties of natural substances, such as microorganisms or an imbalance of hot and cold humours in the body. Treatments of conditions resulting from naturalistic causes are usually pragmatic and empirical and involve medicinal preparations of plant or animal substances.[35] The Aztec believed that the world had been created and destroyed many times. Their pantheon was large and incorporated deities of the peoples they conquered. These deities were seen to be anthropomorphic, animistic and involved with astrological aspects of health and illness. Words were also thought to have the power to harm and heal, and multiple souls had specific roles related to growth, development, function and death. In Aztec religion, the roles of shaman and priest were fused. Shamanic healing centred on the use of hallucinogenic plants such as the morning glory, but with the ultimate aim of reordering the ecological and spiritual balance of the ill person. The Aztec city-state also supported doctors who treated mild, naturalistic illnesses with herbs, and referred sufferers of chronic/severe illness to priests for religious ritual/confessions. Doctors kept botanical gardens in Tenochtitlan where they gave patients free medicinal plants on the condition that they reported results. There were also battle surgeons who used obsidian blades.[36]

Herbal medicines and concepts of efficacy

Medical ethnobotany has advanced the study of naturalistic medicine further by demonstrating that the use of medicinal plants in traditional societies is rational and systematic. Traditional healers and other people who use medicinal plants employ species that are biologically effective and actively experiment with plants to meet evolving social, spiritual and public health needs. Most ethnobotanical inventories (whether drawn from contemporary or historical populations) are excellent sources of raw data that can be used to answer theoretical questions and conduct cross-cultural studies of medicinal plant use. They may also become important leads for pharmaceutical development. However, the way efficacy is measured must be culturally appropriate, if ethnobotany is to contribute to our understanding of the practice of herbal medicine.

Anthropologists and ethnobotanists view efficacy as directly or indirectly producing a set of required, culturally defined outcomes. Etkin suggests that the key to any consideration of efficacy is the distinction between its emic (insider/subjective) and etic (outsider/objective) interpretations. Whether one chooses to adopt an emic or etic perspective, an important gauge of the efficacy of herbal medicines is related to their physiological effects.[37] In the context of Western science, biochemical assays are a common first step in determining the efficacy of medicinal plants. Such an exercise is used to identify physiologic responses to treatment.[38] The efficacy of plant medicines may be judged on their ability to induce full remission of symptoms. However, in many cultures other physical signs such as fever, salivation or emesis (proximate outcomes) are also important, as they indicate that the plant has initiated the healing process.[39] In other medical systems, the alleviation of physical symptoms is not enough. Chinese-style doctors have been known to tell patients that they are still ill, even when they experience complete alleviation of physical symptoms. This occurs because the underlying problem causing the symptoms has not been adequately treated.[40] There are also many examples in the literature that suggest that some medicinal plants are effective based on both emic and etic criteria, even though perceptions of disease aetiology and mode of drug actions may be different. Nettles are externally applied to the body in both New Guinea and Ecuador to reduce pain. The emic understanding of this practice dictates that the plant consolidates the disease substance at some internal locus, and facilitates its expulsion or chases away the pain. The biomedical explanation for the efficacy of this practice is based on the principle of counterirritation (i.e. superficial irritation at the skin that relieves inflammation of underlying structures).[41] Thus, while definitions of what is effective vary across time and space (especially between industrialized and traditional societies), they may also overlap.

As Anderson points out, the attribution of efficacy to 'time-tested' traditional medicines simply because they 'work' is not acceptable for a scientific anthropology. Nor does it comprise rigorous historical or ethnobotanical study.[42] However, pharmacological screening and biochemical assays are also limited in their ability to measure the efficacy of medicinal plants. When medicinal plants are evaluated in a clinical setting and removed from their cultural context, they are transformed into something other than traditional medicine.[43] Laboratory procedures of extraction and purification do not always resemble traditional recipes, and active compounds may likewise vary depending on the methods by which a medicinal plant is processed. Even when extractions with biologically active constituents are the focus of study, the failure of researchers to consider the cultural context within which the plant is used can result in misunderstandings of the plant's efficacy. Etkin points out that one of the most significant obstacles to the full comprehension of efficacy is the failure to understand healing as a process. In order to adequately evaluate efficacy (using either emic or etic criteria), one must understand the cultural expectations and biological outcomes of the medicinal plant in question.[44] For example, the raw tubers of several *Aconitum* spp. contain the alkaloids mesaconitine and hypaconitine. Due to the toxicity of these alkaloids, the use of *Aconitum* in Asian medicine has been criticized as irrational, or ignorant, despite the absence of reported fatalities following the use of these plants. In more recent investigations, it has been shown that when the tubers of *A. japonicum* are heated (the traditional method of processing these plants), the concentration of toxic alkaloids drops from 0.35 per cent to 0.04 per cent.[45]

Ortiz de Montellano was one of the first anthropological ethnobotanists to suggest that traditional medicines must be evaluated according to the standards of their own medical systems, rather than those of biomedicine. He evaluated whether chemical components in 25 Aztec medicinal plants could produce the effects ascribed to them by Aztec physicians. Ortiz de Montellano found that 16 components would produce the effects claimed in native sources, four may possibly be active and five did not appear to possess activity.[46] In a later study, Ortiz de Montellano and Browner developed a method for assessing the efficacy of medicinal plants according to both indigenous understandings of their therapeutic effects and the standards of biomedicine, by placing them in one of four 'confidence levels'. The first level is comprised of reported folk use. Multiple reports of use by populations widely dispersed through space, or persistent reports over long periods of time, increase the probability that a plant will exhibit pharmacological activity. Level II plants meet the criteria of level I and show the desired activity of isolated compounds or extracts in in vitro or in vivo tests. In level III, plants satisfy level II requirements and show a plausible biochemical mechanism by which the active constituents could exert the indicated physiological effect. Finally, level IV plants fulfil the criteria for level III and have been clinically tested, or are commonly used in medicine. Information on a plant's level of confidence is then considered by Ortiz de Montellano and Browner in the light of its emic evaluation of efficacy.[47]

In 1988, Browner, Ortiz de Montellano and Rubel[48] developed a more elaborate model for analyzing ethnomedical data in their own terms, as well as according to the standards of biomedicine. This model builds upon the earlier work of Ortiz de Montellano and Browner described above, and can be applied to both the study of folk illnesses and the assessment of plant medicines. The first step is to identify the phenomena under investigation in emic terms (e.g. the reasons given for using a particular plant for specific symptoms of diseases). In the second step, one determines the extent to which the phenomena described can be understood in terms of biomedical concepts and methods. For example, if the emic explanation for the efficacy of a plant medicine is that it causes bleeding, the biomedical evaluation will assess whether the plant has chemical constituents that will evoke bleeding. Finally, the third step is to identify the areas of convergence and divergence between the emically described phenomena and their biomedical understandings. In this stage, biomedical concepts are not used to examine the phenomena in their own terms (as in the second step), but to see if they are consistent with biomedical assumptions.

These principles were applied in *Aztec Medicine, Health, and Nutrition*, in a study which evaluated a group of 118 medicinal plant species. Eighty-five per cent of these species could be shown to be effective according to Aztec standards. However, concordance with biomedical criteria for efficacy was lower at about 60 per cent. The following examples help to explain these findings. Some Aztec remedies for headaches have no known analgesic properties. However, headaches were thought to be caused by an excess of blood in the head, and treatment required blood to be released through the nose. Thus, plants to treat headaches were selected for their ability to induce nosebleed (which have been confirmed), but not necessarily to provide analgesia. Likewise, Aztecs believed fever to be caused by hot phlegm in the chest, and sweating/purging was the appropriate course of treatment. Thus, while many medicinal plants used for fever do not necessarily reduce inflammation, most do induce sweating.[49] As an ethnobotanical perspective guides the objective assessment of the efficacy of Aztec medicinal plants, both the species used and the reasoning behind their use become more intelligible. This not only allows contemporary medicinal plant scientists to more accurately identify healing applications of species documented in historical texts, but also provides insight on global processes of medical diffusion.

Medical diffusion between the old and new worlds

Eventually, after the conquest of Mesoamerica by the Spanish was firmly established, the Aztec Empire became the colony of New Spain. Ortiz de Montellano's work (complemented by a variety of other sources) sheds light on ethnobotanical continuities throughout pre-colonial, colonial and modern times in this region. By critically assessing historical records and interpreting them within their socio-ecological contexts, this work shows which species, practices and concepts are likely to be artefacts of colonialism and which pre-dated contact between the Old and New Worlds. The remainder of this chapter will show that the Spanish conquest and subsequent colonial rule of Mesoamerica had a dramatic impact on the morbidity and mortality of the indigenous population. However, the colonial reaction to indigenous medicine (and medicine in general) in New Spain was not as repressive as in other parts of the world, where medicine was much more integral to colonial rule. The Church did transform certain Mesoamerican spiritual customs and traditions (including those related to healing), but it seems that their underlying cosmologies received less attention from religious authorities, and the syncretization of Catholicism and indigenous traditions was allowed to flourish. Moreover, as Aztec healing was grounded in an empirical system of medicinal plant use, Mexican plants were adopted into the Spanish pharmacopoeia, in addition to many Old World species being introduced into Mesoamerican herbal medicine. Spain also had strong ties to the Islamic world and there was an enormously powerful medical tradition in Islamic Spain, which filtered into European medical schools and influenced medical learning throughout Europe.[50] Ortiz de Montellano's work has important implications for determining how far the influence of Islamic medicine spread through the Americas, as it helps historians to identify which aspects of Mesoamerican medical thinking are part of a global philosophy of humoral medicine introduced through (Islamic) Spain and which elements of the Aztec medical system were similar to Old World medical theories.

Ethnohistorical data, as well as religious and fiscal documents, have been used to estimate the effect conquest and colonization had on the indigenous population of Mesoamerica. While there is disagreement among scholars about the size of the indigenous Mesoamerican population leading up to the conquest, population estimates suggest a large and rapid decline during the early colonial period.[51] While the indigenous population was declining, the Spanish population in Mesoamerica was increasing (from 63,000 in 1570 to 1,050,000 in 1793). As the Spanish were dependent on indigenous peoples for the production of foods and supplies, the decimation of the indigenous population sent New Spain, as well as other areas in Mesoamerica, into a century of depression.[52] The extent and scale of the Amerindian population decline that followed the Spanish conquest has been the subject of intense debate. However, Whitmore argues that it is most likely that the scale of the population collapse was moderate, and that the population of the Basin of Mexico on the eve of the conquest was 1.59 million. This population was reduced (in an irregular fashion) to 183,000 by 1607. By far the most significant contributor was epidemic disease, although disease-induced famine also played a part. Whitmore also states that epidemics were cause enough for this population decline, even if legends of excessive Spanish brutality and genetic vulnerability to disease are exaggerated. The Amerindian depopulation, along with the introduction of exotic biota and technologies, and the reordering of land and the rural economy, had a severe impact on the Mesoamerican environment.[53]

Early on, the Spanish realized that they could not effectively control people, in terms of tax collection or proselytization, who live scattered about in remote areas. The indigenous population was forced to move to larger, more centralized towns (*congregaciones*). The Spanish tried to claim that moving people to *congregaciones* was for their own good, but indigenous people did not appreciate the policy. Gerhard describes how the concentration of indigenous settlements occurred in two stages: one in 1550–64 and the other in 1593–1605. Both of these stages came after devastating epidemics. Additionally, he suggests that present-day settlements in Mexico are in essence the same towns that were formed in 1550–64.[54] However, it has also been argued that the *pueblos de indios* of the eighteenth-century central Mexican highlands should be seen as the continuation of pre-Hispanic indigenous landed estates. The *pueblos* were highly-stratified entities and were ruled by a small group of elite families (*caciques*). The local-level elite either traced descent from the pre-Hispanic nobility, or had taken the place of that nobility by acquiring parts of early post-conquest grants in which pre-Hispanic claims were recognized. Consequently, Spanish institutions might have changed the form but not the basic substance of indigenous lordship.[55] Likewise, the form and substance of indigenous medicine were not uniformly influenced by colonial medical thought and practice.

The medical system that the Spanish took to the New World drew heavily on Greco-Arab and Islamic medicine, which was developed between the seventh and fifteenth centuries. Islamic medicine was grounded in the work of Hippocrates, Galen and other Greek physicians, along with important Persian, Indian and Chinese medical texts.[56] Greek, Ayurvedic and Chinese medicine are found within a continuous geographical area, throughout which there has been much cultural diffusion. These medical systems share some major theoretical similarities, particularly concepts that relate to balancing various fluids/energies/humours in the body to maintain health.[57] According to these medical systems, disease results from disharmony between body and spirit. Such disharmony was attributed to humoral imbalance (which could be corrected by physicians) rather than supernatural forces. These global medical theories were set within Islamic ethics and, under the umbrella of Islamic, Muslim, Christian and Jewish physicians, became highly influential in Western science and medical education.[58] Great Islamic physicians and scholars helped transform Hippocratic-Galenic-Persian medicine into orthodox medicine in both Western Europe and its colonies.[59] Avicenna's *Canon of Medicine* was the most widely studied medical text in Europe from the twelfth into the seventeenth century and was a major guide to medical science in European universities.[60] Moreover, Avicenna's set of rules for testing the efficacy of new medications still serves as the basis for modern-day clinical trials.[61] Spain became not only an important centre of Islamic culture, but cities such as Seville, Toledo and Granada were especially well known for their contributions to the development of Arab-Islamic medical sciences.[62] However, medical knowledge in Spain at the time of the Mesoamerican conquest was generally restricted to the elite classes, especially clergy and physicians.[63]

Throughout Mexico, missionaries, rather than doctors, were primarily responsible for the care of the sick during the colonial era.[64] The clergy was generally preoccupied with extinguishing models of sickness that related to Mesoamerican deities, spirits and magical entities, although many of these supernatural agents were blended with Catholic saints, and a syncretic shamanistic tradition exists in many parts of Mexico to this day. During the colonial period, Catholic priests shared much of the professional medical models developed by (Spanish-Islamic) physicians, which emphasized naturalistic aspects of health and healing. For three centuries following the conquest, humoral concepts were pervasive among all educated and intellectual people in New Spain. It has been argued that the elite theory was then filtered into popular Latin American medical traditions through missionaries, hospitals, pharmacies and home medical guides. Although a long time has passed since humoral theory was supplanted by other biomedical models of disease (and virtually erased from elite biomedical theory), models of health and healing that focus on balancing hot and cold elements of the body are still popular in Latin America (and other parts of the world). There is evidence of hot–cold data in Sahagún and the *Badianus Codex*, but this is generally dismissed as colonial contamination.[65] The question remains, did humoral theory filter down into the general populace from Spanish missionaries and physicians and become the Latin American hot–cold model of healing, or was there an emphasis on balancing hot and cold in Aztec (and other indigenous Mesoamerican) medicine before the conquest?

Looking at this question in medical history from an ethnobotanical perspective reveals that reverse acculturation (colonists adopting aspects of indigenous culture) occurred in New Spain. While many indigenous cosmological beliefs about health and sickness were lost or transformed by Spanish missionary activity, the empirical use of medicinal plants remained vibrant. In fact, the Spanish were greatly interested in the medicinal plants of the New World and incorporated many Aztec plants into colonial medicine because of the fit of their reported properties with European conceptions of illness and the Greco-Arab/Islamic doctrine of balancing humours. The colonial pharmacopoeia included Aztec (and other indigenous) remedies for Aztec ailments, though indigenous aetiological explanations were rationalized to fit Old World humoral principles.[66] To the indigenous pharmacopoeia, European *materia medica* were added. In modern times, the use of the same medicinal plants (both introduced and native species) for related disease conditions is common among Mexican *mestizos* and Mexican Americans, as well as numerous indigenous Mexican groups.[67] The syncretic nature of Mexican traditional medicine reflects a high degree of medical pluralism, which continues to be a major characteristic of Mexican health care culture, despite the pre-eminence given to biomedicine by the state.[68] During the colonial period, clear evidence for the adoption of Aztec medicinal plants into the pharmacopoeias of both Spain and New Spain suggests that the transmission of medical knowledge flowed in two directions. Thus, scholars cannot conclude that Greco-Arab/Islamic humoral theory was a dominant paradigm that completely displaced indigenous models of balance and healing and is therefore the only possible inspiration for Latin American hot–cold systems.[69] Scholars such as Sahagún certainly took Aztec medicinal plant knowledge seriously and likely had a similar amount of respect for indigenous medical theories, especially if they were based on similar concepts (e.g. hot and cold). There is no conclusive evidence that references to Aztec models of hot–cold equilibrium in the *Florentine* and *Badianus* codices were simply the result of their authors' influence. Rather, the ethnobotanical data suggests that hot, cold and other empirical qualities of Aztec medicinal plants were recognized prior to the conquest.

Conclusion

Ethnobotany has much to contribute to the history of herbal medicine. Specifically, the anthropological and ethnobiological perspectives on the study of people–plant relationships that form the foundations of ethnobotanical research complement traditional historical approaches to understanding the use of herbal medicines in the past. As this chapter has shown, historical sources must be contextualized to illuminate cultural, social, political, cosmological and environmental factors that influence the practice of medicine in a given time and place. In evaluating the empirical efficacy of herbal remedies, we need to understand how the people who first developed them understood and experienced the illnesses they were, or are, used to treat. This is because some species that are empirically effective according to such emic criteria do not measure up to biomedical expectations. To achieve this understanding, herbal/medical texts must be read alongside other historical documents (e.g. colonial) that provide a broader picture of social and political relationships that influence the theory and practice of medicine. By drawing on ethnobotany to better understand alternative models of health, illness and healing, historians can create respect and appreciation for other medical systems throughout space and time. This, in turn, encourages innovation in medicine. Although Mesoamerica may at first seem far removed from the study of the history of Western herbal medicine, ethnobotanical consideration of Aztec medicinal plants shows that many questions remain about what exactly happened when New and Old World medical theories collided. Colonization certainly had a transformative effect on indigenous Mesoamerican medicine, but it is important to bear in mind that there is also evidence of reverse acculturation, especially in the domain of medicinal plants.

On the eve of the conquest, the Valley of Mexico was the seat of an Aztec Empire that controlled and managed much of Postclassic Mesoamerica's biological diversity. The capital cities were cosmopolitan homes to a variety of learned medical professionals, as well as botanical gardens and centres of agricultural innovation. Although most Aztec literature was destroyed, several key medical texts remain. While the very act of writing Nahuatl texts was made possible only through contact with colonial missionaries and physicians, the texts nevertheless provide insight into pre-colonial Aztec cosmology and ethnobotanical practice. The Aztec worldview, similar to that of other Mesoamerican civilizations, is one of multiple material, spiritual and energetic elements that are set into states of balance and/or imbalance. Aztec healing was a sophisticated combination of shamanic practices and naturalistic applications of herbal (and other) medicines. However, there are notable differences between ancient Aztec and contemporary biomedical explanatory models for many conditions and their treatment. There is much to be learned from scientifically assessing medicinal plants documented in historical and ethnohistorical texts, but unless such herbal medicines are evaluated according to their own ethnomedical criteria, important pharmacological properties could be misunderstood or missed altogether. Looking at the history of Mesoamerican herbal medicine from an ethnobotanical perspective provides deeper insight into the history of medicine on a global scale, particularly the relationships between (Islamic) Spain and New Spain and the two-way flow of medical knowledge, practices and materials across the Atlantic. This provides contemporary students and scholars with a more holistic understanding of the history of Western herbal medicine and how to apply it to current questions in health, illness and medicine.

Recommended reading

Foster, George M. *Hippocrates' Latin American Legacy: Humoral Medicine in the New World*. Langhorne, PA: Gordon and Breach, 1994.
Ortiz de Montellano, Bernard R. *Aztec Medicine, Health, and Nutrition*. New Brunswick: Rutgers University Press, 1990.

Schultes, Richard E., and Siri Von Reis. *Ethnobotany: Evolution of a Discipline*. London: Chapman and Hall, 1995.

Notes

1. For recent general work in the field of ethnobotany, see Ulysses P. de Albuquerque and Natalia Hanazaki, *Recent Developments and Case Studies in Ethnobotany* (Recife, Pernambuco, Brazil: Sociedade Brasileira de Etnobiologia [and] Núcleo de Publicaçóes em Eclogia e Etnobotânica Aplicada, 2010); Thomas J. S. Carlson and Luisa Maffi, *Ethnobotany and Conservation of Biocultural Diversity* (Bronx, NY: New York Botanical Garden Press, 2004); and Manuel Pardo de Santayana, Andrea Pieroni and Rajindra K. Puri, eds., *Ethnobotany in the New Europe: People, Health and Wild Plant Resources* (New York: Berghahn Books, 2010).
2. Michael Heinrich et al., 'Ethnobotany and Ethnopharmacology – Interdisciplinary Links with the Historical Sciences', *Journal of Ethnopharmacology* 107 (2006): 157–60.
3. Maria F. Medeiros and Ulysses P. de Albuquerque, 'The Pharmacy of the Benedictine Monks: The Use of Medicinal Plants in Northeast Brazil During the Nineteenth Century (1823–1829)', *Journal of Ethnopharmacology* 139, no. 1 (2012): 280–6.
4. Michael Adams et al., 'Malaria in the Renaissance: Remedies from European Herbals from the 16th and 17th Century', *Journal of Ethnopharmacology* 133, no. 2 (2011): 278–88.
5. Paul Kirchoff, 'Mesoamerica: Its Geographical Limits, Ethnic Composition and Cultural Characteristics', in *Heritage of Conquest: The Ethnology of Middle America*, ed. Sol Tax (Glencoe: Free Press Publishers, 1952), 17–30.
6. Winifred Creamer, 'Mesoamerica as a Concept: An Archaeological View from Central America', *Latin American Research Review* 22, no. 1 (1987): 35–62.
7. Victor M. Toledo, 'Biocultural Diversity and Local Power in Mexico: Challenging Globalization', in *On Biocultural Diversity: Linking Language, Knowledge and the Environment*, ed. Luisa Maffi (Washington, DC: Smithsonian Institution Press, 2001), 472–88.
8. Alejandro Anaya Muñoz, 'The Emergence and Development of the Politics of Recognition of Cultural Diversity and Indigenous Peoples' Rights in Mexico: Chiapas and Oaxaca in Comparative Perspective', *Journal of Latin American Studies* 37 (2005): 585–610.
9. Toledo, 'Biocultural Diversity', 477.
10. B. Frei et al., 'Multiple Screening of Medicinal Plants from Oaxaca, Mexico: Ethnobotany and Bioassays as a Basis for Phytochemical Investigation', *Phytomedicine* 5, no. 3 (1998): 177–86.
11. Bernard Ortiz de Montellano, *Aztec Medicine, Health, and Nutrition* (New Brunswick: Rutgers University Press, 1990), 233.
12. Richard E. Blanton et al., *Ancient Mesoamerica: A Comparison of Change in Three Regions*, 2nd ed. (Cambridge: Cambridge University Press, 1993), 148.
13. Patricia R. Anawalt, 'The Emperors' Cloak: Aztec Pomp, Toltec Circumstances', *American Antiquity* 55, no. 2 (1990): 291–307.
14. Michael E. Smith, 'The Expansion of the Aztec Empire: A Case Study in the Correlation of Diachronic Archaeological and Ethnohistorical Data', *American Antiquity* 52, no. 1 (1987): 37–54.

15 Elizabeth M. Brumfiel, 'Agricultural Development and Class Stratification in the Southern Valley of Mexico', in *Land and Politics in the Valley of Mexico*, ed. H. R. Harvey (Albuquerque: University of New Mexico Press, 1991), 43–61.
16 Anne C. Chapman, 'Port of Trade Enclaves in Aztec and Maya Civilizations', in *Trade and Market in the Early Empires: Economies in History and Theory*, ed. Karl Polanyi, Conrad M. Arensberg, and Harry W. Pearson (New York: Free Press, 1957), 114–53.
17 Susan T. Evans, 'Architecture and Authority in an Aztec Village: Form and Function of the Tecpan', in *Land and Politics in the Valley of Mexico: A Two Thousand-Year Perspective*, ed. Herbert R. Harvey (Albuquerque: University of New Mexico Press, 1991), 63–92.
18 Elizabeth M. Brumfiel, 'Weaving and Cooking: Women's Production in Aztec Mexico', in *Engendering Archaeology*, ed. Joan M. Gero and Margaret Conkey (Oxford: Basil Blackwell, 1991), 224–54.
19 Geoffrey Kimball, 'Aztec Homosexuality: The Textual Evidence. [New Translation and Study of Florentine Codex]', *Journal of Homosexuality* 26, no. 1 (1993): 7–24.
20 Bernal Diaz del Castillo, *The True History of the Conquest of Mexico*, trans. Maurice Keatinge (New York: Robert M. McBride, 1927).
21 See, for example, Jan Ovesen and Ing-Britt Trankell, *Cambodians and Their Doctors: A Medical Anthropology of Colonial and Postcolonial Cambodia* (Copenhagen: NIAS, 2012).
22 Bernardino de Sahagún, *Florentine Codex: General History of the Things of New Spain*, trans. Arthur Anderson and Charles Dibble (Santa Fe, NM: School of American Research: University of Utah, 1950–82).
23 Ortiz de Montellano, *Aztec Medicine*, 27.
24 Ibid., 20–1.
25 Peter T. Furst, 'This Little Book of Herbs: Psychoactive Plants as Therapeutic Agents in the Badianus Manuscript of 1552', in *Ethnobotany: Evolution of a Discipline*, ed. Richard E. Schultes and Siri Von Reis (London: Chapman and Hall, 1995), 108–30.
26 Ortiz de Montellano, *Aztec Medicine*, 24.
27 J. R. Parsons, 'The Role of Chinampa Agriculture in the Food Supply of Aztec Tenochtitlan', in *Cultural Change and Continuity: Essays in Honor of James Bennett Griffin*, ed. Charles E. Cleland (New York: Academic Press, 1976), 233–58.
28 Brumfiel, 'Agricultural Development'.
29 Parsons, 'Role of Chinampa'.
30 Ortiz de Montellano, *Aztec Medicine*, 94.
31 Ibid., 155.
32 George M. Foster, 'On the Origin of Humoral Medicine in Latin America', *Medical Anthropology Quarterly* 1, no. 4 (1987): 355–93.
33 Carole H. Browner, 'Criteria for Selecting Herbal Remedies', *Ethnology* 24, no. 1 (1985): 13–32.
34 George M. Foster, 'Disease Etiologies in Non-Western Medical Systems', *American Anthropologist* 78 (1976): 773–82.
35 Anna Waldstein and Cameron Adams, 'The Interface between Medical Anthropology and Medical Ethnobiology', *Journal of the Royal Anthropological Institute* 12, Supplement 1 (2006): 95–118.
36 Ortiz de Montellano, *Aztec Medicine*, 37–43.
37 Nina L. Etkin, 'Cultural Constructions of Efficacy', in *The Context of Medicines*

in *Developing Countries: Studies in Pharmaceutical Anthropology*, ed. Sjaak Van der Geest and Susan R. Whyte (Dordrecht: Kluwer Academic Publishers, 1988), 299–327.
38 Robert Anderson, 'The Efficacy of Ethnomedicine: Research Methods in Trouble', *Medical Anthropology* 13, no. 1–2 (1991): 1–17.
39 Etkin, 'Cultural Constructions of Efficacy', 302.
40 Arthur Kleinman and Lilias H. Sung, 'Why Do Indigenous Practitioners Successfully Heal?', *Social Science and Medicine* 13B, no. 1 (1979): 7–26.
41 Nina L. Etkin, 'Ethnopharmacology: Biological and Behavioral Perspectives in the Study of Indigenous Medicine', in *Medical Anthropology: Contemporary Theory and Method*, ed. Carolyn F. Sargent and Thomas M. Johnson (Westport, CT: Praeger, 1996), 149–58.
42 Anderson, 'Efficacy of Ethnomedicine', 2.
43 Kleinman and Sung, 'Indigenous Practitioners', 21.
44 Etkin, 'Cultural Constructions of Efficacy', 318.
45 Norman R. Farnsworth, 'The Development of Pharmacological and Chemical Research for Application to Traditional Medicine in Developing Countries', *Journal of Ethnopharmacology* 2, no. 2 (1980): 173–81.
46 Bernard Ortiz de Montellano, 'Empirical Aztec Medicine: Aztec Medicinal Plants Seem to Be Effective If They Are Judged by Aztec Standards', in *Ancient and Modern Medical Practices in Mesoamerica*, ed. Bernard Ortiz de Montellano (Greeley: University of Northern Colorado Press, 1982), 18–22.
47 Bernard Ortiz de Montellano and Carole H. Browner, 'Chemical Bases for Medicinal Plant Use in Oaxaca, Mexico', *Journal of Ethnopharmacology* 13, no. 1 (1985): 57–88.
48 Carole H. Browner, Bernard Ortiz de Montellano and Arthur J. Rubel, 'A Methodology for Cross-Cultural Ethnomedical Research', *Current Anthropology* 29, no. 5 (1988): 681–9.
49 Ortiz de Montellano, *Aztec Medicine*, 189.
50 For more on the Islamic contribution to Western culture, including medicine, see also chs 4 and 6 in this book.
51 Ortiz de Montellano, *Aztec Medicine*, 73.
52 See Woodrow Borah, *New Spain's Century of Depression* (Berkeley: University of California Press, 1951).
53 Thomas M. Whitmore, *Disease and Death in Early Colonial Mexico: Simulating Amerindian Depopulation* (Boulder, CO: Westview Press, 1992).
54 Peter Gerhard, 'Congregaciones de indios en la Nueva España antes de 1570', *Historia Mexicana* 26, no. 3 (1977): 347–89.
55 Arij Ouweneel, 'From *tlahtocayotl* to *gobernadoryotl*: A Critical Examination of Indigenous Rule in 18th-Century Mexico', *American Ethnologist* 22, no. 4 (1995): 756–86.
56 Bashar Saad and Omar Said, 'Tradition and Perspectives of Greco-Arab and Islamic Medicine', in *Herbal Supplements: Efficacy, Toxicity, Interactions with Western Drugs, and Effects on Clinical Laboratory Tests*, ed. Amitava Dasgupta and Catherine A. Hammet-Stabler (Hoboken, NJ: Wiley, 2011), 209–54.
57 Foster, 'Origin of Humoral Medicine', 359. For more on Greek medicine, see also chs 2, 9 and 10 in this book.
58 Saad and Said, 'Tradition and Perspectives', 211.
59 Foster, 'Origin of Humoral Medicine', 361.

60 Sharif K. Al-Ghazal, 'The Influence of Islamic Philosophy and Ethics on the Development of Medicine During the Islamic Renaissance', *Journal of the International Society for the History of Islamic Medicine* 3, no. 6 (2004): 3–9.
61 David Tschanz, 'A Short History of Islamic Pharmacy', *Journal of the International Society for the History of Islamic Medicine* 1, no. 3 (2003): 11–17.
62 Saad and Said, 'Tradition and Perspectives', 210.
63 Foster, 'Origin of Humoral Medicine', 361.
64 Margarita A. Kay, 'The Florilegio Medicinal: Source of Southwest Ethnomedicine', *Ethnohistory* 24, no. 3 (1977): 251–9.
65 Foster, 'Origin of Humoral Medicine', 357.
66 Ortiz de Montellano, *Aztec Medicine*, 204.
67 Kay, 'Florilegio Medicinal', 251.
68 Gustavo Nigenda et al., 'Non-Biomedical Health Care Practices in the State of Morelos, Mexico: Analysis of an Emergent Phenomenon', *Sociology of Health and Illness* 23, no. 1 (2001): 3–23.
69 Ortiz de Montellano, *Aztec Medicine*, 221.

15

Conclusion: The History of Herbal Medicine as a Developing Field

Anne Stobart and Susan Francia

Progress in the history of herbal medicine

In our introduction we discussed issues relating to the fragmentation of research in the history of herbal medicine. In this final chapter we consider progress made in this book in identifying a range of research and making it available, and we look ahead to further challenges and the benefits of research and studies in the history of herbal medicine.

Existing research in the history of herbal medicine

Our initial claim was that the history of herbal medicine could provide a recognizable theme to underpin a range of research. We defined research in the history of herbal medicine as 'systematic enquiry to understand and explain the supply, knowledge and use of plants incorporating people's beliefs, knowledge and involvement in past therapeutic practices in the context of health and illness'. Use of this framework incorporating plants, people and practice helped in structuring an overview of research related to the history of herbal medicine. Our second claim was that there is a range of research relevant to the history of herbal medicine, albeit somewhat fragmented, which needs to be made more accessible. The chapters in this book provide examples which support this observation of a range of research, incorporating findings on many topics of direct relevance, and show how our contributors have come from varied disciplines and backgrounds. In order to make this material more accessible, our contributors have endeavoured to provide a window on original sources that they have used, as well as further resources which might be considered.

Text editions of ancient sources are still much needed in today's work, and John Wilkins provides direct testimony regarding the issues faced in preparing editions of classical texts. In terms of extending the range of sources that might be used, Richard Aspin and Susan Francia have both sought to illuminate archives which deserve more attention, for example testamentary and trade records respectively. Nicky Wesson has noted a variety of possible difficulties in locating suitable sources for considering herbal medicine usage in childbirth, nevertheless finding some household and legal records that might be considered.

Despite the gaps identified by our contributors, a startling array of resources for research in the history of herbal medicine are being explored, from original manuscripts and printed texts to illustrations and physical remains. These chapters may provide only a limited indication of potential sources so far unexplored, from archives to artefacts. More significantly, it is apparent that a treasure trove of digitized texts and images is now becoming readily (sometimes freely) available electronically worldwide. Manuscript sources are continuously being added, with transcriptions, commentaries and context statements, and numerous specialist sites have developed for classical, medieval and early modern texts.

Our contributors have also sought to make their methodologies more explicit. Some of them have gone back to original sources to carry out detailed textual analysis and provide new interpretations. For example, Alison Denham and Midge Whitelegg have compared detailed elements of Dioscorides and other texts to reveal some of the complexities in plant identification in classical times and beyond, especially since texts were continually being recopied, translated and reworded. Graeme Tobyn has sought to clarify the sources used by Nicholas Culpeper, finding that he was not so original in the content of much of his famous herbal. Elaine Hobby has skilfully considered changes in early-modern midwifery texts for indications of herbal elements and how they can be better understood.

A number of approaches in the study of the history of herbal medicine have been further discussed, in terms of beliefs and knowledge in past practice. Vicki Pitman has taken a comparative approach in considering holistic perspectives represented in classical writings and in present-day herbal practice. Explicit recognition of different approaches to investigating the sources is important in the context of researching the history of herbal medicine: there is not one truth and much is implicit, as Anne Van Arsdall discusses in relation to medieval texts. In these and other studies, previous assumptions have been questioned in many ways. For example, in biographical studies, both Marie Addyman and Jill Francis have shown that significant individuals associated with the history of herbal medicine must be carefully reconsidered and understandings of their relative contributions need to be revised.

Explanations of methods and perspectives which are appropriate within other research disciplines can prove revealing. The contribution from Anna Waldstein is valuable in providing an overarching perspective drawn from ethnobotanical studies which highlights the context of plants, people and practice. Painstaking archaeological techniques in concert with other sources have been used by Brian Moffat and his co-workers in uncovering and interpreting remaining evidence of medical practices in a medieval hospital site. Altogether, the historical studies in this book and those drawn from several other disciplines, have provided in-depth examples of investigations in the history of herbal medicine which, it is hoped, will encourage readers who may use these findings in direct ways, or adopt suggestions regarding sources and methodologies in their own fields.

Promoting further research

Our third claim was that there is a need to promote further research in the history of herbal medicine, based on agreed standards of enquiry. Part of the rationale for this book has been to enable the sharing of experience to inform both current and potential researchers. However, there are difficulties facing any individual who wishes to distinguish the quality of research in the history of herbal medicine. How can a reader be assured that they are reading an authoritative and reliable study? While the recommendations of ourselves and contributors may provide useful starting points in identifying important and recent studies, it is apparent that guidelines for critical appraisal of further research in the history of herbal medicine would also be helpful. The relatively recent establishment of a peer-reviewed journal for herbal medicine (*Journal of Herbal Medicine*, Elsevier) might imply that there is already some consensus on 'good' or 'acceptable' research relating to the history of herbal medicine: expectations of research papers in other aspects of herbal medicine, such as clinical therapeutics and pharmacology, are well established and include methodologies such as clinical studies, case reports, literature reviews, laboratory analyses, in vitro experiments, controlled trials, surveys, and so on. These expectations draw on widely understood standards for research in health, social and biological sciences, and provide a way of appraising and comparing research output to ensure minimum standards (even though there may be debates on matters such as the nature of evidence and relevance of various research designs and methodologies).

However, there are no comparable standards particular to research and writing related to the history of herbal medicine. Indeed, the portrayal of events of the past is sometimes regarded as more of an art than a science, and, since history is part of the humanities, selective use of sources is regarded by some as permissible. Perhaps this is not so surprising when we consider that surviving historical evidence can be extremely piecemeal, so that systematic investigation can be very challenging, thus opening the door to creative interpretation. Yet the quality of much research in the history of herbal medicine could be much improved: historians and other scholars do have a range of approaches which can be used to provide evidenced and soundly based interpretations of the past through critical appraisal of the sources available.[1] In order to raise the status of studies in the history of herbal medicine, and to underpin herbal history with more scholarly studies, there is now a need to benefit from the experience of historical and other researchers and to promote higher standards through the production of guidelines and further training opportunities.

The contributions in this volume have raised many issues. For example, in terms of plants there is a need for more reliable identification in classical and later sources, and for evidence about the sourcing and use of specific herbs. In relation to people, continuing studies of significant practitioners are needed as well as further analysis of the users of herbal medicines in lay contexts, including their understandings of the relationships between food and medicine, their ownership and readership of herbal texts, and their means of passing on knowledge and skills. In terms of practice, classical and later texts need further analysis, and studies are needed on the impact of Eastern and other influences and the translation of European beliefs to other cultures.

These topics are starting points which, likely with further suggestions, will repay further investigation.

Interdisciplinary collaboration

Our fourth claim was that interdisciplinary links are needed to provide a way forward for research in the history of herbal medicine. For interdisciplinary work to be effective, a collaborative style of working is needed which incorporates identification of common problems and sharing of expertise and methodologies. Our foray into selected aspects of research relating to the history of herbal medicine has provided much insight into the historical and other problems raised, common to a number of the authors contributing to this book, such as: the lack of authenticity and availability of sources; gaps in the records; inappropriate attribution of meanings of past terms; problematic identification of plant species; and previous assumptions in research. Contributors have shown that they are concerned with accuracy; they endeavour to maintain a systematic approach; they are able to recognize and deal with complexities in their findings; they are keen to link to specialists in related areas; and, above all, they would like to see further research and scholarship in the history of herbal medicine.

Working together on this book has provided a good opportunity to understand the differing expectations and experiences of contributors from a variety of disciplines. On being asked what helps in working in an interdisciplinary way, they have voiced some significant factors. For example, one herbal practitioner commented on the generosity and openness of classical and history scholars in sharing their work and giving advice on relevant sources. In turn, history scholars expressed genuine appreciation for the input from herbal practitioners and others which draws from direct experience of using plants in the present day in both scientific and traditional ways. Some researchers have indicated that their particular interest in the history of herbal medicine has placed them on the fringes of their own academic discipline and so they have welcomed discussion and support related to these topics.

In a way, the compilation of this book could be described as a multidisciplinary project, since many of the individual contributors will return to their 'home' research disciplines. Yet, this underestimates the effects of our collaboration which include changes arising from the process of sharing ideas and knowledge, from which all have benefited in some way. Extension of awareness of sources, methodologies and key issues in the history of herbal medicine has been a particularly valued outcome, bringing both more layered perspectives and sharper technical skills. Thus, the contributors, to varying extents, have acquired further understanding of the techniques and approaches of others, and this experience paves the way for more interdisciplinary and collaborative work.

Looking ahead

Herbal medicine today

Professional practice in herbal medicine today has the odd characteristic of being the complementary therapy which is most similar to mainstream Western medicine. This can be seen in the professional nature of practitioner organizations, with ethical policies and codes of conduct, therapeutic approaches based largely on extensive training in current medical understanding alongside traditional knowledge, and treatment involving physiologically active medications (generally whole plants in combination rather than single extracts). Yet, most traces of the herbal *materia medica* curriculum have been erased from the modern medical practitioner and pharmacy curriculum.[2] For some, herbal medicine is indistinguishable from other kinds of complementary or alternative medicine provision. However, this may be misleading, as herbal medicine practitioners do not necessarily share the precepts of other complementary or alternative approaches to healing. There is much elasticity in definitions of complementary and alternative medicine in the West, ranging from anything not regarded as orthodox, to therapies with a particularly holistic perspective.[3] Both traditional Chinese medicine and Ayurvedic medicine have considerable and cohesive cultural backgrounds whilst Western herbal medicine is rather less well defined in terms of culture or history.[4]

The picture of herbal medicine in the wider world today is varied, both in terms of herbal medications and clinical herbal practitioners. Many medicines currently in use in the context of modern medicine were originally derived from plants, but the use of whole plants and plant extracts has declined as, increasingly, single constituent pharmaceuticals have come to dominate the market. Nevertheless, many plant materials, both whole and in extract form, are still widely available for direct purchase in health food stores and pharmacies, although there may be legal limitations on therapeutic claims for these plants, and there has been a trend towards regulation through licensing of products available, both in European countries and in the US.

Increasing interest in complementary and alternative medicine in the UK has led to the development of professional training and research opportunities in higher education. The practice of herbal medicine in the UK was one of the five main complementary therapies considered by a House of Lords Select Committee in 2000,[5] leading to recommendations for statutory regulation in order to maintain safety and standards based on training and professional codes of behaviour comparable to those of other health care professionals.[6] In the US there are comparable professional groupings, although the regulation of provision varies state by state, as some states offer licences to practitioners whilst others restrict diagnosis and treatment to those with medical qualifications. In Europe there are further variations in practice and regulations: for example, in Germany, many medical practitioners prescribe herbs, whereas in France there are limitations on the range of herbs available for purchase over the counter.[7]

An increasing commercial demand for over-the-counter herbal remedies suggests that the use of 'natural medicines' in the developed world is definitely big business, running into billions of dollars.[8] Thus, in addition to the potential recognition of herbal practitioners, it appears that herbal medicines continue to be a significant element in health care. Alongside this commercial growth, professional motivation and scholarly interest combine to support the need for more and better research relating to the history of herbal medicine.

Some further challenges

Many tasks remain ahead for researchers and others interested in advancing research in the history of herbal medicine, and are summarized here.

Historiographical issues

Both the motivation and the perspective of the researcher can impact on research findings and interpretations of historical sources, and these are issues which need to be considered. For example, Christopher Lloyd has discussed the ahistoricism of many scientists.[9] A challenge for researchers with differing backgrounds in science and history is to improve their understanding of each other's approach. However, researchers may be unable to agree with the view that today's historian must forget the science: rather, as Grmek has noted, a non-presentist history is probably not entirely desirable.[10] It is certainly difficult to disregard knowledge of plant constituents and their effects on human physiology – and a challenge for researchers to clarify when and how they use this knowledge in relation to historical findings.[11]

Technical and training requirements

A number of issues arise in terms of the skills and expertise required for research in the history of herbal medicine. Training in historical methods and botanical knowledge may both be required. There is a particular problem in the lack of common usage of terminology, especially where such terms are poorly defined. For example, the term 'tradition' is readily used to refer to the past but can sometimes be found without clear definition of context, thus raising the question of 'which' past is specifically intended. 'Tradition' is helpfully identified by Huisman and Warner as denoting:

> clusters of practices and values fashioned at particular historical moments to serve specific purposes, constructions that gain in power as they come to be imbued with a sense of timelessness and to be regarded as inbuilt components of a culture rather than contingent creations.[12]

A challenge for researchers is to be more explicit about such terms, particularly in order to be able to promote interdisciplinary understanding and improve networking and access to specialist knowledge. However, training opportunities rarely bridge the gap between science and history research. Herbal practitioners and historical researchers working together can embody the required links and help to synthesize traditions with modern scientific knowledge. More training opportunities are needed to underpin the technical knowledge and skills for research and to promote both a consistent scholarly approach and collaboration between disciplines.

Dissemination opportunities

Further dissemination of research is a challenge, since there are relatively few publications, and no key journals, in the field of the history of herbal medicine. Researchers may need to adapt their work to fit within other fields in order to achieve recognition and publication. Ideally, a focus is needed for publishing research findings so that they are made accessible to others. Frustratingly, there are many potted histories of herbs and herbal medicine[13] which incorporate few references and are not extensive enough for academic interest. This, perhaps, is not the fault of the authors, who probably could supply detailed referencing, but rather the influence of publishers in desiring books of popular interest. Thus, forward-looking publishers perceive that a demand exists for more substantial and scholarly works in the history of herbal medicine. We suggest that there is considerable scope for further publications to address the paucity of published research in the history of herbal medicine.

Conclusion

Recognition of the nature and breadth of research in the history of herbal medicine has helped us to identify a way forward. As discussed above, the provision of a clear definition and framework for history of herbal medicine research, making research studies more widely available, setting the record straight in interpretation of the past, and collaborative approaches are all desirable. But, ultimately, who will benefit from more and 'better' history of herbal medicine? In our view, the list of potential benefits is extensive. (1) Research into the history of herbal medicine can provide benefits to society through improved understanding of complementary and traditional medicine practices, and choices made by modern patients and practitioners. (2) Such research can also contribute to further understanding of the use and range of biomedicine available today, as well as flagging up potential treatments worthy of further investigation. (3) The history of herbal medicine is a topic of wide-ranging popular interest, particularly for those who wish to understand, or recreate, the past in living history contexts, museums, gardens and other archives.[14] Thus, study of the history of herbal medicine can enhance the accuracy of interpretations of sources on the past use of herbal medicine. (4) For patients and practitioners of herbal medicine, research in the history of herbal medicine can help to underpin the tradition of Western herbal medicine, correcting assumptions and misunderstandings about past developments. Such research may also extend the clinical practitioner's repertoire. (5) Research in the history of herbal medicine provides a further benefit of scholarly interest in enhancing the interpretation of the past. Increased availability and better-evidenced knowledge of the history of herbal medicine will support other historical studies and studies in a wide range of disciplines from arts to archaeology, from botany to literature.

As bio-medical provision has developed in the West, often relying on reductionist approaches to treatment, perspectives on herbal medicine have changed, leading to exclusion and fragmentation of research. In turn, this affects the motivations of writers and researchers. However, there is now more likelihood of cultural and economic drivers influencing the move of many aspects of herbal medicine back within the wider margins of medicine and society. Yet, without scholarly research, the history of herbal medicine will continue to be re-imagined with a limited evidence base. We hope that this book will promote further interest and interdisciplinary activity in research into the history of herbal medicine.

Notes

1. Jeremy Black and Donald D. MacRaild, *Studying History*, 2nd ed. (Basingstoke: Palgrave, 2000). Provides a general overview of differing approaches and methodologies in history.
2. L. Dvorkin, P. Gardiner and J. S. Whelan, 'Herbal Medicine Course within [the] Pharmacy Curriculum', *Journal of Herbal Pharmacotherapy* 4, no. 2 (2004): 47–58.
3. Catherine Zollman and Andrew Vickers, 'What Is Complementary Medicine?', *British Medical Journal* 319, no. 721 (1999): 693–6. See also Deborah Brunton, ed., *Health, Disease and Society in Europe 1800–1930: A Source Book* (Manchester: Manchester University Press in association with the Open University, 2004), 'Introduction', xii.
4. This can be seen in agreements on curriculum content regarding professional practice with herbal medicines, and medical and botanical sciences required for accreditation of programmes of degree status (see 'EHTPA Accreditation', available at http://ehtpa.eu/standards/accreditation/index.html [accessed 16 June 2013]). This is not to suggest that other countries rely solely on traditional medicine practices. See Hormoz Ebrahimnejad, ed., *Development of Modern Medicine in Non-Western Countries: Historical Perspectives* (Abingdon: Routledge, 2008).
5. House of Lords Select Committee on Science and Technology, *Sixth Report: Complementary and Alternative Medicine* (London: HMSO, 2000).
6. Leading professional bodies in the UK, including the National Institute of Medical Herbalists (NIMH), College of Phytotherapy Practitioners (CPP) and Unified Register of Herbal Practitioners (URHP), have united with Chinese and Ayurvedic medicine practitioner organizations under the umbrella of the European Herbal and Traditional Practitioner's Association (EHTPA) in order to work towards statutory regulation of herbal practitioners.
7. World Health Organization, *National Policy on Traditional Medicine and Regulation of Herbal Medicines: Report of a WHO Global Survey* (Geneva: World Health Organization, 2005).
8. World Health Organization, *WHO Traditional Medicine Strategy: 2002–2005* (Geneva: World Health Organization, 2002). Mintel reported expenditure of $5 billion in the USA on complementary and alternative medicine, largely herbal and homoeopathic products, in 2006, http://oxygen.mintel.com/sinatra/oxygen/display/id=223497 (accessed 15 June 2013). See also Richard L. Nahin et al., 'Costs of Complementary and Alternative Medicine Use and Frequency of Visits to CAM Practitioners: United States 2007', *National Health Statistics Reports* 18 (2009): 1–14.

9   Christopher Lloyd, 'History and the Social Sciences', in *Writing History: Theory and Practice*, ed. Stefan Berger, Heiko Feldner and Kevin Passmore (London: Hodder Arnold, 2003), 83–103.
10 Mirko D. Grmek, ed., *Western Medical Thought from Antiquity to the Middle Ages* (Cambridge, MA: Harvard University Press, 1998), 17.
11 For example, at least 60 per cent of remedies for rheumatic disorders in sixteenth- and seventeenth-century herbals are considered likely to have had some effect, based on relevant assays. See Michael Adams et al., 'Medicinal Herbs for the Treatment of Rheumatic Disorders – a Survey of European Herbals From the 16th and 17th Century', *Journal of Ethnopharmacology* 121, no. 3 (2009): 287.
12 Frank Huisman and John H. Warner, 'Medical Histories', in *Locating Medical History: The Stories and Their Meanings*, ed. Frank Huisman and John H. Warner (Baltimore and London: Johns Hopkins University Press, 2004), 4.
13 For example, Judith Sumner, *The Natural History of Medicinal Plants* (Portland, OR: Timber Press, 2000); Christine Stockwell, *Nature's Pharmacy: A History of Plants and Healing* (London: Arrow Books, 1988).
14 Jerome De Groot has provided a thoughtful assessment of the potentially positive links for scholarly historians with public engagement opportunities. See Jerome De Groot, *Consuming History: Historians and Heritage in Contemporary Popular Culture* (London: Routledge, 2009), 122.

Select Glossary

Aconitum Used in the sixteenth century to refer to a number of poisonous plants such as monkshood (*Aconitum* spp.) and leopard's bane (*Doronicum pardalianches*).
Aither See ether.
Alembic See still.
Apothecary A person who prepared and dispensed medicines based on a physician's prescription, although later treated patients directly.
Archaeo-ethnopharmacology The study of the medications of a specific group of people, and medical practice in that society, using archaeological and other methods.
Barber-surgeon A person to whom the physicians in early modern England delegated surgery and treatment of skin conditions, a forerunner to the modern surgeon.
Bezoar A mass of animal or vegetable matter found as an accretion in the stomach of an animal, especially a goat, and used as an antidote or medicine.
Bile Both yellow and black bile were cardinal humours.
Biomedicine Modern medicine concerned with the application of the principles and methods of biological and biochemical sciences to clinical practice.
Caudle A hot sweetened drink, usually made with ale or wine and used in childbirth.
Choler A form of bile. An excess of this humour was thought to cause anger.
Chumos See humour. Term for juice or sap (plural is chumoi) which physicians used for fluid elements of the body, primarily choler (bile), phlegm, haima (blood), melancholy (black bile).
Clyster An enema or suppository injected into the rectum as a medicine.
Diaita Diet in a broad sense, referring to way of living. See also regimen.
Dynamis The potential property, quality or power of a food or medicine (plural is dynameis).
Early modern Generally refers to the period from 1500 CE to 1800 CE.
Emic In anthropology, this refers to the point of view of the people one is studying; the subjective, insider's perspective.
Emmenagogue A substance which stimulates menstrual flow.
Empiric An irregular medical practitioner, giving treatment on the basis of experience, and not regarded as trained or licensed.
Energeia The activated property of a food or medicine.
Ether A primordial element in nature, of complex meaning, which differed among ancient authors: it denoted the divine air of heaven in contrast to the lower, moister air.
Ethnobotany The scientific study of the traditional knowledge and customs of a people concerning plants.
Ethnographic Anthropological data about a given culture that has been collected through long-term field research where the ethnographer lives and works with the people being studied.
Ethnohistory The reconstruction of past ways of life based on historical documents (both oral and written) that are produced by the people under study.

Ethnomedicine System of healing and curing as understood from the perspective of the people or group who practise those medical traditions and customs.

Etic In anthropology, this refers to the anthropologist's objective (outsider's) view of cultural phenomena.

God-sib Old English for godparent. See also gossip.

Gossip Person invited to be present at a birth, usually referring to women who were friends, relatives or neighbours.

Haima Blood, blood humour.

Harmonia Harmony.

Herbal A book that contains details of plants, with names and descriptions, often listing their habitat, time to harvest, medicinal properties and virtues, uses, and so on.

Herbal practitioner Also known as a medical herbalist. A modern Western herbal practitioner knows how to identify and prepare medicinal herbs and how to use them in treatment. The professional herbal practitioner uses a holistic approach in conjunction with modern diagnostic skills. Today, most UK professional herbalists have training and clinical experience at university degree level in medical and botanical sciences.

Herbalism The study or practice of herbal medicine.

Herbalist One who prepares, provides or administers herbal remedies.

Herbarium A collection of preserved botanical specimens.

Hippocratic Corpus A collection of works by different physician-writers spanning the period roughly 450–230 BCE, and ascribed to Hippocrates, the ideas of which were widely used in medicine until the nineteenth century.

Holistic An approach to medical treatment which aims to deal with the whole person.

Holon, holos Whole; in the cosmological sense, the wholeness of the universe; in health, the healthy wholeness of the body.

Humanism Intellectual movement of the Renaissance with a focus on classical scholarship and rediscovering ancient texts.

Humour In classical and medieval medicine, a vital fluid of the body such as blood, phlegm, yellow bile and black bile. The relative proportions of these humours determined a person's physical and mental state.

Katastasis Constitution; constitution or make-up of an individual person, sometimes of disease; sometimes the climate and environment of a particular place.

Kosmos Order, good order; the world or universe of perfect order.

Krasis Blending, mingling; inherent mingling of the constituent elements, or humours, or individual tissues of a body; eukrasis is a healthy balance or harmony.

Limbeck See still.

Lochia The discharge from the uterus and vagina following a birth which includes blood, mucus and placental tissue.

Materia medica Remedies including plant medicines and their preparations used in the practice of medicine.

Matrix The womb or uterus.

Medical herbalist See herbal practitioner.

Medico-pharmaceutical text A term used to describe many classical and early-medieval technical texts on healing because they did not usually differentiate between medicine, surgery and pharmacy.

Medicus See physician.

Medieval Referring to the Middle Ages, between the classical and early modern periods, approximately 500–1500 CE.

Medieval medical practitioners The training and skills of such people is largely unknown, and they appear to have combined knowledge of medicine, pharmacy and surgery. Thus, a more generalized term for medical personnel is preferred to the more specific physician, surgeon, etc. which emerged later in the Middle Ages (post-1100 CE).

Medieval medicine Two periods can be identified, early (up to 1100 CE) and late (from about 1100 CE TO 1500 CE), encompassing new university training in rational medicine, with specializations emerging.

Melancholic Relating to black (melan) bile (chole), one of the cardinal humours; an excess of black bile was linked to disease and mental conditions such as melancholy, which we know today as depression.

Mestizo A person of mixed racial origin, used to refer to one with indigenous and European (especially Spanish and Portuguese) heritage.

Metria Moderate, balanced; adverbial form of metrios, used for balanced or well balanced.

Mother See matrix. Diseases of the mother were thought to be connected to noxious vapours arising from the womb, or movement of the womb around the body.

Necessary activity One of the six bodily activities regarded as essential to health, namely breathing air, eating and drinking, exercise and rest, sleep, physiological balance and mental well-being (later a 'non-natural').

Nesynge powder The name used by Turner and his contemporaries for both *Helleborus* and *Veratrum* spp.; 'sneezing powder' was believed to encourage purgation by inducing vomit.

Nitre Saltpetre or potassium nitrate, used in gunpowder and soap-making. May also refer to other mineral compounds, especially alkaline salts.

Non-naturals The six external factors thought to be necessary for health: air, diet, sleep, exercise, excretion and emotional well-being.

One berrye William Turner's early name for the plant which he first identified and which is more usually referred to as 'herb paris' (*Paris quadrifolia*).

Oxymel A medicinal drink prepared from vinegar and honey with other ingredients.

Pan All, everything.

Pepsis The process of coction or 'cooking', the chief means by which humours or other factors are rendered blended and harmonized.

Perissoma A food residue from poor digestion that unbalances the body; impurity.

Pharmacopoeia An authoritative or official treatise containing lists of approved medicines, their formulations, dosages and uses.

Phlegm One of the cardinal humours, regarded as cold and moist. In excess, the phlegmatic humour was thought to produce dullness and sluggishness.

Phusai Another term for breaths, winds (not etymologically related to phusis).

Phusis Nature; may refer to nature in a universal, cosmological sense, or to a person's individual nature or constitutional make-up; also the nature of an individual disease or condition.

Physic or physick The practice of healing based largely on the authority of the writings of the ancients which viewed illness as an imbalance of the humours in the body. Also refers to medicines taken as treatment.

Physician A person trained and qualified to practise medicine, usually distinct from a surgeon or apothecary. A regular physician would have had degree-level training and be eligible to join an organization like the College of Physicians based in London.

Plant hunter A term retrospectively applied to adventurers who travelled overseas to seek out new plants to collect and bring back to England.

Plethora An overabundance of one or more humours, particularly blood, and thought to be unhealthy.

Pneuma Used to refer to breath, wind or air in ancient texts and known to be important for the heart and brain to function.

Poultice A moist preparation with a soft constituency, often of herbs, applied direct to skin and to sore or aching parts of the body, to help healing, reduce swelling and pain. Similar to a fomentation or a cataplasm.

Probate The formal legal process for inspecting, validating and executing wills and disposing of the effects of deceased property-holders.

Ptisane See tisane.

Quack A medical imposter, who dishonestly claims to have medical or surgical skills, or who advertises and sells fake remedies.

Regimen A plan for living which may include foods, exercise, medicines and other daily elements.

Renaissance European intellectual movement of the fourteenth to the sixteenth centuries based on the revival of classical elements in arts and literature. Focusing on the rediscovery of ancient texts, these were copied, printed and distributed widely, forming the basis of a new system of humanist learning which spread throughout Europe.

Rickets Disorder of infancy and early childhood, caused by lack of vitamin D, resulting in softened and misshapen bones.

Royal Society Founded in London in 1660, the Royal Society is a fellowship of eminent scientists and is one of the oldest scientific acadamies in continuous existence.

Shamanic Refers to spiritual systems in which specialists (shamans) consult with the spirit world in order to maintain and restore balance within and between individuals.

Simple Medicine composed of only one constituent, especially of one herb or plant; hence, a plant or herb employed for medical purposes.

Still A specially constructed apparatus for distillation, in which heated liquid is placed and from which its vapour is extracted.

Strangled by the mother A disorder of the uterus, a disease previously thought only to affect women, producing a sense of fullness in the abdomen and chest with difficulty breathing or choking, later described as hysteria (the word 'mother' here means womb).

Succedanea The legitimate substitutes used by apothecaries when the herbs recommended by the physician were unavailable.

Sympathetic remedy A remedy which is believed to act by some form of affinity or correspondence with the disease or complaint suffered.

Techne Art, skill, craft or method by which something is created.

Theriac An ancient medicinal preparation with many ingredients, used as an antidote to poisons and also as a panacea against all diseases.

Tisane A wholesome or medicinal drink, originally made with barley, and subsequently made as an infusion with herbs.

Unguentum An ointment.

Bibliography

Manuscript sources

British Library, London, UK

Western Manuscripts. Barthollomew Glanvill. *De proprietatibus rerum*, in 19 books; translated into English by John de Trevisa.

National Archives, Kew, UK

Prerogative Court of Canterbury Wills. Will of Elizabeth Okeover, 1670 (registered copy).

Oxfordshire Record Office, Oxford, UK

Deeds for Parishes in South-east Oxfordshire. Gift [Charter of Ralph Russel].

Staffordshire Record Office, Stafford, UK

The Stafford Family Collection: Jerningham Papers. Medical Recipe Book, late seventeenth century.

Wellcome Library, London, UK

Western MS 169. Recipe Book of Elizabeth Bulkeley [1627].
Western MS 751. Sleigh, Elizabeth and Felicia Whitfeld. Collection of Medical Receipts, with Some Cookery Receipts, 1647–1722.
Western MSS 3712 and 7391. Recipe Books of the Okeover Family, c. 1675–c. 1725.

Printed Primary Sources

Amigues, Suzanne, ed. *Théophraste: Recherches sur les plantes*. 5 vols. Paris: Les Belles Lettres, 1988–2006.
Arons, Wendy. *When Midwifery Became the Male Physician's Province: The Sixteenth Century Handbook: The Rose Garden for Pregnant Women and Midwives*. London: McFarland, 1994.
Avicenna. *Liber tertius naturalium. De generatione et corruptione*. Translated by S. van Riet and introduction by Gérard Verbeke. Leiden: Brill, 1987.

Best, Michael R., and Frank H. Brightman, eds. *The Book of Secrets of Albertus Magnus of the Virtues of Herbs, Stones and Certain Beasts*. Revised ed. Boston: Samuel Weiser, 1999.

Boudon-Millot, Véronique, and Jacques Jouanna, eds. *Ne pas se chagriner/Galien*. Paris: Belles Lettres, 2010.

Bourgeois, Louise. *Observations diuerses, sur la sterilité, perte de fruict, foecondité, accouchements, et maladies des femmes*. Paris: A. Sougrain, 1609.

Brock, Arthur J., ed. *Galen. On the Natural Faculties*. Cambridge, MA: Harvard University Press, 1916.

Brodin, Gösta, ed. *Agnus Castus: A Middle English Herbal Reconstructed from Various Manuscripts*. Vol. 6. Essays and Studies on English Language and Literature. Uppsala: Lundequist, 1950.

A Calendar of Grants of Probate and Administration and of Other Testamentary Records of the Commissary Court of the Venerable the Dean and Chapter of Westminster... 1504–1858. London, 1864.

Calendar of the Close Rolls... Vol. 3 Richard II. A.D. 1385–1389. London: HMSO, 1921.

[Calendar of the] Close Rolls Preserved in the Public Record Office... Henry III, A.D. 1227–[1272]. London: HMSO, 1902–38.

Carmichael, Alexander, ed. *Carmina Gadelica: Hymns and Incantations with Illustrative Notes on Words, Rites and Customs, Dying and Obsolete: Orally Collected in the Highlands and Islands of Scotland and Translated into English*. 2nd ed. Vol. II. Edinburgh: Oliver and Boyd, 1928.

Castelveltro, Giacomo. *The Fruit, Herbs and Vegetables of Italy: An Offering to Lucy, Countess of Bedford*. Translated by Gillian Riley. London: Viking, 1989.

A Catalogue of the Plants Growing in the University of Oxford Botanic Garden and Harcourt Arboretum. Oxford: University of Oxford Botanic Garden, 1999.

Chamberlayne, Thomas. *The Complete Midwife's Practice Enlarged*. London: Printed for Obadiah Blagrave, 1680.

Cockayne, Thomas O. *Leechdoms, Wortcunning and Starcraft of Early England*. 3 vols. London: Kraus Reprint, 1965.

Coleman, Olive, ed. *The Brokerage Book of Southampton, 1443–1444*. Vol. 1. Southampton: Southampton University, 1960.

Coles, William. *The Art of Simpling. An Introduction to the Knowledge and Gathering of Plants*. London: Printed by J. G. for Nathaniel Brook, 1656.

The Compleat Midwifes Practice... By T.C. I.D. M.S. T.B. Practitioners. London: Printed for Nathaniel Brooke at the Angell in Cornhill, 1656.

Conybeare, Frederick C., ed. *Letters and Exercises of the Elizabethan Schoolmaster John Conybeare: Schoolmaster at Molton, Devon, 1580 and at Swimbridge, 1594*. London: Henry Frowde, 1905.

Craster, Herbert H. E., and Mary E. Thornton, eds. *The Chronicle of St. Mary's Abbey, York, from Bodley MS. 39*. Vol. CXLVIII. Durham: Surtees Society, 1934.

Culpeper, Nicholas. *Culpeper's Complete Herbal*. London: W. Foulsham and Co, n.d.

—*A Physical Directory or a Translation of the London Dispensatory, Made by the College of Physicians in London*. London: Printed for Peter Cole, 1649.

—*A Physical Directory, or, a Translation of the Dispensatory Made by the Colledge of Physitians of London*. London: Printed by Peter Cole, 1650.

—*A Directory for Midwives, or, a Guide for Women, in Their Conception, Bearing and Suckling Their Children*. London: Printed by Peter Cole, 1651.

—*Semeiotica Uranica or, an Astrological Judgment of Diseases from the Decumbiture of the Sick*. London: Printed for Nathaniell Brookes, 1651.
—*The English Physician*. London: W. Bentley, 1652.
—*The English Physitian*. London: Printed by Peter Cole, 1652.
—*Galen's Art of Physick*. London: Printed by Peter Cole, 1652.
—*The English Physitian Enlarged*. London: Printed by Peter Cole, 1653.
—*Pharmacopoeia Londinensis; or, the London Dispensatory*. London: Printed for Peter Cole, 1653.
Culpeper's Complete Herbal: A Book of Natural Remedies for Ancient Ills. Ware: Wordsworth Editions, 1995.
D'Alechamps, Jacques. *Historia generalis plantarum*. Lugdini: Apud Gulielmum Rouillium, 1586.
D'Aronco, Maria A., and M. L. Cameron, eds. *The Old English Illustrated Pharmacopoeia: British Library Cotton Vitellius C III*. Copenhagen: Rosenkilde and Bagger, 1998.
Dawson, Warren R., ed. *A Leechbook or Collection of Medical Recipes of the Fifteenth Century: The Text of Ms. No. 136 of the Medical Society of London, Together with a Transcript into Modern Spelling*. London: Macmillan, 1934.
De Lacy, Phillip, ed. *Galen: On the Elements According to Hippocrates*. Vol. 5, part 1. Corpus Medicorum Graecorum. Berlin: Akademie Verlag, 1996.
Diaz del Castillo, Bernal. *The True History of the Conquest of Mexico*. Translated by Maurice Keatinge. New York: Robert M. McBride, 1927.
Dioscorides. *Pedanius Dioscorides of Anazarbus De materia medica*. Translated by Lily Y. Beck. Hildesheim: Olms, 2005.
—*Pedanius Dioscorides of Anazarbus De materia medica*. Translated by Lily Y. Beck. Altertumswissenschaftliche Texte und Studien, 2nd revised and enlarged ed. Vol. 38. Hildesheim: Olms, 2011.
Dodoens, Rembert. *A New Herbal, or Historie of Plants*. Translated by Henry Lyte. London: Edward Griffin, 1619.
Dr. Chamberlain's Midwifes Practice. London: Printed for Thomas Rooks, 1665.
Edelstein, Emma J. and Ludwig Edelstein. *Asclepius: A Collection and Interpretation of the Testimonies*. Baltimore, MD: Johns Hopkins University Press, 1998.
Emmison, Frederick G. *Elizabethan Life: Wills of Essex Gentry and Merchants Proved in the Prerogative Court of Canterbury*. Chelmsford: Essex County Council, 1978.
—ed. *Essex Wills. The Bishop of London's Commissary Court, 1569–1578*. Vol. 9 (no. 127). Chelmsford: Essex Record Office, 1994.
—ed. *Essex Wills: The Bishop of London's Commissary Court, 1578–1588*. Vol. 10 (no. 129). Chelmsford: Essex Record Office, 1995.
—ed. *Essex Wills: The Archdeaconry Courts, 1591–1597*. Vol. 6 (no. 114). Chelmsford: Essex Record Office, 1998.
—ed. *Essex Wills: The Bishop of London's Commissary Court, 1587–1599*. Vol. 11 (no. 137). Chelmsford: Essex Record Office, 1998.
Empericus, Marcellus. *Marcellus über Heilmittel*. Corpus Medicorum Latinorum; 5. Edited by Max Niedermann. 2 vols. Berlin: Akademie-Verlag, 1968.
Erotianus. *Erotiani vocum Hippocraticarum collectio: Cum fragmentis*. Edited by Ernst Nachmanson. Uppsala: Appelbergs Boktryckeri, 1918.
Estienne, Charles. *L'agriculture et maison rustique*. Paris: For Iaques Du-Puys, 1564.
—*Maison rustique, or the Countrie Farme*. London: Edm. Bollifant for Bonham Norton, 1600.

Evans, Arthur H., ed. *Turner on Birds*. Kessinger reprint ed. Cambridge: Cambridge University Press, 1903.
Fabricius, Cajus. *Galens Exzerpte aus älteren Pharmakologen*. Berlin: De Gruyter, 1972.
Foster, Brian, ed. *The Local Port Book of Southampton for 1435-36*. Vol. 7, Southampton Record Series. Southampton: Southampton University, 1963.
Foster, Charles W., ed. *Final Concords of the County of Lincoln from the Feet of Fines Preserved in the Public Record Office*. Vol. II. Lincoln: Lincoln Record Society, 1920.
Frisk, Gösta, ed. *A Middle English Translation of Macer Floridus' De viribus herbarum*. Vol. 3, Essays and Studies on English Language and Literature. Uppsala: Lundequist, 1949.
Fuchs, Leonhart. *De historia stirpium*. Basileae: In Officina Isingriniana, 1545.
Furnivall, F. J., ed. *The Fyrst Boke of the Introduction of Knowledge Made by Andrew Borde, of Physycke Doctor: A Compendyous Regyment; or, a Dyetary of Helth Made in Mountpyllier*. London: Published for the Early English Text Society, by N. T. Trübner and Co., 1870.
Galen. *Claudii Galeni opera omnia*. Edited by Carolus G. Kühn. Leipzig: C. Cnobloch, 1821-33.
Gerard, John. *The Herball or, Generall Historie of Plantes*. London: Edm. Bollifont for John Norton, 1597.
—*The Herball or Generall Historie of Plantes... Very Much Enlarged and Amended by Thomas Iohnson Citizen and Apothecarye of London*. London: Printed by Adam Islip, Ioice Norton and Richard Whitakers, 1633.
—*The Herbal: Or, General History of Plants, the Complete 1633 Edition*. Edited by Thomas D. Johnson. New York: Dover Publications, 1975.
Getz, Faye M., ed. *Healing and Society in Medieval England: A Middle English Translation of the Pharmaceutical Writings of Gilbertus Anglicus*. Madison, WI: University of Wisconsin Press, 1991.
Goodyer, John. *The Greek Herbal of Dioscorides*. Edited by Robert T. Gunther. Oxford: Oxford University Press, 1934.
Grant, Mark, ed. *Galen: On Food and Diet*. London: Routledge, 2002.
Green, Monica H., ed. *The Trotula: A Medieval Compendium of Women's Medicine*. Philadelphia: University of Pennsylvania Press, 2001.
Green, Robert M. *A Translation of Galen's Hygiene: (De sanitate tuenda)*. Springfield, IL: Charles C. Thomas, 1951.
The Grete Herball. Southwark: Peter Treueris for L. Andrewe, 1529.
Guillemeau, Jacques. *Child-birth, or, the Happie Deliverie of Women*. London: A. Hatfield, 1612.
—*Child-birth; or, the Happy Delivery of Women*. 2nd ed. London: Anne Griffin, for Ioyce Norton and Richard Whitaker, 1635.
Harrison, William. *The Description of England: The Classic Contemporary Account of Tudor Life*. Edited by Georges Edelen. New ed. Washington: Folger Shakespeare Library and Dover Publications, 1994.
Harvey, Gideon. *The Family Physician and the House Apothecary*. London: T. Rooks, 1676.
Heimat- und Kulturverein Lorsch. *Das Lorscher Arzneibuch: Klostermedizin in der Karolingerzeit; ausgewählte Texte und Beiträge*. Lorsch, Germany: Laurissa, 2002.
Henslow, George. *Medical Works of the Fourteenth Century: Together with a List of Plants Recorded in Contemporary Writings, with Their Identifications*. London: Chapman and Hall, 1899.

Herridge, D. M., ed. *Surrey Probate Inventories, 1558–1603*. Vol. 39. Surrey Record Society Publications (New Series). Woking: Surrey Record Society, 2005.
Hieatt, Constance B., and Sharon Butler, eds. *Curye on Inglysch: English Culinary Manuscripts of the Fourteenth Century (Including the Forme of Cury)*. London: Published for The Early English Text Society by the Oxford University Press, 1985.
Hill, Thomas. *A Most Briefe and Pleasaunte Treatise, Teachyng How to Dresse, Sowe and Set a Garden*. London: John Day, 1558.
—*The Proffitable Art of Gardening*. London: Thomas Marshe, 1568.
—*The Gardeners Labyrinth*. London: Henry Bynneman, 1577.
—*The Proffitable Art of Gardening: Now the Third Tyme Set Fourth*. London: Henry Bynneman, 1579.
Hippocrate. Vol. 13. Des lieux dans l'homme [and other works]. Translated by Robert Joly. Paris: Belles Lettres, 1978.
Hippocrates. Vol. I. Translated by W. H. S. Jones. London: William Heinemann, 1972.
—*Vol. II*. Translated by W. H. S. Jones. Cambridge, MA: Harvard University Press, 1981.
—*Vol. IV*. Translated by W. H. S. Jones. Cambridge, MA: Harvard University Press, 1979.
—*Vol. V*. Translated by Paul Potter. Cambridge, MA: Harvard University Press, 1988.
—*Vol. VI*. Translated by Paul Potter. Cambridge, MA: Harvard University Press, 1988.
—*Vol. VII*. Translated by Wesley D. Smith. London: William Heinemann, 1994.
—*Vol. VIII*. Translated by Paul Potter. Cambridge, MA: Harvard University Press, 1995.
Hodgett, Gerald A. J., ed. *The Cartulary of Holy Trinity, Aldgate*. Leicester: London Record Society, 1971.
Hunger, F. W. T., ed. *The Herbal of Pseudo-Apuleius: From the Ninth-Century Manuscript in the Abbey of Monte Cassino (Codex Casinensis 97)*. Leiden: Brill, 1935.
Hunt, Tony. *Popular Medicine in Thirteenth-Century England: Introduction and Texts*. Cambridge: D. S. Brewer, 1990.
Hunt, Tony, and Michael Benskin, eds. *Three Receptaria from Medieval England: The Languages of Medicine in the Fourteenth Century*. Oxford: The Society for the Study of Medieval Languages and Literature, 2001.
Jacques, Jean-Marie, ed. *Oeuvres. Tome 2: Les thériaques, fragments iologiques antérieures à Nicandre*. Paris: Les Belles Lettres, 2002.
Johnstone, Ian, and G. H. R. Horsley, eds. *Method of Medicine/Galen*. 3 vols, Loeb Classical Library. Cambridge, MA: Harvard University Press, 2011.
Jones, W. H. S., ed. *The Medical Writings of Anonymus Londinensis*. Cambridge: Cambridge University Press, 1947.
Jouanna, Jacques, ed. *La nature de l'homme/Hippocrate*. Vol. I, parts 1, 3, Corpus Medicorum Graecorum. Berlin: Akademie-Verlag, 1975.
Laing, David, ed. *Registrum Domus de Soltre necnon Ecclesie Collegiate S. Trinitatis prope Edinburgh... Charters of the Hospital of Soltre, of Trinity College, Edinburgh and Other Collegiate Churches in Mid-Lothian*. Vol. 109. Edinburgh: Bannatyne Club, 1861.
Larkey, Sanford V., and Thomas Piles, eds. *An Herbal [1525] Edited and Transcribed into Modern English*. New York: Scholars Facsimiles and Reprints, 1941.
Lawson, William. *A New Orchard and Garden: with, The Country-Houswifes Garden*. London: Bar. Alsop for Roger Jackson, 1618. Facsimile edition, with an introduction by Malcolm Thick. Totnes: Prospect Books, 2003.
Littré, Emile, ed. *Oeuvres complètes d'Hippocrate*. Vol. 8. Paris: J. B. Baillière, 1839 [–1861].

Manly, John M., and Edith Rickert, eds. *The Text of the Canterbury Tales Studied on the Basis of All Known Manuscripts. Vol. 4. Text and Critical Notes, Part 2*. Chicago: University of Chicago Press, 1940.

Markham, Gervase. *The English Husbandman*. London: T. S. for John Browne, 1613.

—*Maison rustique, or, the Countrey Farme*. London: Adam Islip for John Bill, 1616.

Marland, Hilary, ed. *Mother and Child Were Saved: The Memoirs (1693–1740) of the Frisian Midwife, Catharina Schrader*. Amsterdam: Rodopi, 1987.

Marwick, James D., ed. *Extracts from the Records of the Burgh of Edinburgh. A.D. 1403–1528*. Edinburgh: Printed for the Scottish Burgh Records Society, 1869.

Mascall, Leonard. *A Booke of the Arte and Maner, Howe to Plant and Graffe All Sortes of Trees*. London: Henrie Denham for John Wight, 1572.

Matthioli, Pietro A. *Commentarii, in libros sex Pedacii Dioscoridis Anazarbei, De materia medica*. Venice: In Officina Erasmiana, apud Vincentium Valgrisium, 1554.

Mauriceau, François. *The Diseases of Women with Child*. Translated by Hugh Chamberlen. London: Printed by John Darby, sold by R. Clavel, W. Cooper, Benjamin Billingsley and W. Cadman, 1672.

—*The Accomplisht Midwife*. London: J. Darby for B. Billingsley, 1673.

May, Margaret T., ed. *Galen, on the Usefulness of the Parts of the Body*. 2 vols. Ithaca, NY: Cornell University Press, 1968.

Meyer, Frederick G., Emily E. Trueblood, and John L. Heller, eds. *The Great Herbal of Leonhart Fuchs: De historia stirpium commentarii insignes, 1542*. Vol. 2, reprint, facsimile. Stanford: Stanford University Press, 1999.

Morris, Richard, ed. *Liber cure cocorum*. Berlin: Published for the Philological Society by A. Asher and Co., 1862.

Mowat, J. L. G., ed. *Sinonoma Bartholomei: A Glossary from a Fourteenth-Century Manuscript in the Library of Pembroke College, Oxford*. Anecdota Oxoniensia, Medieval and Modern Series. Vol. 1, part 1. Oxford: Clarendon Press, 1882.

—ed. *Alphita: A Medico-Botanical Glossary from the Bodleian Manuscript, Selden B.35*. Anecdota Oxoniensia, Medieval and Modern Series. Vol. 1, part 2. Oxford: Clarendon Press, 1887.

Napier, Robina, ed. *A Noble Boke off Cookry ffor a Prynce Houssolde or Eny Other Estately Houssholde Reprinted Verbatim from a Rare Ms. In the Holkham Collection*. London: Elliot Stock, 1882.

Nicholson, Marjorie H., ed. *Conway Letters: The Correspondence of Anne, Viscountess Conway, Henry More and Their Friends, 1642–1684*. New Haven, CT: Yale University Press, 1930.

Ogden, Margaret S., ed. *The Cyrurgie of Guy De Chauliac. [Volume I Text]*. Vol. 265, Early English Text Society Series. London: Published for the Early English Text Society by the Oxford University Press, 1971.

Paré, Ambroise. *The Workes of That Famous Chirurgion Ambrose Parey*. Translated by Thomas Johnson. London: Printed by Thomas Cotes and R. Young, 1634.

—*The Works of That Famous Chirurgeon, Ambroise Parey*. Translated by Th. Johnson. London: Printed by Mary Clark and to be sold by John Clark, 1678.

Parkinson, John. *Paradisi in sole paradisus terrestris*. London: H. Lownes and R. Young, 1629.

—*Theatrum botanicum: The Theater of Plants, or, an Herball of a Large Extent*. London: Tho. Cotes, 1640.

Partliz, Simeon. *A New Method of Physick, or, a Short View of Paracelsus and Galen's Physic*. Translated by Nicholas Culpeper. London: Peter Cole, 1654.

Pegge, Samuel. *The Forme of Cury: A Roll of Ancient English Cookery Compiled, About A.D. 1390*. London: J. Nichols, 1780.
Pettit, Edward. *Anglo-Saxon Remedies, Charms and Prayers from British Library MS Harley 585, the Lacnunga*. 2 vols. Lewiston, NY: Edwin Mellen Press, 2001.
Plato. *Charmides*. Translated by Donald Watt. In *Early Socratic Dialogues*, edited by Trevor J. Saunders. Harmondsworth: Penguin, 1987.
—*The Symposium*. Translated by Walter Hamilton. First published 1951. Harmondsworth: Penguin, 1972.
Pliny the Elder. *Natural History. Vol. 1 Preface and Books I–II*. Translated and edited by H. Rackham. Cambridge, MA: Harvard University Press, 1949.
—*Natural History: In Ten Volumes. Vol. 6 Libri XX–XXIII*. Translated by W. H. S. Jones. Cambridge, MA: Harvard University Press, 1969.
—*Natural History: In Ten Volumes. Vol. 7 Libri XXIV–XXVII*. 2nd ed. Translated by W. H. S. Jones. Cambridge, MA: Harvard University Press, 1956.
Powell, Owen, ed. *Galen: On the Properties of Foodstuffs*. Cambridge: Cambridge University Press, 2003.
Power, Eileen, ed. *The Goodman of Paris (Le ménagier de Paris): A Treatise on Moral and Domestic Economy by a Citizen of Paris c. 1393*. [London]: The Folio Society, 1992.
The Queens Closet Opened. London: Nathaniel Brook, 1655.
Raynalde, Thomas. *The Birth of Mankind: Otherwise Named the Woman's Book*. Edited by Elaine Hobby. Farnham: Ashgate, 2009.
Record Commissioners. *Rotuli hundredorum: temp. Hen. III. and Edw. I. In Turr' Lond' et in curia receptæ scaccarij Westm. Asservati*. Vol. 2. London: George Eyre and Andrew Strahan, 1818.
Rivière, Lazare. *The Practice of Physick in Seventeen Several Books*. Translated by Nicholas Culpeper, Abdiah Cole and William Rowland. London: Printed by Peter Cole, 1655.
Rösslin, Eucharius. *The Byrth of Mankynde Newly Translated out of Laten into Englysshe*. Translated by Richard Jonas. London: T[homas] R[aynald], 1540.
Royal College of Physicians of London. *Pharmacopœia Londinensis*. London: Printed [by E. Griffin] for Iohn Marriot and are to be sould at his shop in Fleetstreete in St Dunstons Churchyarde, 1618.
Ruf, Jakob. *The Expert Midwife, or an Excellent and Most Necessary Treatise of the Generation and Birth of Man*. London: Printed by E. Griffin for S. Burton, 1637.
Salter, Herbert E., ed. *The Feet of Fines for Oxfordshire, 1195–1291*. Vol. 12. Oxford: Oxford Record Society, 1930.
Schneider, Reinhard, ed. *Kapitularien*. Historische Texte Mittelalter 5. Göttingen: Vandenhoeck and Ruprecht, 1968.
Scully, Terence, ed. *The Viandier of Taillevent: An Edition of All Extant Manuscripts by Taillevent*. Ottawa: University of Ottawa Press, 1988.
Sennert, Daniel. *Practical Physick*. Translated by Nicholas Culpeper. London: Printed by Peter Cole and Edward Cole, 1661.
Sermon, William. *The Ladies Companion or the English Midwife*. London: Edward Thomas, 1671.
Sharp, Jane. *The Midwives Book, or, the Whole Art of Midwifry Discovered*. Edited by Elaine Hobby. New York: Oxford University Press, 1999.
Sharp, J. E. E. S., ed. *Calendar of Inquisitions Post Mortem and Other Analogous Documents Preserved in the Public Record Office. Vol. I. Henry III*. London: His Majesty's Stationery Office, 1904.

Sharpe, Reginald R., ed. *Calendar of Letter-Books in the City of London*. London: J. E. Francis, 1899.

Singer, P. N., ed. *Galen: Selected Works*. Oxford: Oxford University Press, 1997.

Stone, Eric, ed. *Oxfordshire Hundred Rolls of 1279*. [Oxford]: Oxfordshire Record Society, 1968.

Strype, John. *Annals of the Reformation and Establishment of Religion and Other Various Occurrences in the Church of England, During Queen Elizabeth's Happy Reign*. 3 vols. Oxford: Clarendon Press, 1824.

Thomas, Arthur H., ed. *Calendar of the Plea and Memoranda Rolls Preserved among the Archives of the Corporation of the City of London at the Guildhall*. Vol. 1. Cambridge: The University Press, 1926.

Thornton, Alice. *The Autobiography of Mrs. Alice Thornton of East Newton, Co. York*. Edited by Charles Jackson. Durham: Andrews for Surtees Society, 1875.

Turner, William. *Libellus de re herbaria, 1538: [and] the Names of Herbes, 1548*. Facsimiles with introductory matter. Edited by James Britten, B. Daydon Jackson and W. T. Stearn. London: The Ray Society, 1965.

—*A New Herball*. London: Steven Mierdman [1551].

—*A Booke of the Natures and Properties... of... Bathes*. Cologne [1562/1568].

—*The Seconde Parte of William Turners Herball*. Cologne: Arnold Birckman [1562].

—*A Book of Wines... [a Facsimile of the Edition of 1568.]*. Edited by Sanford V. Larkey and Philip M. Wagner. New York: Scholars' Facsimiles and Reprints, 1941.

—*The First and Seconde Partes of the Herbal of William Turner Doctor in Phisick Lately Oversene, Corrected and Enlarged*. Cologne: By [the heirs of] Arnold Birckman, [1568].

—*A New Herball, Part 1*. Vol. 1. Edited by George T. L. Chapman and Marilyn N. Tweddle and with indexes compiled by Frank McCombie. Cambridge: Cambridge University Press, 1995.

—*A New Herball, Parts II and III*. Edited by George T. L. Chapman, Frank McCombie and Anne U. Wesencraft. Cambridge: Cambridge University Press, 1995.

Van Arsdall, Anne. *Medieval Herbal Remedies: The Old English Herbarium and Anglo-Saxon Medicine*. New York: Routledge, 2002.

Vicary, Thomas. *The Anatomie of the Bodie of Man*. Edited by F. J. Furnivall and P. Furnivall. London: Early English Text Society, 1888.

Wallner, Björn, ed. *The Middle English Translation of Guy de Chauliac's Treatise on 'Apostemes': Book II of the Great Surgery/Edited from MS. New York Academy of Medicine 12 and Related MSS*. Lund: Lund University Press, 1988-9.

Wellmann, Max, ed. *Pedanii Dioscuridis Anazarbei De materia medica libri quinque*. 3 vols. Berlin: Weidmann, 1906-14.

Willughby, Percival. *Observations in Midwifery: As Also the Country Midwifes Opusculum or Vade Mecum*. Edited by Henry Blenkinsop. Warwick: H. T. Cooke, 1863.

Wolveridge, James. *Speculum matricis; or, the Expert Midwives Handmaid*. London: Printed by E. Okes, sold by Rowland Reynolds, 1671.

Wright, M. R., ed. *Empedocles, the Extant Fragments*. London: Bristol Classical Press, 1995.

Wright, Thomas, ed. *The Latin Poems Commonly Attributed to Walter Mapes*. London: Printed for the Camden Society, by John Bowyer Nichols and Son, 1841.

Zink, Michel, ed. *Oeuvres complètes. [Rutebeuf]*. 2 vols. Paris: Bordas, 1990.

Secondary Sources

Adams, Michael, Wandana Alther, Michael Kessler, Martin Kluge, and Matthias Hamburger. 'Malaria in the Renaissance: Remedies from European Herbals from the 16th and 17th Century'. *Journal of Ethnopharmacology* 133, no. 2 (2011): 278–88.

Adams, Michael, Caroline Berset, Michael Kessler, and Matthias Hamburger. 'Medicinal Herbs for the Treatment of Rheumatic Disorders – a Survey of European Herbals From the 16th and 17th Century'. *Journal of Ethnopharmacology* 121, no. 3 (2009): 343–59.

Adamson, Melitta W. *Food in Medieval Times*. Westport, CT: Greenwood Press, 2004.

Addyman, Marie. *William Turner: Father of English Botany*. Morpeth: Castle Morpeth Borough Council, 2008.

—*Physic and Philosophy: William Turner's Botanical Medicine* (forthcoming).

Albuquerque, Ulysses P. de, and Natalia Hanazaki. *Recent Developments and Case Studies in Ethnobotany*. Recife, Pernambuco, Brazil: Sociedade Brasileira de Etnobiologia [and] Núcleo de Publicações em Eclogia e Etnobotânica Aplicada, 2010.

Al-Ghazal, Sharif K. 'The Influence of Islamic Philosophy and Ethics on the Development of Medicine During the Islamic Renaissance'. *Journal of the International Society for the History of Islamic Medicine* 3, no. 6 (2004): 3–9.

Aliotta, Giovanni. *Le piante medicinali del corpus Hippocraticum*. Milan and Naples: Guerini e Associati; Istituto Italiano per gli Studi Filosofici, 2003.

Allahghadri, Tolou, Iraj Rasooli, Parviz Owlia, Mohammadreza J. Nadooshan, Tooba Ghazanfari, Massoud Taghizadeh, and Shakiba D. A. Astaneh. 'Antimicrobial Property, Antioxidant Capacity and Cytotoxicity of Essential Oil from Cumin Produced in Iran'. *Journal of Food Science* 75, no. 2 (2010): H54–61.

Allen, David E., and Gabrielle Hatfield. *Medicinal Plants in Folk Tradition: An Ethnobotany of Britain and Ireland*. Portland: Timber Press, 2004.

Anawalt, Patricia R. 'The Emperor's Cloak: Aztec Pomp, Toltec Circumstances'. *American Antiquity* 55, no. 2 (1990): 291–307.

Anaya Muñoz, Alejandro. 'The Emergence and Development of the Politics of Recognition of Cultural Diversity and Indigenous Peoples' Rights in Mexico: Chiapas and Oaxaca in Comparative Perspective'. *Journal of Latin American Studies* 37 (2005): 585–610.

Anderson, Robert. 'The Efficacy of Ethnomedicine: Research Methods in Trouble'. *Medical Anthropology* 13, no. 1–2 (1991): 1–17.

André, Jacques. *Les noms de plantes dans la Rome antique*. Paris: Belles Lettres, 1985.

Andrews, Alfred C. 'The Carrot as a Food in the Classical Era'. *Classical Philology* 44, no. 3 (1949): 182–96.

—'Hyssop in the Classical Era'. *Classical Philology* 56, no. 4 (1961): 230–48.

Arber, Agnes. *Herbals, Their Origin and Evolution: A Chapter in the History of Botany, 1470–1670*. 3rd ed. Cambridge: Cambridge University Press, 1986.

Arikha, Noga. *Passions and Tempers: A History of the Humours*. New York: Harper Perennial, 2007.

Arkell, Tom. 'Interpreting Probate Inventories'. In *When Death Us Do Part*, edited by Tom Arkell, Nesta Evans and Nigel Goose, 72–102. Oxford: Leopard's Head Press, 2000.

—'The Probate Process'. In *When Death Us Do Part*, edited by Tom Arkell, Nesta Evans and Nigel Goose, 3–13. Oxford: Leopard's Head Press, 2000.

Arkell, Tom, Nesta Evans, and Nigel Goose, eds. *When Death Us Do Part*. Oxford: Leopard's Head Press, 2000.
Aspin, Richard. 'Who Was Elizabeth Okeover?'. *Medical History* 44, no. 4 (2000): 531–40.
Atkinson, Colin B., and William P. Stoneman. '"These Gripping Greefes and Pinching Pangs": Attitudes to Childbirth, in Thomas Bentley's *The Monument of Matrones* (1582)'. *The Sixteenth Century Journal* 21, no. 2 (1990): 193–203.
Atran, Scott. *The Cognitive Foundations of Natural History*. Cambridge: Cambridge University Press, 1990.
Avila, Elena. *Woman Who Glows in the Dark: A Curandera Reveals Traditional Aztec Health Secrets of Physical and Spiritual Health*. New York: Putnam, 1998.
Bakx, Keith. 'The "Eclipse" of Folk Medicine in Western Society'. *Sociology of Health and Illness* 13, no. 1 (1991): 20–38.
Baldwin, Barry. 'The Career and Works of Scribonius Largus'. *Rheinisches Museum für Philologie* 135 (1992): 75–82.
Baldwin, Martha. 'Review of *Nicholas Culpeper: English Physician and Astrologer*, by Olav Thulesius'. *Journal of the History of Medicine and Allied Sciences* 49, no. 1 (1994): 120–2.
Ball, Philip. *The Devil's Doctor: Paracelsus and the World of Renaissance Magic and Science*. London: W. Heinemann, 2006.
Bardsley, Charles W. E. *English Surnames: Their Sources and Significations*. 2nd ed. London: Chatto and Windus, 1875.
Barnard, John, D. F. McKenzie, and Maureen Bell, eds. *The Cambridge History of the Book in Britain. Vol. 4, 1557–1695*. Cambridge: Cambridge University Press, 2002.
Bartram, Thomas. *Bartram's Encyclopedia of Herbal Medicine*. London: Robinson, 1998.
Baugh, G. C., ed. *A History of Shropshire. Vol. 4. Agriculture*. The Victoria History of the Counties of England. Oxford: Oxford University Press for the Institute of Historical Research, 1989.
Beagon, Mary. *Roman Nature: The Thought of Pliny the Elder*. Oxford: Clarendon Press, 1992.
Beccaria, Augusto. *I codici di medicina del periodo presalernitano (secoli IX, X, e XI)*. Storia e Letteratura. Rome: Edizioni di Storia e Letteratura, 1956.
Beith, Mary. *Healing Threads: Traditional Medicines of the Highlands and Islands*. Repr. 1995 ed. Edinburgh: Polygon, 2004.
Benedek, Thomas G. 'The Changing Relationship between Midwives and Physicians During the Renaissance'. *Bulletin of the History of Medicine* 51, no. 4 (1977): 550–64.
Bennett, Henry S. *English Books and Readers, 1475 to 1557: Being a Study in the History of the Book Trade from Caxton to the Incorporation of the Stationers' Company*. Cambridge: Cambridge University Press, 1952.
—*Life on the English Manor: A Study of Peasant Conditions 1150–1400*. Cambridge: Cambridge University Press, 1960.
Bergdolt, Klaus. *Wellbeing: A Cultural History of Healthy Living*. Translated by Jane Dewhurst. Cambridge: Polity, 2008.
Bierbaumer, Peter, and Helmut W. Klug, eds. *Old Names – New Growth: Proceedings of the Second Anglo Saxon Plant Name Society Conference, University of Graz, 6–10 June 2007*. Frankfurt: Peter Lang, 2009.
Biller, Peter, and Joseph Ziegler, eds. *Religion and Medicine in the Middle Ages*. Woodbridge: York Medieval Press in association with Boydell Press, 2001.
Bivins, Roberta. 'Histories of Heterodoxy'. In *The Oxford Handbook of the History of Medicine*, edited by Mark Jackson, 578–97. Oxford: Oxford University Press, 2011.

Black, Jeremy, and Donald D. MacRaild. *Studying History*. 2nd ed. Basingstoke: Palgrave, 2000.
Blanton, Richard E., Stephen A. Kowalewski, Gary M. Feinman, and Laura M. Finsten. *Ancient Mesoamerica: A Comparison of Change in Three Regions*. 2nd ed. Cambridge: Cambridge University Press, 1993.
Blumenthal, Mark, Alicia Goldberg, and Josef Brinkman, eds. *Herbal Medicine: Expanded Commission E Monographs*. Austin, TX: American Botanical Council, 2000.
Blunt, Wilfrid, and Sandra Raphael. *The Illustrated Herbal*. New York: Metropolitan Museum of Art, 1979.
Blunt, Wilfrid, and William T. Stearn. *The Art of Botanical Illustration*. Revised 1994 ed. Woodbridge: Antique Collectors' Club in association with Royal Botanic Gardens, 1950.
Bober, Phyllis P. *Art, Culture and Cuisine: Ancient and Medieval Gastronomy*. Chicago: University of Chicago Press, 1999.
Bone, Kerry. *A Clinical Guide to Blending Liquid Herbs: Herbal Formulations for the Individual Patient*. St Louis, MO: Churchill Livingstone, 2003.
Bone, Kerry, and Simon Mills. *The Principles and Practice of Phytotherapy: Modern Herbal Medicine*. Edinburgh: Churchill Livingstone, 2000.
Bonser, Wilfrid. *The Medical Background of Anglo-Saxon England: A Study in History, Psychology and Folklore*. London: Wellcome Historical Medical Library, 1963.
Borah, Woodrow. *New Spain's Century of Depression*. Berkeley: University of California Press, 1951.
Brooks, Chandler M., Jerome L. Gilbert, Harold A. Levey, and David R. Curtis. *Humors, Hormones and Neurosecretions: The Origins and Development of Man's Present Knowledge of the Humoral Control of Body Function*. New York: State University of New York, 1962.
Browner, Carole H. 'Criteria for Selecting Herbal Remedies'. *Ethnology* 24, no. 1 (1985): 13–32.
Browner, Carole H., Bernard Ortiz de Montellano, and Arthur J. Rubel. 'A Methodology for Cross-Cultural Ethnomedical Research'. *Current Anthropology* 29, no. 5 (1988): 681–9.
Brumfiel, Elizabeth M. 'Agricultural Development and Class Stratification in the Southern Valley of Mexico'. In *Land and Politics in the Valley of Mexico*, edited by H. R. Harvey, 43–61. Albuquerque, NM: University of New Mexico Press, 1991.
— 'Weaving and Cooking: Women's Production in Aztec Mexico'. In *Engendering Archaeology*, edited by Joan M. Gero and Margaret Conkey, 224–51. Oxford: Basil Blackwell, 1991.
Brunton, Deborah, ed. *Health, Disease and Society in Europe 1800–1930: A Source Book*. Manchester: Manchester University Press in association with the Open University, 2004.
Bryce, Derek, ed. *The Herbal Remedies of the Physicians of Myddfai*. Felinfach, Wales: Llanerch Enterprises, 1988.
Buenz, Eric J., Brent A. Bauer, Holly E. Johnson, Gaugau Tavana, Eric M. Beekman, Kristi L. Frank, and Charles L. Howe. 'Searching Historical Herbal Texts for Potential New Drugs'. *British Medical Journal* 333, no. 7582 (2006): 1314–15.
Burnby, Juanita. 'The Herb Women of the London Markets'. *Pharmaceutical Historian* 13, no. 1 (1983): 5–6.
— *A Study of the English Apothecary from 1660–1760*. Medical History Supplement, vol. 3. London: Wellcome Institute for the History of Medicine, 1983.

Burnham, John C. *What Is Medical History?* Cambridge: Polity, 2005.
Bushnell, Rebecca. *Green Desire: Imagining Early Modern English Gardens.* New York: Cornell University Press, 2003.
Bynum, W. F., and Helen Bynum, eds. *Dictionary of Medical Biography.* 5 vols. Westport, CT: Greenwood Press, 2007.
Calixto, Joao B. 'Twenty-Five Years of Research on Medicinal Plants in Latin America: A Personal View'. *Journal of Ethnopharmacology* 100, no. 1-2 (2005): 131-4.
Cameron, Donald. *The Field of Sighing: A Highland Boyhood.* Edinburgh: Birlinn, 2003.
Cameron, M. L. 'The Sources of Medical Knowledge in Anglo-Saxon England'. *Anglo-Saxon England* 11 (1982): 135-55.
Camp, Anthony J. *Wills and Their Whereabouts.* 4th ed. London: A. J. Camp, 1974.
Campbell, John L. *Edward Lhuyd in the Scottish Highlands, 1699-1700.* Oxford: Clarendon Press, 1963.
Camporesi, Piero. *The Incorruptible Flesh: Bodily Mutation and Mortification in Religion and Folklore.* Translated by Tania Croft-Murray. Cambridge: Cambridge University Press, 1988.
—*Bread of Dreams: Food and Fantasy in Early Modern Europe.* Translated by David Gentilcore. Cambridge: Polity Press in association with B. Blackwell, 1989.
Carlin, Martha, and Joel T. Rosenthal, eds. *Food and Eating in Medieval Europe.* London: Hambledon, 1998.
Carlson, Thomas J. S., and Luisa Maffi. *Ethnobotany and Conservation of Biocultural Diversity.* Bronx, NY: New York Botanical Garden Press, 2004.
Cave, Roy C., and Herbert Henry Coulson. *A Source Book for Medieval Economic History.* New York: Biblo and Tannen, 1965.
Chance, Burton. 'Seventeenth Century Ophthalmology as Gleaned from Works of Nicholas Culpeper Physician-Astrologer (1616-1653)'. *Journal of the History of Medicine and Allied Sciences* 8, no. 2 (1953): 197-209.
Chapman, Anne C. 'Port of Trade Enclaves in Aztec and Maya Civilizations'. In *Trade and Market in the Early Empires: Economies in History and Theory*, edited by Karl Polanyi, Conrad M. Arensberg and Harry W. Pearson, 114-53. New York: Free Press, 1957.
Chapman, George T. L. 'William Turner of Morpeth, Northumberland (1508-1568)'. *The Scottish Naturalist* (1986): 11-27.
Cheng, Eileen K. *Historiography: An Introductory Guide.* London: Continuum, 2012.
Chevallier, Andrew. *The Encyclopedia of Medicinal Plants.* London: Dorling Kindersley, 1996.
Christie, John R. R. 'The Paracelsian Body'. In *Paracelsus: The Man and His Reputation, His Ideas and Their Transformations*, edited by Ole P. Grell, 269-91. Leiden: Brill, 1998.
Christopher, John R. *School of Natural Healing.* Provo, UT: Bi-World Publishers, 1976.
Clark, Alice. *Working Life of Women in the Seventeenth Century.* 3rd ed. London: Routledge, 1992.
Clark, George. *A History of the Royal College of Physicians of London.* Vol. 1. Oxford: Clarendon Press for the Royal College of Physicians, 1964.
Cockayne, Oswald. *Spoon and Sparrow, Spendein and Psar, Fundere and Passer: Or, English Roots in the Greek, Latin and Hebrew.* London: Parker, Son and Bourn, 1861.
Collins, Harry M. *Changing Order: Replication and Induction in Scientific Practice.* Chicago: University of Chicago Press, 1992.
—*Tacit and Explicit Knowledge.* Chicago: University of Chicago Press, 2010.

Collins, Minta. *Medieval Herbals: The Illustrative Traditions*. London: British Library, 2003.
Colquhoun, Kate. *Taste: The Story of Britain through Its Cooking*. London: Bloomsbury, 2007.
Connolly, Peter. *The Ancient City: Life in Classical Athens and Rome*. Oxford: Oxford University Press, 1998.
Conrad, Lawrence I., Michael Neve, Vivian Nutton, Roy Porter, and Andrew Wear. *The Western Medical Tradition: 800 BC to AD 1800*. Cambridge: Cambridge University Press, 1995.
Conway, Peter. *Tree Medicine: A Comprehensive Guide to the Healing Power of Over 170 Trees*. London: Piatkus, 2001.
—*The Consultation in Phytotherapy: The Herbal Practitioner's Approach to the Patient*. Edinburgh: Churchill Livingstone, 2010.
Cook, Harold J. *Trials of an Ordinary Doctor: Joannes Groenevelt in Seventeenth-Century London*. Baltimore, MD: Johns Hopkins University Press, 1994.
Cooper, Alix. *Inventing the Indigenous: Local Knowledge and Natural History in Early Modern Europe*. Cambridge: Cambridge University Press, 2007.
Cooper, Marion R., and Anthony W. Johnson. *Poisonous Plants and Fungi in Britain: Animal and Human Poisoning*. London: Stationery Office, 1998.
Cooter, Roger. '"Framing" the End of the Social History of Medicine'. In *Locating Medical History: The Stories and Their Meanings*, edited by Frank Huisman and John H. Warner, 310–37. Baltimore, MD: Johns Hopkins University Press, 2004.
—ed. *Studies in the History of Alternative Medicine*. Basingstoke: Macmillan in association with St Antony's College, Oxford, 1988.
Copenhaver, Brian P. 'Natural Magic, Hermetism and Occultism'. In *Reappraisals of the Scientific Revolution*, edited by David C. Lindberg and Robert S. Westman, 261–302. Cambridge: Cambridge University Press, 1990.
Cowan, Ian B., and David E. Easson. *Medieval Religious Houses, Scotland*, 2nd ed. London: Longman, 1976.
Cox, Jeff, and Nancy Cox. 'Probate 1500–1800: A System in Transition'. In *When Death Us Do Part*, edited by Tom Arkell, Nesta Evans and Nigel Goose, 14–37. Oxford: Leopard's Head Press, 2000.
Creamer, Winifred. 'Mesoamerica as a Concept: An Archaeological View from Central America'. *Latin American Research Review* 22, no. 1 (1987): 35–62.
Crellin, John K. 'Revisiting Eve's Herbs: Reflections on Therapeutic Uncertainties'. In *Herbs and Healers from the Ancient Mediterranean through the Medieval West: Essays in Honour of John M. Riddle*, edited by Anne Van Arsdall and Timothy Graham, 307–28. Farnham: Ashgate, 2012.
Cressy, David. *Birth, Marriage, and Death: Ritual, Religion and the Life-Cyle in Tudor and Stuart England*. Oxford: Oxford University Press, 1997.
Cronier, Marie. 'Recherches sur l'histoire du texte du De materia medica de Dioscoride'. Unpublished PhD thesis, University of Paris IV–Sorbonne, 2007.
Crossley, Alan, ed. *A History of the County of Oxford, Vol. 12. Woolton Hundred (South), Including Woodstock*. The Victoria History of the Counties of England. Oxford: Published for the Institute of Historical Research by Oxford University Press, 1990.
Culbreth, David M. R. *A Manual of Materia Medica and Pharmacology*. Philadelphia: Lea Brothers and Co., 1906.
Cunningham, Anthony B. *Applied Ethnobotany: People, Wild Plant Use and Conservation*. London: Earthscan, 2001.

Curry, Patrick. *Prophecy and Power: Astrology in Early Modern England*. Cambridge: Polity Press, 1989.
Curtin, Leonora S. M. *Healing Herbs of the Upper Rio Grande*. Los Angeles: Southwest Museum, 1965.
Curtin, Philip D. 'Overspecialization and Remedies'. In *The Backbone of History: Health and Nutrition in the Western Hemisphere*, edited by Richard H. Steckel and Jerome C. Rose, 603–8. Cambridge: Cambridge University Press, 2002.
Dalby, Andrew. *Cheese, a Global History*. London: Reaktion, 2009.
D'Aronco, Maria A. 'The Botanical Lexicon of the Old English Herbarium'. *Anglo-Saxon England* 17 (1988): 15–33.
Daston, Lorraine, and Katherine Park. *Wonders and the Order of Nature 1150–1750*. New York: Zone Books, 1998.
Davidson, Alan. *The Oxford Companion to Food*. Oxford: Oxford University Press, 1999.
Davies, Roy W. *Service in the Roman Army*. Edited by David Breeze and Valerie A. Maxfield. Edinburgh: Edinburgh University Press, 1989.
Davis, Peter H., James Cullen, and M. J. E. Coode. *Flora of Turkey and the East Aegean Islands*. Edinburgh: Edinburgh University Press, 1965.
Debru, Armelle, ed. *Galen on Pharmacology: Philosophy, History and Medicine: Proceedings of the Vth International Galen Colloquium, Lille, 16–18 March 1995*. Leiden: Brill, 1997.
Debus, Allen. *The English Paracelsians*. London: Oldbourne, 1965.
—'The Medico-Chemical World of the Paracelsians'. In *Changing Perspectives in the History of Science: Essays in Honour of Joseph Needham*, edited by Mikulas Teich and Robert Young, 85–99. London: Heinemann, 1973.
Deegan, Marylin, and D. G. Scragg. *Medicine in Early Medieval England*. Manchester: University of Manchester Centre for Anglo-Saxon Studies, 1989.
De Groot, Jerome. *Consuming History: Historians and Heritage in Contemporary Popular Culture*. London: Routledge, 2009.
Dendle, Peter, and Alain Touwaide. *Health and Healing from the Medieval Garden*. Woodbridge: Boydell and Brewer, 2008.
De Smet, P. A. G. M., and W. A. Nolen. 'St. John's Wort as an Anti-Depressant'. *British Medical Journal* 313, no. 7052 (1996): 241–2.
De Vos, Paula. 'European Materia Medica in Historical Texts: Longevity of a Tradition and Implications for Future Use'. *Journal of Ethnopharmacology* 132, no. 1 (2010): 28–47.
Drummond, J. C., and Anne Wilbraham. *The Englishman's Food: A History of Five Centuries of English Diet*. Revised by Dorothy Hollingsworth. London: Pimlico, 1991.
Duffin, Jacalyn. *History of Medicine: A Scandalously Short Introduction*. Toronto: University of Toronto Press, 1999.
—*Lovers and Livers: Disease Concepts in History*. Toronto: University of Toronto Press, 2005.
Duffy, Eamon. *The Voices of Morebath: Reformation and Rebellion in an English Village*. New Haven, CT: Yale University Press, 2003.
Duke, James A. *Herbs of the Bible: 2000 Years of Plant Medicine*. Edited by Mary A. Telatnik. Loveland, CO: Interweave Press, 1999.
Dvorkin, L., P. Gardiner, and J. S. Whelan. 'Herbal Medicine Course within [the] Pharmacy Curriculum'. *Journal of Herbal Pharmacotherapy* 4, no. 2 (2004): 47–58.
Dyer, Christopher. *Standards of Living in the Later Middle Ages: Social Change in England, c. 1200–1500*. Cambridge: Cambridge University Press, 1989.

—*Making a Living in the Middle Ages: The People of Britain, 850–1520*. New Haven, CT: Yale University Press, 2002.
Eadie, Mervyn J. 'The Antiepileptic Materia Medica of Pediacus Dioscorides'. *Journal of Clinical Neurosciences* 11, no. 7 (2004): 697–701.
Eamon, William. *Science and the Secrets of Nature: Books of Secrets in Medieval and Early Modern Culture*. Princeton, NJ: Princeton University Press, 1994.
Ebrahimnejad, Hormoz, ed. *Development of Modern Medicine in Non-Western Countries: Historical Perspectives*. Abingdon: Routledge, 2008.
Eccles, Audrey. *Obstetrics and Gynaecology in Tudor and Stuart England*. London: Croom Helm, 1982.
Elmer, Peter, ed. *The Healing Arts: Health, Disease and Society in Europe, 1500–1800: A Source Book*. Manchester: Manchester University Press in association with the Open University, 2004.
Erickson, Amy. 'Using Probate Accounts'. In *When Death Us Do Part*, edited by Tom Arkell, Nesta Evans and Nigel Goose, 103–19. Oxford: Leopard's Head Press, 2000.
Etkin, Nina L. 'Cultural Constructions of Efficacy'. In *The Context of Medicines in Developing Countries: Studies in Pharmaceutical Anthropology*, edited by Sjaak Van der Geest and Susan R. Whyte, 299–327. Dordrecht: Kluwer Academic Publishers, 1988.
—'Ethnopharmacology: Biological and Behavioral Perspectives in the Study of Indigenous Medicine'. In *Medical Anthropology: Contemporary Theory and Method*, edited by Carolyn F. Sargent and Thomas M. Johnson, 149–58. Westport, CT: Praeger, 1996.
—ed. *Eating on the Wild Side: The Pharmacologic, Ecologic and Social Implications of Using Noncultigens*. Tucson, AZ: University of Arizona Press, 1994.
European Herbal and Traditional Medicine Practitioners Association. *The Core Curriculum for Herbal and Traditional Medicine: Producing Safe and Competent Practitioners*. Tewkesbury: EHTPA, 2007.
Evans, Susan T. 'Architecture and Authority in an Aztec Village: Form and Function of the Tecpan'. In *Land and Politics in the Valley of Mexico: A Two Thousand-Year Perspective*, edited by Herbert R. Harvey, 63–92. Albuquerque, NM: University of New Mexico Press, 1991.
Evans, William C. *Trease and Evans' Pharmacognosy*. 14th ed. London: W. B. Saunders, 1998.
Evenden, Doreen. *The Midwives of Seventeenth-Century London*. Cambridge: Cambridge University Press, 2000.
Eyton, R. W. *Antiquities of Shropshire*. Vol. 6. London: John Russell Smith, 1858.
Farnsworth, Norman R. 'The Development of Pharmacological and Chemical Research for Application to Traditional Medicine in Developing Countries'. *Journal of Ethnopharmacology* 2, no. 2 (1980): 173–81.
Farrar, Linda. *Ancient Roman Gardens*. Stroud: Budding Books, 2000.
Featherstone, Cornelia, and Lori Forsyth. *Medical Marriage: The New Partnership between Orthodox and Complementary Medicine*. Findhorn: Findhorn Press, 1997.
Finberg, Herbert P. R. *Tavistock Abbey: A Study in the Social and Economic History of Devon*. Cambridge: Cambridge University Press, 1951.
Findlen, Paula. 'Francis Bacon and the Reform of Natural History in the Seventeenth Century'. In *History and the Disciplines: The Reclassification of Knowledge in Early Modern Europe*, edited by Donald R. Kelley, 239–60. Woodbridge: University of Rochester Press, 1997.
—'The Formation of a Scientific Community: Natural History in Sixteenth-Century Italy'.

In *Natural Particulars: Nature and the Disciplines in Renaissance Europe*, edited by Anthony Grafton and Nancy Siraisi, 369–400. Cambridge, MA: MIT Press, 1999.

Firth, Catherine B. 'Village Gilds of Norfolk in the Fifteenth Century'. *Norfolk Archaeology* 18 (1914): 161–208.

Fissell, Mary E. *Patients, Power and the Poor in Eighteenth-Century Bristol*. Cambridge: Cambridge University Press, 1991.

Flemming, Rebecca. *Medicine and the Making of Roman Women: Gender, Nature and Authority from Celsus to Galen*. Oxford: Oxford University Press, 2000.

Fluckiger, Friedrich A., and Daniel Hanbury. *Pharmacographia: A History of the Principal Drugs of Vegetable Origin, Met with in Great Britain and British India*. London: Macmillan, 1874.

Forbes, Thomas R. 'The Regulation of English Midwives in the Sixteenth and Seventeenth Centuries'. *Medical History* 8, no. 3 (1964): 235–44.

Foster, George M. 'Disease Etiologies in Non-Western Medical Systems'. *American Anthropologist* 78 (1976): 773–82.

—'On the Origin of Humoral Medicine in Latin America'. *Medical Anthropology Quarterly* 1, no. 4 (1987): 355–93.

—*Hippocrates' Latin American Legacy: Humoral Medicine in the New World*. Langhorne, PA: Gordon and Breach, 1994.

Foust, Clifford M. *Rhubarb: The Wondrous Drug*. Princeton, NJ: Princeton University Press, 1992.

Francis, Jill. '"A Ffitt Place for any Gentleman"? Gardens, Gardeners and Gardening in England and Wales, c. 1560–1660'. Unpublished PhD thesis, University of Birmingham, 2011.

Frangos, Constantinos C. 'Towards a Realistic Approach to Medical Biography'. *Journal of Medical Biography* 18, no. 1 (2010): 1.

Fraser, Antonia. *The Weaker Vessel: Woman's Lot in Seventeenth-Century England*. London: Mandarin, 1993.

Freedman, Paul H. *Out of the East: Spices and the Medieval Imagination*. New Haven, CT: Yale University Press, 2008.

Frei, B., M. Heinrich, P. M. Bork, D. Hermann, B. Jaki, T. Kato, M. Kuhnt, J. Schmitt, W. Schuhly, C. Volken, and O. Sticher. 'Multiple Screening of Medicinal Plants from Oaxaca, Mexico: Ethnobotany and Bioassays as a Basis for Phytochemical Investigation'. *Phytomedicine* 5, no. 3 (1998): 177–86.

Furdell, Elizabeth L. *The Royal Doctors: Medical Personnel at the Tudor and Stuart Courts*. Rochester, NY: Rochester University Press, 2001.

—*Publishing and Medicine in Early Modern England*. Rochester, NY: Rochester University Press, 2002.

Furst, Peter T. 'This Little Book of Herbs: Psychoactive Plants as Therapeutic Agents in the Badianus Manuscript of 1552'. In *Ethnobotany: Evolution of a Discipline*, edited by Richard E. Schultes and Siri Von Reis, 108–30. London: Chapman and Hall, 1995.

Gardner-Medwin, David. 'Down the Long Series of Eventful Time'. In *Medicine in Northumbria: Essays in the History of Medicine in the North East of England*, edited by David Gardner-Medwin, Anne Hargreaves and Elizabeth Lazenby, 1–23. Newcastle-upon-Tyne: The Pybus Society for the History and Bibliography of Medicine, 1993.

—'William Turner and Medicine'. Paper presented at Turner 500 and Hancock 200: Naturalists in North-East England, Newcastle University, 6–8 September 2008.

Gelis, Jacques. *History of Childbirth: Fertility, Pregnancy and Birth in Early Modern Europe*. Cambridge: Polity Press, 1991.

Gerhard, Peter. 'Congregaciones de indios en la Nueva España antes de 1570'. *Historia Mexicana* 26, no. 3 (1977): 347–89.
Gerrard, Christopher M. *Medieval Archaeology: Understanding Traditions and Contemporary Approaches*. London: Routledge, 2003.
Gertsch, Jürg. 'How Scientific Is the Science of Ethnopharmacology? Historical Perspectives and Epistemological Problems'. *Journal of Ethnopharmacology* 122, no. 2 (2009): 177–83.
Gibson, Gail M. 'Scene and Obscene: Seeing and Performing Late Medieval Childbirth'. *Journal of Medieval and Early Modern Studies* 21, no. 1 (1999): 7–24.
Gibson, Jeremy S. W. *Wills and Where to Find Them*. 4th ed. Chichester: Phillimore for the British Record Society, 1974.
Gill, Christopher, Tim Whitmarsh, and John Wilkins, eds. *Galen and the World of Knowledge*. Cambridge: Cambridge University Press, 2009.
Giorgetti, Melina G., and Eliana Rodrigues. 'Brazilian Plants with Possible Action on the Central Nervous System – a Study of Historical Sources from the 16th to 19th Century'. *Journal of Ethnopharmacology* 109, no. 19 (2007): 338–47.
Givens, Jean A., Karen M. Reeds, and Alain Touwaide, eds. *Visualizing Medieval Medicine and Natural History, 1200–1500*. Aldershot: Ashgate, 2006.
Glaze, Florence E. 'Prolegomena: Scholastic Openings to Gariopontus of Salerno's Passionarius'. In *Between Text and Patient: The Medical Enterprise in Medieval and Early Modern Europe*, edited by Florence E. Glaze and Brian K. Nance, 57–86. Florence: SISMEL, 2011.
—'Speaking in Tongues: Medical Wisdom and Glossing Practices in and around Salerno, c. 1040–1200'. In *Herbs and Healers from the Ancient Mediterranean through the Medieval West: Essays in Honour of John M. Riddle*, edited by Anne Van Arsdall and Timothy Graham, 63–106. Farnham: Ashgate, 2012.
Glaze, Florence E., and Brian K. Nance, eds. *Between Text and Patient: The Medical Enterprise in Medieval and Early Modern Europe*. Florence: SISMEL, 2011.
Goodman, Jordan, and Vivien Walsh. *The Story of Taxol: Nature and Politics in the Pursuit of an Anti-Cancer Drug*. Cambridge: Cambridge University Press, 2001.
Goose, Nigel, and Nesta Evans. 'Wills as an Historical Source'. In *When Death Us Do Part*, edited by Tom Arkell, Nesta Evans and Nigel Goose, 30–71. Oxford: Leopard's Head Press, 2000.
Gowing, Laura. *Common Bodies: Women, Touch and Power in Seventeenth-Century England*. New Haven, CT: Yale University Press, 2003.
Granshaw, Lindsay, and Roy Porter, eds. *The Hospital in History*. London: Routledge, 1990.
Grant, Edward. *A History of Natural Philosophy: From the Ancient World to the Nineteenth Century*. Cambridge: Cambridge University Press, 2007.
Green, Monica H. *Women's Healthcare in the Medieval West: Texts and Contexts*. Aldershot: Ashgate, 2000.
—'Gendering the History of Women's Healthcare'. *Gender and History* 20, no. 3 (2008): 487–518.
Greene, J. Patrick. *Medieval Monasteries*. Leicester: Leicester University Press, 1992.
Greenslade, Michael W. *The Victoria History of the Counties of England. Vol. 3. A History of the County of Stafford*. London: Oxford University Press for the Institute of Historical Research, 1970.
Grieve, Maud. *A Modern Herbal: The Medicinal, Culinary, Cosmetic and Economic Properties, Cultivation and Folklore of Herbs, Grasses, Fungi, Shrubs and Trees with

All Their Modern Scientific Uses. Edited by C. F. Leyel. Reprint of the 1931 ed. London: Peregrine Books, 1976.
Griggs, Barbara. *Green Pharmacy: A History of Herbal Medicine*. London: Jill Norman and Hobhouse, 1981.
—*New Green Pharmacy*. London: Vermillion, 1997.
Grigson, Geoffrey. *The Englishman's Flora*. Facsimile of 1955 ed. London: Phoenix House, 1987.
Grmek, Mirko D., ed. *Western Medical Thought from Antiquity to the Middle Ages*. Cambridge, MA: Harvard University Press, 1998.
Gutas, Dimitri. *Greek Thought, Arab Culture: The Graeco-Arabic Translation Movement in Baghdad and Early 'Abbāsid Society (2nd-4th/5th-10th c.)*. London: Routledge, 1998.
Guthrie, Douglas. 'Plants as Remedies: The Debt of Medicine to Botany'. *Transactions of the Botanical Society of Edinburgh* 39, no. 2 (1961): 184–95.
Guthrie, William K. C. *A History of Greek Philosophy: The Earlier Presocratics and the Pythagoreans*. Vol. 1. London: Cambridge University Press, 1962.
Hadfield, Miles. *A History of British Gardening*. London: Spring Books, 1960.
Hammond, E. A. 'The Westminster Abbey Infirmarer's Rolls as a Source of Medical History'. *Bulletin of the History of Medicine* 39 (1965): 261–76.
Hammond, Nicholas G. L., ed. *Atlas of the Greek and Roman World in Antiquity*. Park Ridge, NJ: Noyes Press, 1981.
Hanawalt, Barbara A. *The Ties That Bound: Peasant Families in Medieval England*. New York: Oxford University Press, 1986.
Hankinson, R. J., ed. *The Cambridge Companion to Galen*. Cambridge: Cambridge University Press, 2008.
Harig, Georg. *Bestimmung der Intensität im medizinischen System Galens: Ein Beitrag zur theoretiscchen Pharmakologie, Nosologie und Therapie in der Galenischen Medizin*. Berlin: Akademie-Verlag, 1974.
Harkness, Deborah E. *The Jewel House: Elizabethan London and the Scientific Revolution*. New Haven, CT: Yale University Press, 2007.
Harley, David. 'Historians as Demonologists: The Myth of the Midwife-Witch'. *Social History of Medicine Bulletin* 3, no. 1 (1990): 1–26.
—'English Archives, Local History and the Study of Early Modern Midwifery'. *Archives (British Records Association)* 21, no. 92 (1994): 145–54.
Harris, Stephen J., and Bryon L. Grigsby, eds. *Misconceptions About the Middle Ages*. New York: Routledge, 2008.
Harvey, John H. 'Garden Plants of Moorish Spain: A Fresh Look'. *Garden History* 20, no. 1 (1992): 71–82.
—'Westminster Abbey: The Infirmarer's Garden'. *Garden History* 20, no. 2 (1992): 1–97.
—*Mediaeval Gardens*. London: B. T. Batsford, 1981.
Hatfield, Gabrielle. *Country Remedies: Traditional East Anglian Plant Remedies of the Twentieth Century*. Woodbridge: Boydell Press, 1994.
—*Hatfield's Herbal: The Secret History of British Plants*. London: Allen Lane, 2007.
Haycock, David B., and Patrick Wallis. *Quackery and Commerce in Seventeenth-Century London: The Proprietary Medicine Business of Anthony Daffy*. London: The Wellcome Trust Centre for the History of Medicine at UCL, 2005.
Healy, John F. *Pliny the Elder on Science and Technology*. New York: Oxford University Press, 1999.
Heinrich, Michael, Joanne Barnes, Simon Gibbons, and Elizabeth M. Williamson.

Fundamentals of Pharmacognosy and Phytotherapy. Edinburgh: Churchill Livingstone, 2004.
Heinrich, Michael, Johanna Kufer, Marco Leonti and Manuel Pardo-de-Santayana. 'Ethnobotany and Ethnopharmacology – Interdisciplinary Links with the Historical Sciences'. *Journal of Ethnopharmacology* 107, no. 2 (2006): 157–60.
Henderson, Paula. *The Tudor House and Garden: Architecture and Landscape in the Sixteenth and Early Seventeenth Centuries*. London: Yale University Press, 2005.
Henrey, Blanche. *British Botanical and Horticultural Literature before 1800: Comprising a History and Bibliography of Botanical and Horticultural Books Printed in England, Scotland and Ireland from the Earliest Times until 1800. Vol. 1: The Sixteenth and Seventeenth Centuries*. Oxford: Oxford University Press, 1975.
Hensel, Wolfgang. *Medicinal Plants of Britain and Europe*. Black's Nature Guides. London: A. and C. Black, 2008.
Hieatt, Constance B. 'Making Sense of Medieval Culinary Records'. In *Food and Eating in Medieval Europe*, edited by Martha Carlin and Joel T. Rosenthal, 101–16. London: Hambledon, 1998.
—'Medieval Britain'. In *Regional Cuisines of Medieval Europe: A Book of Essays*, edited by Melitta W. Adamson, 19–46. New York: Routledge, 2002.
Higgit, John, ed. *Scottish Libraries*. Vol. 12. Corpus of British Medieval Library Catalogues. London: British Library in association with the British Academy, 2006.
Hili, Pauline, C. S. Evans, and R. G. Veness. 'Antimicrobial Action of Essential Oils: The Effect of Dimethylsulphoxide on the Activity of Cinnamon Oil'. *Letters in Applied Microbiology* 24, no. 4 (1997): 269–75.
Hitchcock, James. 'A Sixteenth-Century Midwife's License'. *Bulletin of the History of Medicine* 41, no. 1 (1967): 75–6.
Holland, Bart K., ed. *Prospecting for Drugs in Ancient and Medieval European Texts: A Scientific Approach*. Amsterdam: Harwood Academic Publishers, 1996.
Hollis, Stephanie. 'The Social Milieu of Bald's Leechbook'. *Avista Forum Journal* 14, no. 1 (2004): 11–16.
Holloway, S. W. F. 'The Year 1000: Pharmacy at the Turn of the First Millennium'. *The Pharmaceutical Journal* 264, no. 7077 (2000): 32–4.
Holman, Joan, and Marion Herridge, eds. *Index of Surrey Probate Inventories: 16th–19th Centuries*. Epsom: Domestic Buildings Research Group, 1986.
Holmes, Urban T. *Daily Living in the Twelfth Century Based on the Observations of Alexander Neckam in London and Paris*. Madison, WI: University of Wisconsin Press, 1952.
Horden, Peregrine. 'What's Wrong with Early Medieval Medicine?'. *Social History of Medicine* 24, no. 1 (2011): 5–25.
House of Lords Select Committee on Science and Technology. *Sixth Report: Complementary and Alternative Medicine*. London: HMSO, 2000.
Howard, Sharon. 'Imagining the Pain and Peril of Seventeenth-Century Childbirth: Travail and Deliverance in the Making of an Early Modern World'. *Social History of Medicine* 16, no. 3 (2003): 367–82.
Hozeski, Bruce W., ed. *Hildegard's Healing Plants: From Her Medieval Classic Physica*. Boston: Beacon Press, 2001.
Huisman, Frank, and John H. Warner, eds. *Locating Medical History: The Stories and Their Meanings*. Baltimore, MD: Johns Hopkins University Press, 2004.
Humphreys, Keith W., ed. *The Friars' Libraries*. Vol. 1. Corpus of British Medieval Library Catalogues. London: British Library in association with the British Academy, 1990.

Hunt, Tony. *Plant Names of Medieval England*. Cambridge: D. S. Brewer, 1989.
Hunter, Michael. *Establishing the New Science: The Experience of the Early Royal Society*. Woodbridge: Boydell Press, 1989.
Hyams, Edward. *A History of Gardens and Gardening*. London: Dent, 1971.
Irving, Miles. *The Forager Handbook: A Guide to the Edible Plants of Britain*. London: Ebury Press, 2008.
Jackson, Mark, ed. *The Oxford Handbook of the History of Medicine*. Oxford: Oxford University Press, 2011.
Jackson, Ralph. *Doctors and Diseases in the Roman Empire*. London: British Museum Press, 1988.
Jackson, Stanley W. *Melancholia and Depression: From Hippocratic Times to Modern Times*. New Haven, CT: Yale University Press, 1986.
Jansen-Sieben, Ria, ed. *Artes mechanicae en Europe medievale en middeleeuws Europa*. Brussels: Archives et bibliothèques de Belgique, 1989.
Jashemski, Wilhelmina F. *The Gardens of Pompeii: Herculaneum and the Villas Destroyed by Vesuvius*. Vols 1 and 2. New Rochelle, NY: Caratzas Bros, 1979, 1993.
—*A Pompeian Herbal: Ancient and Modern Medicinal Plants*. Austin, TX: University of Texas Press, 1999.
Jenner, Mark S. R., and Patrick Wallis. 'The Medical Marketplace'. In *Medicine and the Market in England and Its Colonies, c. 1450–c. 1850*, edited by Mark S. R. Jenner and Patrick Wallis, 1–23. Basingstoke: Palgrave Macmillan, 2007.
Johnson, Francis R. 'Thomas Hill: An Elizabethan Huxley'. *Huntington Library Quarterly* 7, no. 4 (1944): 329–51.
Jones, Whitney R. D. *William Turner: Tudor Naturalist, Physician and Divine*. London: Routledge, 1988.
Jordanova, Ludmilla. 'The Social Construction of Medical Knowledge'. In *Locating Medical History: The Stories and Their Meanings*, edited by Frank Huisman and John H. Warner, 338–63. Baltimore, MD: Johns Hopkins University Press, 2004.
Jotischky, Andrew. *A Hermit's Cookbook: Monks, Food and Fasting in the Middle Ages*. London: Continuum, 2011.
Kassell, Lauren. *Medicine and Magic in Elizabethan London: Simon Forman; Astrologer, Alchemist and Physician*. Oxford: Clarendon Press, 2005.
Kay, Margarita A. 'The Florilegio Medicinal: Source of Southwest Ethnomedicine'. *Ethnohistory* 24, no. 3 (1977): 251–9.
Keevill, Graham, Mick Aston, and Teresa Hall, eds. *Monastic Archaeology: Papers on the Study of Medieval Monasteries*. Oxford: Oxbow Books, 2001.
Keil, Gundolf, and Paul Schnitzer, eds. *Das Lorscher Arzneibuch und die frühmittelalterliche Medizin*. Lorsch: Verlag Laurissa, 1991.
Keiser, George. 'Rosemary: Not Just for Remembrance'. In *Health and Healing from the Medieval Garden*, edited by Peter Dendle and Alain Touwaide, 180–204. Woodbridge: Boydell and Brewer, 2008.
Keller, Hildegard E. and Hubert Steinke. 'Jakob Ruf's *Trostbüchlein* and *De conceptu* (Zürich, 1554): A Textbook for Midwives and Physicians'. In *Scholarly Knowledge: Textbooks in Early Modern Europe*, edited by Emidio Campi, Simone de Angelis, Anja-Silvia Goenig and Anthony Grafton, 307–32. Geneva: Librairie Droz, 2008.
Kennedy, David L., ed. *The Roman Army in the East*. Supplementary Series No. 18. Ann Arbor, MI: Journal of Roman Archaeology, 1996.
Keyser, Paul T., and Georgia Irby-Massie, eds. *The Encyclopaedia of Ancient Natural Scientists: The Greek Tradition and Its Many Heirs*. London: Routledge, 2008.

Kimball, Geoffrey. 'Aztec Homosexuality: The Textual Evidence [New Translation and Study of Florentine Codex]'. *Journal of Homosexuality* 26, no. 1 (1993): 7-24.
King, Helen. *Hippocrates' Woman: Reading the Female Body in Ancient Greece*. London: Routledge, 1998.
King, Steven. 'Accessing Drugs in the Eighteenth-Century Regions'. In *From Physick to Pharmacology: Five Hundred Years of British Drug Retailing*, edited by Louise H. Curth, 49-78. Aldershot: Ashgate, 2006.
Kingsley, Peter. *Ancient Philosophy, Mystery and Magic: Empedocles and Pythagorean Tradition*. Oxford: Clarendon Press, 1995.
Kirchoff, Paul. 'Mesoamerica: Its Geographical Limits, Ethnic Composition and Cultural Characteristics'. In *Heritage of Conquest: The Ethnology of Middle America*, edited by Sol Tax, 17-30. Glencoe: Free Press Publishers, 1952.
Kirk, Geoffrey S., and John E. Raven. *The Presocratic Philosophers: A Critical History with a Selection of Texts*. Cambridge: Cambridge University Press, 1962.
Kitching, Christopher J. 'Probate During the Civil War and Interregnum'. *Journal of the Society of Archivists* 5, no. 5-6 (1976): 283-93, 346-56.
Klebs, Arnold C. 'Balneology in the Middle Ages'. *Transactions of the American Climatological and Clinical Association* 32 (1916): 15-37.
Kleinman, Arthur and Lilias H. Sung. 'Why Do Indigenous Practitioners Successfully Heal?'. *Social Science and Medicine* 13B, no. 1 (1979): 7-26.
Klug, Helmet W., and Roman Weinberger. 'Modding Medievalists: Designing a Web-Based Portal for the Medieval Plant Survey/Portal der Pflanzen Des Mittelalters'. In *Herbs and Healers from the Ancient Mediterranean through the Medieval West: Essays in Honour of John M. Riddle*, edited by Anne Van Arsdall and Timothy Graham, 329-57. Farnham: Ashgate, 2012.
Knight, Leah. *Of Books and Botany in Early Modern England: Sixteenth-Century Plants and Print Culture*. Farnham: Ashgate, 2009.
Laín Entralgo, Pedro. *The Therapy of the Word in Classical Antiquity*. New Haven, CT: Yale University Press, 1970.
Lane, Joan. '"The Doctor Scolds Me": The Diaries and Correspondence of Patients in Eighteenth-Century England'. In *Patients and Practitioners: Lay Perceptions of Medicine in Pre-Industrial Society*, edited by Roy Porter, 205-48. Cambridge and New York: Cambridge University Press, 1985.
—*A Social History of Medicine: Health, Healing and Disease in England, 1750-1950*. London: Routledge, 2001.
Laroche, Rebecca. *Medical Authority and Englishwomen's Herbal Texts, 1550-1650*. Farnham: Ashgate, 2009.
Latimer, John. *Sixteenth-Century Bristol*. Reprint of 1908 ed. Charleston, SC: Bibliolife LLC, 2009.
Laurence, Anne. *Women in England, 1500-1760: A Social History*. London: Weidenfeld and Nicolson, 1994.
Lawless, Julia. *The Encyclopaedia of Essential Oils*. Shaftesbury, Dorset: Element, 1992.
Lawlor, Clark. *From Melancholia to Prozac: A History of Depression*. Oxford: Oxford University Press, 2012.
Leighton, Ann. *Early English Gardens in New England*. London: Cassell, 1970.
Leonard, Dorothy, and Sylvia Sensiper. 'The Role of Tacit Knowledge in Group Innovation'. *California Management Review* 40, no. 3 (1998): 112-32.
Leong, Elaine, and Sara Pennell. 'Recipe Collections and the Currency of Medical Knowledge in the Early Modern "Medical Marketplace"'. In *Medicine and the Market*

in England and Its Colonies, c. 1450–c. 1850, edited by Mark S. R. Jenner and Patrick Wallis, 133–52. Basingstoke: Palgrave Macmillan, 2007.

Leonti, Marco. 'The Future Is Written: Impact of Scripts on the Cognition, Selection, Knowledge and Transmission of Medicinal Plant Use and Its Implications for Ethnobotany and Ethnopharmacology'. *Journal of Ethnopharmacology* 134, no. 3 (2011): 542–55.

Leonti, Marco, Stefano Cabras, Caroline S. Weckerle, Maria N. Solinas, and Laura Casu. 'The Causal Dependence of Present Plant Knowledge on Herbals – Contemporary Medicinal Plant Use in Campania (Italy) Compared to Matthioli (1568)'. *Journal of Ethnopharmacology* 130, no. 2 (2010): 379–91.

Leonti, Marco, Laura Casu, Francesca Sanna, and Leonardo Bonsignore. 'A Comparison of Medicinal Plant Use in Sardinia and Sicily – De Materia Medica Revisited?'. *Journal of Ethnopharmacology* 121, no. 2 (2009): 255–67.

Lewis, Bernard. *The Muslim Discovery of Europe*. London: Weidenfeld and Nicolson, 1982.

Liddell, Henry, and Robert Scott. *An Intermediate Greek-English Lexicon Founded Upon the Seventh Edition of Liddell and Scott's Greek-English Lexicon*. Oxford: Clarendon Press, 1991.

Liddell, Henry G., Robert Scott, and H. Stuart Jones. *A Greek-English Lexicon: A Supplement*. 9th ed. Oxford: Clarendon Press, 1968.

Linde, Klaus, Gilbert Ramirez, Cynthia D. Mulrow, Andrej Pauls, Wolfgang Wedenhammer, and Dieter Melchart. 'St. John's Wort for Depression – an Overview and Meta-Analysis of Randomised Clinical Trials'. *British Medical Journal* 313, no. 7052 (1996): 253–8.

Lindemann, Mary. *Medicine and Society in Early Modern Europe*. Cambridge: Cambridge University Press, 1999.

Little, Andrew G. *The Grey Friars in Oxford*. Oxford: Printed for the Oxford Historical Society at the Clarendon Press, 1892.

Lloyd, Christopher. 'History and the Social Sciences'. In *Writing History: Theory and Practice*, edited by Stefan Berger, Heiko Feldner and Kevin Passmore, 83–103. London: Hodder Arnold, 2003.

Lloyd, Geoffrey E. R. *The Revolutions of Wisdom: Studies in the Claims and Practice of Ancient Greek Science*. Berkeley: University of California Press, 1995.

Lobel, Mary D., ed. *A History of the County of Oxford. Vol. 7. Dorchester and Thame Hundreds*. London: Oxford University Press for the Institute of Historical Research, 1962.

MacKinney, Loren C. *Early Medieval Medicine: With Special Reference to France and Chartres*. 1937 ed. New York: Arno Press, 1979.

MacLean, Ian. *Logic, Signs and Nature in the Renaissance: The Case of Learned Medicine*. Cambridge: Cambridge University Press, 2002.

Maehle, Andreas-Holger. 'Peruvian Bark: From Specific Febrifuge to Universal Remedy'. *Clio Medica* 87 (1999): 223–309.

Magie, David. *Roman Rule in Asia Minor to the End of the Third Century after Christ*. Princeton, NJ and Oxford: Princeton University Press and Oxford University Press, 1950.

Majno, Guido. *The Healing Hand: Man and Wound in the Ancient World*. Cambridge, MA: Harvard University Press, 1975.

Mannish, Lise. *An Ancient Egyptian Herbal*. London: British Museum Publications, 1989.

Marcombe, David. *Leper Knights: The Order of St Lazarus of Jerusalem in England, c. 1150-1544*. Woodbridge: Boydell Press, 2004.
Marganne, Marie-Hélène. 'Les références a l'Égypte dans la *matière médicale* de Dioscoride'. In *Serta Leodiensia secunda: mélanges publiés par les classiques de Liège à l'occasion du 175e anniversaire de l'Université*. 309-22. Liège: Université de Liège, 1992.
Masschaele, James. *Peasants, Merchants and Markets: Inland Trade in Medieval England, 1150-1350*. New York: St. Martin's Press, 1997.
Masson, Madeleine, and Anthony Vaughan, eds. *The Compleat Cook, or Secrets of a Seventeenth-Century Housewife*. London: Routledge and Kegan Paul, 1974.
Matthew, H. C. G., and Brian Harrison, eds. *Oxford Dictionary of National Biography*. Oxford: Oxford University Press, 2004.
Matthews, Leslie G. 'Royal Apothecaries of the Tudor Period'. *Medical History* 8, no. 2 (1964): 170-80.
McCarl, Mary R. 'Publishing the Works of Nicholas Culpeper, Astrological Herbalist and Translator of Latin Medical Works in Seventeenth-Century London'. *Canadian Bulletin of Medical History* 13, no. 2 (1996): 225-76.
McConchie, R. W. *Lexicography and Physicke: The Record of Sixteenth-Century English Medical Terminology*. Oxford: Clarendon Press, 1997.
McLaren, Angus. *Reproductive Rituals: The Perception of Fertility in England from the Sixteenth to the Nineteenth Century*. London: Methuen, 1984.
McLean, Antonia. *Humanism and the Rise of Science in Tudor England*. London: Heinemann Educational, 1972.
McLean, G. R. D. *Poems of the Western Highlanders: From the Gaelic*. London: S. P. C. K., 1961.
McLean, Teresa. *Medieval English Gardens*. London: Barrie and Jenkins, 1989.
McQuay, T. A. I. 'Childbirth Deaths in Shipton-under-Wychwood, 1565-1665'. *Local Population Studies* 42 (1989): 54-6.
McVaugh, Michael R. *Medicine before the Plague: Practitioners and Their Patients in the Crown of Aragon 1285-1345*. Cambridge: Cambridge University Press, 1993.
Meaney, Audrey L. 'Variant Versions of Old English Medical Remedies and the Compilation of Bald's Leechbook'. *Anglo-Saxon England* 13 (December 1984): 235-68.
Medeiros, Maria F., and Ulysses P. de Albuquerque. 'The Pharmacy of the Benedictine Monks: The Use of Medicinal Plants in Northeast Brazil During the Nineteenth Century (1823-1829)'. *Journal of Ethnopharmacology* 139, no. 1 (2012): 280-6.
Mills, Simon. *Out of the Earth: The Essential Book of Herbal Medicine*. London: Arkana, 1991.
Mills, Simon, and Kerry Bone. *The Essential Guide to Herbal Safety*. St Louis, MO: Elsevier/Churchill Livingstone, 2005.
Minter, Sue. *The Apothecaries Garden: A History of Chelsea Physic Garden*. Stroud: Sutton, 2000.
Mitchell, Piers D. *Medicine in the Crusades: Warfare, Wounds and the Medieval Surgeon*. Cambridge: Cambridge University Press, 2004.
Moffat, Brian. 'A Curious Assemblage of Seeds from a Pit at Waltham Abbey, Essex: A Study of Medieval Medication'. *Essex Archaeology and History* 18 (1987): 121-3.
—'Investigations into Medieval Medical Practice: The Remnants of Some Herbal Treatments, on Archaeological Sites and in Archives'. In *Medicine in Early Medieval England: Four Papers*, edited by Marilyn Deegan and D. G. Scragg, 33-40. Manchester: University of Manchester Centre for Anglo-Saxon Studies, 1989.

—'The Seeds of Narcosis in Medieval Medicine: The Prehistory of Anaesthesia in Practice?'. *The History of Anaesthesia Society Proceedings* 22 (1999): 7–12.
—'"A Marvellous Plant": The Place of the Heath Pea in the Scottish Ethnobotanical Tradition'. *Folio (National Library of Scotland)* 1 (Autumn 2000): 13–15.
—ed. *SHARP Practice 1. First Report on Researches into the Medieval Hospital at Soutra, Lothian*. Fala: SHARP, 1986.
—ed. *SHARP Practice 2: The Second Report on Researches into the Medieval Hospital at Soutra, Lothian Region*. Edinburgh: SHARP, 1988.
—ed. *SHARP Practice 3: The Third Report on Researches into the Medieval Hospital at Soutra, Lothian/Borders Region, Scotland*. Edinburgh: SHARP, 1989.
—ed. *SHARP Practice 4: Fourth Report on Researches into the Medieval Hospital at Soutra, Lothian Region, Scotland*. Edinburgh: SHARP, 1992.
—ed. *SHARP Practice 5: The Fifth Report on Researches into the Medieval Hospital at Soutra, Lothian/Borders Region, Scotland*. Edinburgh: SHARP, 1995.
—ed. *SHARP Practice 6. The Sixth Report on Researches into the Medieval Hospital at Soutra, Scottish Borders/Lothian, Scotland*. Fala: SHARP, 1998.
Moody, Joanna. *The Private Life of an Elizabethan Lady: The Diary of Lady Margaret Hoby 1599–1605*. Stroud: Sutton, 1998.
Moore, Michael. *Los Remedios: Traditional Herbal Remedies of the Southwest*. Santa Fe, NM: Red Crane Books, 1990.
Mortimer, Ian. *The Dying and the Doctors: The Medical Revolution in Seventeenth-Century England*. Woodbridge: Royal Historical Society/Boydell, 2009.
Morton, Leslie T., and Robert J. Moore. *A Bibliography of Medical and Biomedical Biography*. 2nd ed. Aldershot: Scholar Press, 1994.
Moulinier, Laurence. 'Abbesse et agronome: Hildegarde et le savoir botanique de son temps'. In *Hildegard of Bingen: The Context of Her Thought and Art*, edited by Charles Burnett and Peter Dronke, 135–56. London: Warburg Institute, University of London, 1998.
Musselman, Lytton J. *A Dictionary of Bible Plants*. Cambridge: Cambridge University Press, 2011.
Nahin, Richard L., P. M. Barnes, B. J. Stussman, and B. Bloom. 'Costs of Complementary and Alternative Medicine Use and Frequency of Visits to CAM Practitioners: United States 2007'. *National Health Statistics Reports* 18 (2009): 1–14.
Nartey, L., K. Huwiler-Müntener, A. Shang, K. Liewald, P. Jüni, and M. Egger. 'Matched-Pair Study Showed Higher Quality of Placebo-Controlled Trials in Western Phytotherapy Than Conventional Medicine'. *Journal of Clinical Epidemiology* 60, no. 8 (2007): 787–94.
Nauert, Charles G., Jr. 'Humanists, Scientists and Pliny: Changing Approaches to a Classical Author'. *The American Historical Review* 84, no. 1 (1979): 72–85.
Nelson, George A. 'William Turner's Contribution to the First Records of British Plants'. In *Proceedings of the Leeds Philosophical and Literary Society, Scientific Section*, 109–38. Leeds: Leeds Philosophical and Literary Society, 1959.
Newall, Carol A., Linda A. Anderson, and J. David Phillipson. *Herbal Medicines: A Guide for Healthcare Professionals*. 2nd ed. London: Pharmaceutical Press, 2002.
Newman, William R., and Anthony Grafton. *Secrets of Nature: Astrology and Alchemy in Early Modern Europe*. Cambridge, MA: MIT Press, 2001.
Nigenda, Gustavo, Lejeune Lockett, Cristina Manca, and Gerardo Mora. 'Non-Biomedical Health Care Practices in the State of Morelos, Mexico: Analysis of an Emergent Phenomenon'. *Sociology of Health and Illness* 23, no. 1 (2001): 3–23.

Norri, Juhani. *Names of Sicknesses in English, 1400–1550: An Exploration of the Lexical Field.* Helsinki: Suomalainen Tiedeakatemia, 1992.
Nutton, Vivian. 'Humoralism'. In *Companion Encyclopedia of the History of Medicine*, edited by W. F. Bynum and Roy Porter, 281–91. London: Routledge, 1993.
—'Scribonius Largus, the Unknown Pharmacologist'. *Pharmaceutical Historian* 25, no. 1 (1995): 5–8.
—'The Rise of Medical Humanism: Ferrara, 1464–1555'. *Renaissance Studies* 11, no. 1 (1997): 2–19.
—*Ancient Medicine.* London: Routledge, 2004.
—ed. *The Unknown Galen.* London: Institute of Classical Studies, University of London, 2002.
O'Dowd, Michael J. *The History of Medications for Women: Materia Medica Woman.* New York: Parthenon Publishing Group, 2001.
Ody, Penelope. *Complete Guide to Medicinal Herbs.* New York: Dorling Kindersley, 1993.
Ogilvie, Brian W. *The Science of Describing: Natural History in Renaissance Europe.* Chicago: University of Chicago Press, 2006.
O'Hara-May, Jane. 'Foods or Medicines? A Study in the Relationship between Foodstuffs and materia medica from the Sixteenth to the Nineteenth Century'. *Transactions of the British Society for the History of Pharmacy* 1, no. 2 (1971): 61–97.
Opie, Ionie, and Moira Tatem. *A Dictionary of Superstitions.* Oxford: Oxford University Press, 1989.
Ortiz de Montellano, Bernard. 'Empirical Aztec Medicine: Aztec Medicinal Plants Seem to Be Effective If They Are Judged by Aztec Standards'. In *Ancient and Modern Medical Practices in Mesoamerica*, edited by Bernard Ortiz de Montellano, 18–22. Greeley: University of Northern Colorado, 1982.
—*Aztec Medicine, Health, and Nutrition.* New Brunswick, NJ: Rutgers University Press, 1990.
Ortiz de Montellano, Bernard, and Carole H. Browner. 'Chemical Bases for Medicinal Plant Use in Oaxaca, Mexico'. *Journal of Ethnopharmacology* 13, no. 1 (1985): 57–88.
Ouweneel, Arij. 'From *tlahtocayotl* to *gobernadoryotl*: A Critical Examination of Indigenous Rule in 18th-Century Mexico'. *American Ethnologist* 22, no. 4 (1995): 756–85.
Overton, Mark, Jane Whittle, Darron Dean, and Andrew Hann. *Production and Consumption in English Households, 1600–1750.* London: Routledge, 2004.
Ovesen, Jan, and Ing-Britt Trankell. *Cambodians and Their Doctors: A Medical Anthropology of Colonial and Postcolonial Cambodia.* Copenhagen: NIAS, 2012.
Page, William. *The Victoria History of the Counties of England. Vol. 2. A History of the County of Oxford.* London: Constable, 1907.
Palmer, Roy. 'In Our Lyghte and Learned Tyme'. In *The Medicinal History of Waters and Spas*, edited by Roy Porter. Medical History Supplement No. 10, 14–22. London: Wellcome Institute for the History of Medicine, 1990.
Pardo de Santayana, Manuel, Andrea Pieroni, and Rajindra K. Puri, eds. *Ethnobotany in the New Europe: People, Health and Wild Plant Resources.* New York: Berghahn Books, 2010.
Parkinson, Anna. *Nature's Alchemist: John Parkinson, Herbalist to Charles I.* London: Frances Lincoln, 2007.
Parsons, J. R. 'The Role of Chinampa Agriculture in the Food Supply of Aztec Tenochtitlan'. In *Cultural Change and Continuity: Essays in Honor of James Bennett Griffin*, edited by Charles E. Cleland, 233–58. New York: Academic Press, 1976.

Pavord, Anna. *The Naming of Names: The Search for Order in the World of Plants.* London: Bloomsbury, 2005.
Pearsall, Judy, ed. *The New Oxford Dictionary of English.* Oxford: Oxford University Press, 1998.
Peck, Harry T. *Harper's Dictionary of Classical Antiquities.* London: Harper and Brothers, 1898.
Peck, Linda L. *Consuming Splendor: Society and Culture in Seventeenth-Century England.* Cambridge: Cambridge University Press, 2005.
Pelling, Margaret. *The Common Lot: Sickness, Medical Occupations and the Urban Poor in Early Modern England.* London: Longman, 1998.
—*Medical Conflicts in Early Modern London: Patronage, Physicians and Irregular Practitioners 1550–1640.* Oxford: Clarendon, 2003.
Pelling, Margaret, and Charles Webster. 'Medical Practitioners'. In *Health, Medicine and Mortality in the Sixteenth Century,* edited by Charles Webster, 165–235. Cambridge: Cambridge University Press, 1979.
Pennell, Sara. 'Material Culture, Micro-Histories and the Problem of Scale'. In *History and Material Culture: A Student's Guide to Approaching Alternative Sources,* edited by Karen Harvey, 173–91. London: Routledge, 2009.
—ed. *Women and Medicine: Remedy Books, 1533–1865: From the Wellcome Library for the History and Understanding of Medicine, London.* Reading: Primary Source Microfilm, Thomson Gale, 2004.
Pennington, David. 'Beyond the Moral Economy: Economic Change, Ideology and the 1621 House of Commons'. *Parliamentary History* 25, no. 2 (2006): 214–31.
Petit, C. 'Theorie et pratique: connaissance et diffusion du traité des Simples de Galien au Moyen Age'. In *Fito-zooterapia antigua y altomedieval: Textos y doctrinas,* edited by Arsenio Ferraces Rodriguez, 79–95. Coruña: Universidade da Coruña, 2009.
Pettegree, Andrew. *Foreign Protestant Communities in Sixteenth-Century London.* Oxford: Clarendon Press, 1986.
Pietroni, Patrick. *The Greening of Medicine.* London: Gollancz, 1990.
Pitman, Vicki. *The Nature of the Whole: Holism in Ancient Greek and Indian Medicine.* Delhi: Motilal Barnasidass, 2006.
Pollard, Tanya. *Drugs and Theater in Early Modern England.* Oxford: Oxford University Press, 2005.
Pollington, Stephen. *Leechcraft: Early English Charms, Plant Lore and Healing.* Norfolk: Anglo-Saxon Books, 2000.
Pollock, Linda A. *With Faith and Physic: The Life of a Tudor Gentlewoman, Lady Grace Mildmay, 1552–1620.* London: Collins and Brown, 1993.
—'Childbearing and Female Bonding in Early Modern England'. *Social History* 22, no. 3 (1997): 286–306.
Pormann, Peter, and Emilie Savage-Smith. *Medieval Islamic Medicine.* Edinburgh: Edinburgh University Press, 2007.
Porter, Enid. *Cambridgeshire Customs and Folklore: With Fenland Material Provided by W. H. Barrett.* London: Routledge and Kegan Paul, 1969.
Porter, Roy. *The Greatest Benefit to Mankind: A Medical History of Humanity from Antiquity to the Present.* London: Fontana Press, 1999.
—ed. *Patients and Practitioners: Lay Perceptions of Medicine in Pre-Industrial Society.* Cambridge: Cambridge University Press, 1985.
—ed. *The Medical History of Waters and Spas.* Medical History Supplement No. 10. London: Wellcome Institute for the History of Medicine, 1990.

Potterton, David, ed. *Culpeper's Color Herbal.* New York: Sterling Publishing, 1983.
Poynter, F. N. L. 'Nicholas Culpeper and His Books'. *Journal of the History of Medicine and Allied Sciences* XVII, no. 1 (1962): 152–67.
Pressman, Jack D. 'Concepts of Mental Illness in the West'. In *The Cambridge World History of Human Disease,* edited by Kenneth F. Kiple, 59–85. Cambridge: Cambridge University Press, 1993.
Priest, Albert W., and Lilian R. Priest. *Herbal Medication: A Clinical and Dispensary Handbook.* Saffron Walden: C. W. Daniel Company, 2000.
Radden, Jennifer, ed. *The Nature of Melancholy: From Aristotle to Kristeva.* Oxford: Oxford University Press, 2000.
Rappaport, Steven. *Worlds within Worlds: Structures of Life in Sixteenth-Century London.* Cambridge: Cambridge University Press, 1989.
Raskin, Ilya, David M. Ribnicky, Slavko Komarnytsky, Nebojsa Ilic, Alexander Poulev, Nikolai Borisjuk, Anita Brinker, Diego A. Morenoa, Christophe Ripolla, Nir Yakobya, Joseph M. O'Neal, Teresa Cornwell, Ira Pastor, and Bertold Fridlender. 'Plants and Human Health in the Twenty-First Century'. *Trends in Biotechnology* 20, no. 12 (2002): 522–31.
Raven, Charles E. *Early Naturalists from Neckam to Ray: A Study of the Making of the Modern World.* Cambridge: Cambridge University Press, 1947.
Raven, John E. *Plants and Plant Lore in Ancient Greece.* Oxford: Leopard's Head Press, 2000.
Rawcliffe, Carole. *The Hospitals of Medieval Norwich.* Studies in East Anglian History, vol. 2. Norwich: Centre of East Anglian Studies, University of East Anglia, 1995.
—*Medicine and Society in Later Medieval England.* Stroud: Sutton, 1995.
—'"On the Threshold of Eternity": Care for the Sick in East Anglian Monasteries'. In *East Anglia's History: Studies in Honour of Norman Scarfe,* edited by Christopher Harper-Bill, Carole Rawcliffe and Richard G. Wilson, 41–72. Woodbridge: Boydell Press, 2002.
—*Leprosy in Medieval England.* Woodbridge: Boydell and Brewer, 2006.
—'"Delectable Sightes and Fragrant Smelles": Gardens and Health in Late Medieval and Early Modern England'. *Garden History* 36, no. 1 (2008): 3–21.
Reeds, Karen M. *Botany in Medieval and Renaissance Universities.* New York: Garland, 1991.
—'Saint John's Wort (*Hypericum perforatum* L.) in the Age of Paracelsus and the Great Herbals: Assessing the Historical Claims for a Traditional Remedy'. In *Herbs and Healers from the Ancient Mediterranean through the Medieval West: Essays in Honour of John M. Riddle,* edited by Anne Van Arsdall and Timothy Graham, 265–305. Farnham: Ashgate, 2012.
Reid, Daniel P. *Chinese Herbal Medicine.* Wellingborough: Thorsons, 1987.
Renner, S. S., J. Scarborough, H. Schaefer, H. S. Paris, and J. Janick. 'Dioscorides's *bruonia melaina* Is *Bryonia alba,* Not *Tamus communis* and an Illustration Labeled *bruonia melaina* in the *Codex Vindobonensis* Is *Humulus lupulus* Not *Bryonia dioica*'. In *Proceedings of the IXth EUCARPIA Meeting on Genetics and Breeding of Cucurbitaceae,* edited by M. Pitrat, 273–80. Avignon: Inra, Centre de Recherche d'Avignon, Génétique et Amélioration des Fruits et Légumes, Montfavet (France), 2008.
Reverby, Susan M., and David Rosner. '"Beyond the Great Doctors" Revisited: A Generation of the "New" Social History of Medicine'. In *Locating Medical History: The Stories and Their Meanings,* edited by Frank Huisman and John H. Warner, 167–93. Baltimore, MD: Johns Hopkins University Press, 2004.

Riddell, John N. D. 'John Parkinson's Long Acre Garden 1600-1650'. *Journal of Garden History* 6, no. 2 (1986): 112-24.
Riddle, John M. 'Dioscorides'. In *Catalogus translationum et commentariorum: Mediaeval and Renaissance Latin Translations and Commentaries: Annotated Lists and Guides, Vol. 4*, edited by F. Edward Cranz and Paul O. Kristeller, 1-143. Washington, DC: Catholic University of America Press, 1980.
—*Dioscorides on Pharmacy and Medicine*. Austin, TX: University of Texas Press, 1985.
—*Eve's Herbs: A History of Contraception and Abortion in the West*. Cambridge: Harvard University Press, 1997.
—'Research Procedures in Evaluating Medieval Medicine'. In *The Medieval Hospital and Medical Practice*, edited by Barbara S. Bowers, 3-18. Aldershot: Ashgate, 2007.
—*A History of the Middle Ages, 300-1500*. Lanham, MD: Rowman and Littlefield, 2008.
—*Goddesses, Elixirs and Witches: Plants and Sexuality Throughout Human History*. New York: Palgrave Macmillan, 2010.
Robbins, Rossel H. 'Science and Information in English Writings of the Fifteenth Century'. *Modern Language Review* 39 (1944): 1-8.
Roberts, R. S. 'The Personnel and Practice of Medicine in Tudor and Stuart England. Part II: London'. *Medical History* 8, no. 3 (1964): 217-33.
Rocco, Fiametta. *The Miraculous Fever Tree: Malaria, Medicine and the Cure That Changed the World*. New York: HarperCollins, 2003.
Rohde, Eleanour S. *The Old English Herbals*. Reprint of the 1922 ed. New York: Dover Publications, 1971.
—*Shakespeare's Wild Flowers, Fairy Lore, Gardens, Herbs, Gatherers of Simples and Bee Lore*. London: Medici Society, 1935.
—*Herbs and Herb Gardening*. London: Medici Society, 1936.
Saad, Bashar, and Omar Said. 'Tradition and Perspectives of Greco-Arab and Islamic Medicine'. In *Herbal Supplements: Efficacy, Toxicity, Interactions with Western Drugs and Effects on Clinical Laboratory Tests*, edited by Amitava Dasgupta and Catherine A. Hammet-Stabler, 209-54. Hoboken, NJ: Wiley, 2011.
Sahagún, Bernardino de. *Florentine Codex: General History of the Things of New Spain*. Translated by Arthur Anderson and Charles Dibble. Santa Fe, NM: School of American Research: University of Utah, 1950-82.
Salazar, Christine F., ed. *Brill's New Pauly: Encyclopaedia of the Ancient World: Antiquity*. Edited by Hubert Cancik and Helmut Schneider. English ed. Leiden: Brill, 2002-10.
Sampson, Alexander. '*Locus amoenus*: Gardens and Horticulture in the Renaissance'. *Renaissance Studies* 25, no. 1 (2011): 1-23.
Sanderson, Jonathan. 'Nicholas Culpeper and the Book Trade: Print and the Promotion of Vernacular Medical Knowledge 1649-65'. Unpublished PhD thesis, University of Leeds, 1999.
Savage, Frederick G. *Shakespeare's Flora and Folk-Lore*. Stratford-upon-Avon: Shakespeare Press, 1923.
Sawday, Jonathan. *The Body Emblazoned: Dissection and the Human Body in Renaissance Culture*. London: Routledge, 1995.
Scarborough, John. *Roman Medicine*. Ithaca, NY: Cornell University Press, 1969.
—'Early Byzantine Pharmacology'. In *Symposium on Byzantine Medicine*, edited by John Scarborough, chs 213-32. Washington, DC: Dumbarton Oaks, 1984.
—'Dioscorides of Anazarbus for Moderns – an Essay Review'. *Pharmacy History* 49, no. 2 (2007): 76-80.

—*Pharmacy and Drug Lore in Antiquity: Greece, Rome, Byzantium*. Farnham: Ashgate, 2010.
Scarborough, John, and Vivian Nutton. 'The Preface of Dioscorides' Materia Medica: Introduction, Translation and Commentary'. *Transactions and Studies of the College of Physicians of Philadelphia (5th series)* 4, no. 3 (1982): 187–227.
Schiebinger, Londa, ed. *Plants and Empire: Colonial Bioprospecting in the Atlantic World*. Cambridge, MA: Harvard University Press, 2004.
Schleissner, Margaret R. *Manuscript Sources of Medieval Medicine: A Book of Essays*. New York: Garland, 1995.
Schöner, Erich. *Das Viererschema in der antiken Humoralpathologie*. Archiv für Geschichte der Medizin und der Naturwissenschaften, Supp. 4. Wiesbaden: F. Steiner, 1964.
Schuckner, Robert. 'The English Puritans and Pregnancy, Delivery and Breast Feeding'. *History of Childhood Quarterly* 1, no. 4 (1974): 637–58.
Schultes, Richard E., and Siri Von Reis. *Ethnobotany: Evolution of a Discipline*. London: Chapman and Hall, 1995.
Scully, Terence. *The Art of Cookery in the Middle Ages*. Woodbridge: Boydell Press, 1995.
Seelig, Sharon. *Autobiography and Gender in Early Modern Literature: Reading Women's Lives, 1600–1800*. Cambridge: Cambridge University Press, 2006.
Shorter, Edward. *Women's Bodies: A Social History of Women's Encounter with Health, Ill-Health and Medicine*. New Brunswick, NJ: Transaction Publishers, 1991.
Sigerist, Henry E. *A History of Medicine. Vol. 2. Early Greek Hindu and Persian Medicine*. New York: Oxford University Press, 1961.
Sim, Alison. *Food and Feast in Tudor England*. Stroud: Sutton, 1997.
Singer, Charles. *From Magic to Science: Essays on the Scientific Twilight*. Unabridged 1928 ed. New York: Dover Publications, 1958.
Siraisi, Nancy G. *Medieval and Early Renaissance Medicine: An Introduction to Knowledge and Practice*. Chicago: University of Chicago Press, 1990.
—'Theory, Experience and Customary Practice in the Medical Writings of Francesco Sanches'. In *Between Text and Patient: The Medical Enterprise in Medieval and Early Modern Europe*, edited by Florence E. Glaze and Brian K. Nance, 441–63. Florence: SISMEL, 2011.
Skenderi, Gazmend. *Herbal Vade Mecum*. Rutherford, NJ: Herbacy Press, 2003.
Smith, Lisa W. 'The Relative Duties of a Man: Domestic Medicine in England and France, ca. 1685–1740'. *Journal of Family History* 31, no. 3 (2006): 237–56.
Smith, Michael E. 'The Expansion of the Aztec Empire: A Case Study in the Correlation of Diachronic Archaeological and Ethnohistorical Data'. *American Antiquity* 52, no. 1 (1987): 37–54.
Smith, Pamela and Paula Findlen. *Merchants and Marvels: Commerce, Science and Art in Early Modern Europe*. London: Routledge, 2002.
Smith, Wesley D. *The Hippocratic Tradition*. Ithaca, NY: Cornell University Press, 1979.
Smuts, Jan C. *Holism and Evolution*. London: Macmillan, 1927.
Spicksley, Judith M., ed. *The Business and Household Accounts of Joyce Jeffreys Spinster of Hereford 1638–1648*. Oxford: Oxford University Press for the British Academy, 2012.
Spufford, Peter. *Money and Its Use in Medieval Europe*. Cambridge: Cambridge University Press, 1989.
Stace, Clive A. *New Flora of the British Isles*. 3rd ed. Cambridge: Cambridge University Press, 2010.

Stannard, Jerry. 'Hippocratic Pharmacology'. *Bulletin of the History of Medicine* 35 (November–December 1961): 497–518.
—'The Plant Called Moly'. *Osiris* 14 (1962): 254–307.
—'Pliny and Roman Botany'. *Isis* 56, no. 4 (1965): 420–5.
—'Medieval Herbals and Their Development'. In *Herbs and Herbalism in the Middle Ages and Renaissance*, edited by Katherine E. Stannard and Richard Kay. Aldershot: Ashgate, 1999.
Stannard, Jerry, and Richard Kay, eds. *Herbs and Herbalism in the Middle Ages and Renaissance*. Aldershot: Ashgate, 1999.
Stobart, Anne. 'The Making of Domestic Medicine: Gender, Self-Help and Therapeutic Determination in Household Healthcare in South-West England in the Late Seventeenth Century'. Unpublished PhD thesis, Middlesex University, 2008.
—'Challenging Research for the History of Herbal Medicine'. Paper presented at Herbal History Research Network conference on 'Researching the History of Western Herbal Medicine: Appraising Methods and Sources: Branching Out in Early Modern Medicine', London, 16 July 2010.
—'"Lett Her Refrain from All Hott Spices": Medicinal Recipes and Advice in the Treatment of the King's Evil in Seventeenth-Century South-West England'. In *Reading and Writing Recipe Books, 1500–1800*, edited by Michelle DiMeo and Sara Pennell, 203–24. Manchester: Manchester University Press, 2013.
Stock, Brian. *Listening for the Text: On the Uses of the Past*. Philadelphia: University of Pennsylvania Press, 1996.
Stockwell, Christine. *Nature's Pharmacy: A History of Plants and Healing*. London: Arrow Books, 1988.
Strong, Roy. *The Renaissance Garden in England*. London: Thames and Hudson, 1979.
—*The Artist and the Garden*. London: Published for the Paul Mellon Centre for Studies in British Art by Yale University Press, 2000.
Sugg, Richard. *Mummies, Cannibals and Vampires: A History of Corpse Medicine from the Renaissance to the Victorians*. London: Routledge, 2011.
Sumner, Judith. *The Natural History of Medicinal Plants*. Portland, OR: Timber Press, 2000.
Sweet, Victoria. *God's Hotel: A Doctor, a Hospital and a Pilgrimage to the Heart of Medicine*. New York: Riverhead Books, 2012.
Sweetinburgh, Sheila. *The Role of the Hospital in Medieval England: Gift-Giving and the Spiritual Economy*. Dublin: Four Courts Press, 2004.
Swinburne, Layinka. 'My Little Lord's Legs: Lay Treatment of Rickets in Early Modern England'. Paper presented at conference on 'Recipes in Early Modern Europe: The Production of Medicine, Food and Knowledge', Wellcome Unit for the History of Medicine, Oxford, 13 February 2004.
Taavitsainen, Irma, and Päivi Pahta. *Medical Writing in Early Modern English*. Cambridge: Cambridge University Press, 2011.
Tannahill, Reay. *Food in History*. Revised ed. Harmondsworth: Penguin, 1988.
Taylor, Suzanne, and Virginia Berridge. 'Medicinal Plants and Malaria: An Historical Case Study of Research at the London School of Hygiene and Tropical Medicine in the Twentieth Century'. *Transactions of the Royal Society of Tropical Medicine and Hygiene* 100, no. 8 (2006): 707–14.
Temkin, Owsei. *Hippocrates in a World of Pagans and Christians*. Baltimore, MD: Johns Hopkins University Press, 1995.
Thirsk, Joan. 'Making a Fresh Start: Sixteenth-Century Agriculture and the Classical

Inspiration". In *Culture and Cultivation in Early Modern England*, edited by Michael Leslie and Timothy Raylor, 15–34. Leicester: Leicester University Press, 1992.
—*Alternative Agriculture: A History from the Black Death to the Present Day*. Oxford: Oxford University Press, 1997.
—*Food in Early Modern England: Phases, Fads, Fashions, 1500–1760*. London: Hambledon Continuum, 2007.
Thiselton-Dyer, T. F. *The Folk-Lore of Plants*. Facsimile of 1889 ed. Felinfach: Llanerch Publishers, 1994.
Thomas, Keith. *Religion and the Decline of Magic: Studies in Popular Beliefs in Sixteenth and Seventeenth-Century England*. London: Weidenfeld and Nicolson, 1971.
—*Man and the Natural World: Changing Attitudes in England 1500–1800*. Harmondsworth: Penguin, 1984.
—*The Ends of Life: Roads to Fulfilment in Early Modern England*. Oxford: Oxford University Press, 2009.
Thompson, Elizabeth. *The Diary of a Kendal Midwife: 1669–1675*. Edited by Loraine Ashcroft. Cumbria: Curwen Archives Trust, 2001.
Thulesius, Olav. *Nicholas Culpeper, English Physician and Astrologer*. New York: St Martin's Press, 1992.
Tiller, Kate. *English Local History: An Introduction*. 2nd ed. Stroud: Sutton, 2002.
Tillotson, Alan K., Nai-Shing H. Tillotson, and Robert Abel. *The One Earth Herbal Sourcebook: Everything You Need to Know About Chinese, Western and Ayurvedic Herbal Treatments*. New York: Kensington Books, 2002.
Tobyn, Graeme. *Culpeper's Medicine: A Practice of Western Holistic Medicine*. New ed. London: Singing Dragon, 2013.
Tobyn, Graeme, Alison Denham, and Margaret Whitelegg. *The Western Herbal Tradition: 2000 Years of Medicinal Plant Knowledge*. Edinburgh: Churchill Livingstone/Elsevier, 2011.
Toledo, Victor M. 'Biocultural Diversity and Local Power in Mexico: Challenging Globalization'. In *On Biocultural Diversity: Linking Language, Knowledge and the Environment*, edited by Luisa Maffi, 472–88. Washington, DC: Smithsonian Institution Press, 2001.
Tomalin, Claire. *Samuel Pepys: The Unequalled Self*. London: Viking, 2002.
Torres, Eliseo. *The Folk Healer: The Mexican-American Tradition of Curanderismo*. Albuquerque, NM: Nieves Press, n.d.
Tosh, John, with Seán Lang. *The Pursuit of History: Aims, Methods and New Directions in the Study of Modern History*. Harlow: Pearson Longman, 2006.
Totelin, Laurence M. V. *Hippocratic Recipes: Oral and Written Transmission of Pharmacological Knowledge in Fifth- and Fourth-Century Greece*. Boston: Brill, 2009.
—'And to End on a Poetic Note: Galen's Authorial Strategies in the Pharmacological Books'. *Studies in History and Philosophy of Science Part A* 43, no. 2 (2012): 307–15.
Touwaide, Alain. 'Therapeutic Strategies: Drugs'. In *Western Medical Thought from Antiquity to the Middle Ages*, edited by Mirko D. Grmek, 259–73. Cambridge, MA: Harvard University Press, 1998.
—'The Legacy of Classical Antiquity in Byzantium and the West'. In *Health and Healing from the Medieval Garden*, edited by Peter Dendle and Alain Touwaide, 15–28. Woodbridge: Boydell and Brewer, 2008.
—'Quid Pro Quo: Revisiting the Practice of Substitution in Ancient Pharmacy'. In *Herbs and Healers from the Ancient Mediterranean through the Medieval West: Essays in*

Honour of John M. Riddle, edited by Anne Van Arsdall and Timothy Graham, 19–61. Aldershot: Ashgate, 2012.

Trease, Geoffrey. 'The Spicers and Apothecaries of the Royal Household in the Reigns of Henry III, Edward I and Edward II'. *Nottingham Medieval Studies* 3 (1959): 19–52.

Troy, David B., ed. *Remington: The Science and Practice of Pharmacy*. 21st ed. Philadelphia: Lippincott, Williams and Wilkins, 2006.

Tschanz, David. 'A Short History of Islamic Pharmacy'. *Journal of the International Society for the History of Islamic Medicine* 1, no. 3 (2003): 11–17.

Tutin, T. J., ed. *Flora Europaea; Vol. 2. Rosaceae to Umbelliferae*. Cambridge: Cambridge University Press, 1968.

Van Arsdall, Anne. 'The Transmission of Knowledge in Early Medieval Medical Texts: An Exploration'. In *Between Text and Patient: The Medical Enterprise in Medieval and Early Modern Europe*, edited by Florence L. Glaze and Brian K. Nance, 201–15. Florence: SISMEL, 2011.

Van Arsdall, Anne, and Timothy Graham, eds. *Herbs and Healers from the Ancient Mediterranean through the Medieval West: Essays in Honour of John M. Riddle*. Farnham: Ashgate, 2012.

Van Meerbeeck, Philippe J. *Recherches historiques et critiques sur la vie et les ouvrages de Rembert Dodoens (Dodonaeus)*. First ed. 1841. Utrecht: HES, 1980.

Vickery, Roy. *Garlands, Conkers and Mother-Die: British and Irish Plant-Lore*. London: Continuum, 2010.

Vogt, Sabine. 'Drugs and Pharmacology'. In *The Cambridge Companion to Galen*, edited by R. J. Hankinson. 304–22. Cambridge: Cambridge University Press, 2008.

Voigts, Linda E. 'A New Look at the Manuscript Containing the Old English Translation of the Herbarium Apulei'. *Manuscripta* 20, no. 1 (1976): 40–59.

—'Anglo-Saxon Plant Remedies and the Anglo-Saxons'. *Isis* 70, no. 2 (1979): 250–68.

—'Multitudes of Middle English Medical Manuscripts'. In *Manuscript Sources of Medieval Medicine: A Book of Essays*, edited by Margaret R. Schleissner, 183–96. New York: Garland, 1995.

Von Staden, Heinrich. *Herophilus: The Art of Medicine in Early Alexandria*. Cambridge: Cambridge University Press, 1989.

Waldstein, Anna, and Cameron Adams. 'The Interface between Medical Anthropology and Medical Ethnobiology'. *Journal of the Royal Anthropological Institute* 12, Supplement 1 (2006): 95–118.

Wall, Cecil. *A History of the Worshipful Society of Apothecaries: Abstracted and Arranged from the Manuscript Notes of the Late Cecil Wall by the Late H. Charles Cameron. Volume 1: 1617–1815*. Edited by E. Ashworth. London: Oxford University Press for the Wellcome Historical Medical Museum, 1963.

Wallis, Faith, ed. *Medieval Medicine: A Reader*. Toronto: University of Toronto Press, 2010.

Wallis, Patrick. 'Exotic Drugs and English Medicine: England's Drug Trade, c. 1550–c. 1800'. Working Paper No. 143/10. London School of Economics, July 2010.

Watkins, Frances, Barbara Pendry, Olivia Corcoran, and Alberto Sanchez-Medina. 'Anglo-Saxon Pharmacopoeia Revisited: A Potential Treasure in Drug Discovery'. *Drug Discovery Today* 16, no. 23/24 (2011): 1069–75.

Watson, Gilbert. *Theriac and Mithridatum: A Study in Therapeutics*. London: Wellcome Historical Medical Library, 1966.

Watson, Sethina. 'The Origins of the English Hospital'. *Transactions of the Royal Historical Society*, Sixth Series 16 (2006): 75–94.

Wear, Andrew. *Health and Healing in Early Modern England*. Aldershot: Ashgate, 1998.
—*Knowledge and Practice in English Medicine, 1550-1680*. Cambridge: Cambridge University Press, 2000.
Wear, Andrew, Roger K. French, and Iain M. Lonie, eds. *The Medical Renaissance of the Sixteenth Century*. Cambridge: Cambridge University Press, 1985.
Weatherall, Miles. 'Drug Treatment and the Rise in Pharmacology'. In *The Cambridge Illustrated History of Medicine*, edited by Roy Porter, 246-77. Cambridge: Cambridge University Press, 1996.
Webber, Teresa, and Andrew G. Watson, eds. *The Libraries of the Augustinian Canons*. Vol. 6. Corpus of British Medieval Library Catalogues. London: British Library in association with the British Academy, 1998.
Webster, Charles. 'The Medical Faculty and the Physic Garden'. In *The History of the University of Oxford, Vol. V: The Eighteenth Century*, edited by Lucy S. Sutherland and Leslie G. Mitchell, 683-723. Oxford: Clarendon Press, 1986.
—ed. *Health, Medicine and Mortality in the Sixteenth Century*. Cambridge: Cambridge University Press, 1979.
Weigall, Rachel. 'An Elizabethan Gentlewoman: The Journal of Lady Mildmay, Circa 1570-1617'. *Quarterly Review* 215 (1911): 119-38.
Weiss, Rudolf F. *Herbal Medicine*. Beaconsfield: Beaconsfield Publishers, 1988.
Wellmann, Max. 'Sextius Niger, eine Quellenuntersuchung zu Dioscorides'. *Hermes* 24, no. 4 (1889): 530-69.
—'Beiträge zur Quellenanalyse des älteren Plinius'. *Hermes* 59, no. 2 (1924): 129-56.
Wesson, Nicky. 'The Experience of Childbirth for Early Modern Women'. *MIDIRS Midwifery Digest* 15, no. 2 (2005): 151-7.
Wheeler, A., P. Davis, and E. Lazenby. 'William Turner's (c. 1508-68) Notes on Fishes in His Letter to Conrad Gessner'. *Archives of Natural History* 13, no. 3 (1968): 291-305.
Whitmore, Thomas M. *Disease and Death in Early Colonial Mexico: Simulating Amerindian Depopulation*. Boulder, CO: Westview Press, 1992.
Whittle, Jane, and Elizabeth Griffiths. *Consumption and Gender in the Early Seventeenth-Century Household: The World of Alice Le Strange*. Oxford: Oxford University Press, 2012.
Wichtl, M. 'Quality Control and Efficacy Evaluation in Phytochemicals'. In *Plants for Food and Medicine: Proceedings of the Joint Conference of the Society for Economic Botany and the International Society for Ethnopharmacology, London, 1-6 July 1996*, edited by Hew D. V. Prendergast, Nina L. Etkin, David R. Harris and Peter J. Houghton, 309-16. Kew: Royal Botanic Gardens, 1998.
Wilkins, John. 'The Contribution of Galen, *De subtilitante diaeta* (On the Thinning Diet)'. In *The Unknown Galen*, edited by Vivian Nutton, 47-55. London: Institute of Classical Studies, University of London, 2002.
—'Galen and Athenaeus in the Hellenistic Library'. In *Ordering Knowledge in the Roman Empire*, edited by Jason König and Tim Whitmarsh, 69-87. Cambridge: Cambridge University Press, 2007.
Wilkins, John, David Harvey, and Mike Dobson. *Food in Antiquity*. Exeter: University of Exeter Press, 1995.
Willes, Margaret *The Making of the English Gardener: Plants, Books and Inspiration, 1560-1660*. New Haven, CT: Yale University Press, 2011.
Williamson, Elizabeth M. 'Synergy and Other Interactions in Phytomedicines'. *Phytomedicine* 8, no. 5 (2001): 401-9.

Williamson, Elizabeth, Samuel Driver, and Karen Baxter. *Stockley's Herbal Medicines Interactions*. London: Pharmaceutical Press, 2009.
Wilson, Adrian. 'The Ceremony of Childbirth and Its Interpretation'. In *Women as Mothers in Pre-Industrial England: Essays in Memory of Dorothy Mclaren*, edited by Valerie A. Fildes, 68–107. London: Routledge, 1989.
—'The Perils of Early Modern Procreation: Childbirth With or Without Fear?'. *Journal for Eighteenth-Century Studies* 16, no. 1 (1993): 1–19.
—*The Making of Man-Midwifery: Childbirth in England, 1660–1770*. Cambridge, MA: Harvard University Press, 1995.
Wilson, Stephen. *The Magical Universe: Everyday Ritual and Magic in Pre-Modern Europe*. London: Hambledon and London, 2000.
Withey, Alun. *Physick and the Family: Health, Medicine and Care in Wales, 1600–1750*. Manchester: Manchester University Press, 2011.
Wolloch, Nathaniel. *History and Nature in the Enlightenment: Praise of the Mastery of Nature in Eighteenth-Century Historical Literature*. Farnham: Ashgate, 2010.
Woodward, Marcus. *Leaves from Gerard's Herball*. New York: Dover Publications, 1969.
—ed. *Gerard's Herball: The Essence Thereof Distilled by Marcus Woodward from the Edition of Th. Johnson, 1636*. London: Minerva, 1971.
Woolf, Daniel R. 'The "Common Voice": History, Folklore and Oral Tradition in Early Modern England'. *Past and Present* 120, no. 1 (1988): 26–52.
Woolgar, Christopher. 'Diet and Consumption in Gentry and Noble Households: A Case Study from around the Wash'. In *Rulers and Ruled in Late Medieval England: Essays Presented to Gerald Harris*, edited by Rowena E. Archer and Simon Walker, 17–32. London: Hambledon, 1995.
—ed. *Household Accounts from Medieval England, Part 1, Introduction, Glossary, Diet Accounts (I)*. Oxford: Oxford University Press for the British Academy, 1992.
Woolgar, Christopher M., Dale Serjeantson, and Tony Waldron, eds. *Food in Medieval England: Diet and Nutrition*. Oxford: Oxford University Press, 2006.
Woolley, Benjamin. *The Herbalist: Nicholas Culpeper and the Fight for Medical Freedom*. London: HarperCollins, 2004.
Wootton, David. *Bad Medicine: Doctors Doing Harm since Hippocrates*. Oxford: Oxford University Press, 2006.
World Health Organization. *WHO Traditional Medicine Strategy: 2002–2005*. Geneva: World Health Organization, 2002.
—*National Policy on Traditional Medicine and Regulation of Herbal Medicines: Report of a WHO Global Survey*. Geneva: World Health Organization, 2005.
Wren, R. C. *Potter's New Cyclopaedia of Botanical Drugs and Preparations*. 2nd ed. Edited by Elizabeth M. Williamson and Fred J. Evans. Saffron Walden: C. W. Daniel, 1988.
Wrigley, Edward A., and Roger S. Schofield. *The Population History of England 1541–1871*. Cambridge: Cambridge University Press, 1981.
Yance, Donald. *Herbal Medicine, Healing and Cancer: A Comprehensive Program for Prevention and Treatment*. Lincolnwood, Chicago: Keats Publishing, 1999.
Zollman, Catherine, and Andrew Vickers. 'What Is Complementary Medicine?'. *British Medical Journal* 319, no. 721 (1999): 693–6.

Index

Abingdon Abbey 112
abortifacients 132, 140
abortion 133
abrotonon 183
accounts 151–2
Achillea millefolium 92
achrades 179–80
Aconitum napellus 222
Aconitum spp. 278
Adamnan 262
adder's tongue 92
Aegineta 91
Affections 31, 33, 34, 34
Agnus castus 262
Agriculture et maison rustique 236
Airs, Waters and Places 28, 30
aither 30
Alarcón, Hernando Ruiz de 274
    Treatise on Superstitions 274–5
Albertus Magnus
    Book of Secrets, The 218
Alcmaeon 29
Alexander of Neckham 123
alkaloids 141, 278
Alliaria petiolata 92
alliums 185
almshouses 111
Alphita 258, 260, 262
analgesia 279
anatomy 217
Ancient Medicine 29, 32
Andromachus 197
anemones 241
angelica 92
Angelica archangelica 92
Anglo-Saxon sources 13
Anna of Oldenburg 212
Anonymus Londinensis 34
    perissomata 32
anthropologists 277
anthropology 57, 249, 271

antimony 213
antirrhinon 179
antirrhinum 179
aparine 180
Aphorisms 182
apion 180
apothecaries 111, 118, 123, 136, 159, 215, 219
apprenticeship 59
Arber, Agnes 5, 89
arbrotinum *see* southernwood
archaeology 249, 250, 253–65, 271, 290
archives 108, 150, 289
Arctium lappa 141
Aristolochia clematitis 221
Aristolochia longa 221
Aristolochia spp. 140
Aristotle 238
Ars medica 88
Artemisia abrotanum 218
Artemisia absinthium 92
Artemisia arborescens 183
Artemisia vulgaris 140
Asclepius 33
asepsis 142
ash (tree) 98
asparagus 95–6, 99
Asparagus officinalis 95–6
Aster linosiris 203
astrology 87, 89, 91, 92–3, 96, 98
astronomy 275
Athamanta 202
Athamanta cretensis 201
Atriplex foetida 98
Atropa belladonna 141
Atran 220
Augustinian Order 250, 253, 254
Averroes 261
Avicenna 69, 72, 96, 261
    Canon of Medicine 78, 281
Ayurvedic medicine 142, 281, 293

Ayurvedic system 2, 3
Aztec 273
   chinampa system 275
   cosmology 275–6, 283
   ethnohistorical sources 273–5
   healing ceremonies 276
   human sacrifice 276
   medicine 272
   religion 276
Aztec Empire 238, 279

baby's pet 219
Bacon, Francis 234, 238
   Novum organum 238
Badiano, Juan 274
balme 141
Bampton
   Hundred Rolls 114
Banckes' Herbal 218, 219
banewort 219
barley 249
barley gruel 33
baronial records 114
Bartholomaeus Anglicus 120, 261
   De proprietatibus rerum 120
bathing 36, 214
Battle Abbey 115
Bauhin, Jean 204
bay 92
Bedlam 261
beef 185
beer 123, 124
Bellis perennis 219
Bernardino de Sahagún 274, 281
Bethlemite foundation 261
bias 51–2
Bible 249
Bibliothèque interuniversitaire de médicine (BIUM) 174–5
Bicester Priory 119
bilberries 93–5, 99
bile 30
biographical approaches 9
biographical studies 169
biomedicine 39, 295
Birth of Mankind, The 67, 68, 69, 71, 72, 74, 75, 76, 77, 79
   editions 78
birthworts 140

bishoprics 114
BIUM *see* Bibliothèque interuniversitaire de médicine
black bile 30, 37, 174
black hellebore 33
black nightshade 38, 39
black pepper 35
black poplar 141
black poppy 141
bleeding 71, 279
blessed thistle 92
blood 30, 37, 174
bloodletting 36, 214, 257
Bock, Hieronymus 95
Boel, William 239
Bolton Abbey 115
Book of Secrets, The 218
book trade 149
Boston
   St Botolph's Fair 115
botanical history 3, 5–6
botanical identification 39
botany 24, 176, 211, 271
   folk 220
bowel function 33
bramble 141
Brasavola, Antonio Musa 220
Brassica nigra 92
breads 123, 124
breast feeding 79–81
Breaths 28, 32
Brief and Pleasaunt Treatise How to Dresse, Sowe and Set a Garden 235–6
Broughton Manor 114
burdock 141
butcher's broom 98

cacao 274
caciques 280
Camerarius, Joachim 95
cannibalism 275
Canon of Medicine 78, 281
Canterbury
   archdeaconry 153
   Prerogative Court of 153
cardamom 35
Carmina Gadelica 261
cartularies 114
Carum carvi 215

Cassia acutifolia 215
Cassington 113
cathedral records 114
Catholicism 279
cautery 36
CBMLC *see* Corpus of British Medieval Library Catalogues
Cecil, Robert 213
Centaurium erythraea 215
Centaurium magnum 215
cervix 139
Chamberlen, Hugh 68
    Diseases of Women, The 68
chamomile 98
Charlemagne 115
Charles I 235
Charles V (of Spain) 274
Charmides 28-9
charms 60
Charter Rolls
    Calendar 114
Chaucer, Geoffrey 123
Chauliac, Guy de 263, 264
    Chirurgia magna 263, 264
cheeses 123, 124
Chelidonium majus 98, 221
Chelsea Physic Garden 6
cherry 141
childbirth 108-9, 131-43, 290
    complications 134-5
    contractions 142
    mortality rates 135
    pain relief 132, 133, 134, 136, 138, 140, 143
    remedies 137-43
Child-birth; or, the Happie Deliverie of Women 68, 69, 71, 139
Chinese system 2, 3
Chinese traditional medicine 142, 281, 298
Chirurgia magna 263, 264
Chrysippus of Cnidos 96
chrysocome 203
chumoi 30
Church courts 151, 153, 157, 160
Cinchona spp. 108
Cinnamomum spp. 114, 140
cinnamon 114, 140, 141-3, 177, 239
city records 114
clary 98

classical languages 37
Claudii Galeni opera omnia 174
cleavers 98, 180
clinical therapeutics 291
clivers *see* cleavers
Close Rolls
    Calendar 114
cloves 114, 119, 239, 249
Cnicus benedictus 92
Cnidian berry 33, 34
Cockayne, T. O. 52
Codex Badianus 274, 281, 282
Codex Florentinus 282
Cole, Peter 89
Coles, William 89
College of Physicians 88, 92, 142, 235
    prosecutions 136
comfrey 141
Commiphora spp. 140
common valerian 258
Company of Grocers 234
Compendium medicinae 264
Compendium of Medicine, The 120
Compleat Midwife, The 136, 139
Compleat Midwife's Practice, The 73
Compleat Midwifes Practice, The 68, 74
complementary therapy 11, 293
Compound Medicines According to Kind 175
Compound Medicines According to Place 175
confectionery 123, 124
Conium maculatum 34, 96
conniseed 119
conservation projects 7
Constantinus Africanus 261
constipation 71
contra yerva 141
Convolvulus scammonia 33
Conybeare, John 121
cookery manuals 122, 123
coriander 200
Cornwall
    archdeaconry 153
Corpus of British Medieval Library Catalogues (CBMLC) 257, 258, 261, 264
Cortes, Hernan 274
cosmetics 213-14

cosmos 29
county record offices 107
courts
    ecclesiastical 151, 153, 157, 160
    inventories 153
Creake Abbey 119
Cretan dittany 140
crocus 237, 241
Crocus sativus 92, 119, 140
Crowne Imperiall 240
culinary history 7
Culpeper, Nicholas 68, 72, 73, 74, 75, 87–100, 141, 169, 200, 220, 290
    biographies 90
    Directory for Midwives 68, 69, 76
    English Physitian 24
    posthumous reputation 89–90
    sources 88
    translation of Senner 76
cultural history 3
cumin 108, 111–24
    affordability 123–4
    as aid to digestion 120, 122
    as stimulant 122
    culinary uses 121–3
    cultivation 115
    trade 117–18
Cuminum cyminum 112, 115
cummin *see* cumin
cupping 36, 71
curanderos 48, 58, 59
Cuscuta europaea 221

D'Alechamps, Jean 203
daffodil 222
daisy 219
dandelion 92, 98
Daniel, Henry 118
Daphne cnidium 33
dates 119
datura 274
Datura stramonium 274
Daucus carota 192
De alimentorum facultatibus 177, 178
De materia medica 27, 34, 170, 180, 191, 192, 194–7, 198, 199, 204, 259
    places named 194–5
    publication 196–7
    translations 79, 192

De medicamentis liber 53–4
De proprietatibus rerum 120
De viribus herbarum 258, 259–60
dementia 261
Dentition 72
depression 260, 263
    treatment 263
diacyminum 120
diaita 32
Dianthus barbatus 234
diaries 107, 111
    midwives 136
Diaz, Bernal 273, 274
dictionaries
    online 24
diet 32, 33, 34, 77, 119, 184, 214
digestion 28, 32, 33, 120
Digitalis purpurea 92
Diocles 177
Diodotus 201
Dioscorides 5, 11, 34, 40, 53, 72, 88, 92, 170, 173, 177, 179, 180, 183, 186, 191–205, 216, 219, 221, 222, 290
    biography 193–4
    De materia medica 27, 34, 79, 170, 180, 191, 192
    pharmacopoeia 38, 69
    translations 220
    travels 194
Directory for Midwives, A 68, 69, 76, 88
disease
    causal factors 32–3
Diseases I 33
Diseases II 33
Diseases of Women, The 68, 69, 72
    preface 75
disequilibrium 276
distilling 159
Dit de l'Herberie, Le 118
Dr Chamberlain's Midwifes Practice 68, 69, 73, 75
doctrine of signatures 98
dodder 221
Dodoens, Rembert 199, 201, 202, 203, 239
Dogmatists 33
drug plants 257
druggists 159
drugs 6, 170, 178, 179, 180, 183
    consumption 6

Dublin
  Holy Trinity Priory 119
Dunstall, John 71
Duret, Noel 88
Durham 115
Durham Cathedral Priory 119
Dyer, Lady
  death 213
dynameis 30, 34, 180–1

Ecballium elaterium 33, 39
Ecluse, Charles de l' 199
economic history 3, 6
Ecuador 277
Edinburgh 118
Edward the Confessor 117
elecampane 192, 198–200
  Dioscorides' description 198–200
electuaries 120
elements 40
Elements and Mixtures 177
Elettaria spp. 35
emesis therapy 33
Empedocles 29
Empiricists 32, 174
enemas 71, 72, 74
English Husbandsman, The 236
English Physitian, The 24, 87–100
  editions 88–9
  originality 93–8
English Physitian Enlarged, The 99
English tobacco 92
Ephesus 196
Epidemics treatises 31, 32
  Epidemics 1 32
  Epidemics 2 34
  Epidemics 6 29
epilepsy 11
epistemology 12
Erasistratus 174
Erotian 197
Eryximachus 29
Estienne, Charles
  L'agriculture et maison rustique 236
ethnobotanists 277
  anthropological 278
ethnobotany 3, 7, 204, 249, 250, 271–83, 290
  medical 271, 277

Ethnomedia project 250
ethnopharmacology 3, 6–7
eukrasia 32
Euonymus europaeus 222
ewe-gollan 219
exercise 28, 33, 77, 119, 184
exorcisms 215
Expert Midwife, The 68, 138–9

Fabius Columna 203–4
fatigue 184
Ficino, Marsilio 214
figs 249
Fleshes 30
Florentine Codex 274
fluellin 96–7
folk botany 220
folklore 8, 51, 261
  studies 10
food 28, 121, 149, 291
  history 3, 7
  preparation 156
Forme of Cury, The 122
Fortescue, Bridget 108
foxglove 92
fractures 263
Fraxinus excelsior 98
Fritillaria imperialis 240
fruit 214
Fuchs, Leonhart 199, 201, 204, 212, 217, 220
Fuga Demonum 262
fumigation 139
fungi 140

Gaeltacht 261
Galen 28, 31, 32, 40, 50, 68, 69, 71, 72, 92, 169–70, 173–86, 202, 203, 219, 281
  Ars medica 88
  humours 175–6, 180
  On Simple Medicines 170, 173, 174–7, 179–83
  pharmacology 175–6, 177, 178, 180
  theory of drugs 178
Galen's Art of Physick 88
Galenism 211
Galium aparine 98, 180
gallnut 114
garden history 3, 6, 230–1, 249

Gardeners' Labyrinth, The 236
gardens 24
garlic 179, 185
garlic mustard 92
Gerard, John 91, 95, 202, 216, 220, 221, 237, 240
   Herball 10, 88, 115, 150, 199, 235, 237
Gessner, Konrad 212, 220
Gilbertus Anglicus 120, 121, 264
ginger 38, 117, 237, 249
gingerbread 123
Global Price and Income History Group 123
Glycyrrhiza glabra 123
Goodyer, John 88, 220
   translation of Dioscorides 79
goosegrass *see* cleavers
Gortys 36
gout 33
grains of paradise 249
Granada 281
grape-hyacinth 185
Great Milton Manor 113
greater celandine 98, 221
greater houseleek 141
Greek medicine 50, 281
Grete Herball, The 150, 218
grocers 117
Grocers' Company 234
gruel 33–4
Guaiacum officinale 220
Guillemeau, Jacques 68, 72, 73, 74, 75, 76
   Child-birth 69

hagnos 183
hallucinogenic plants 276
harmonia 30
Harrison, William 211, 239
Hartlib, Samuel 136
Harvey, Gideon 141
headache
   remedies 279
healing 278
healing ceremonies 276
healthy living 183–4, 186
heartsease 98
hellebore 215
Helleborus cyclophyllus 33
Helleborus niger 215

hemlock 34, 96–7
henbane 34, 38, 141
Henry III 119, 120
Heracleitus 29
herb paris 215
Herba Iohannis 262
herbal knowledge
   transmission 191
herbals 9, 47–61, 150, 154, 272
Herbarium of Pseudo-Apuleius 53
herbariums 4, 108
Hernández, Francisco 274
Herophilus 174
Hildegard of Bingen 261
Hill, Thomas
   Brief and Pleasaunt Treatise How to Dresse, Sowe and Set a Garden 235–6
hippocras 123
Hippocrates 27–8, 32, 69, 71, 72, 173, 178, 183, 186, 281
   Aphorisms 182
Hippocratic authors 40
Hippocratic corpus 24, 27–8, 34, 36, 68, 71, 78, 173, 198, 204
Hippocratic physicians 27, 32, 33, 35, 36
Historia natural de la Nueva España 274
historiography 9, 10, 294
history of science 8, 11–12
Hoby, Lady Margaret 132, 169
holism 28–9, 32, 36–7, 40
holos 28–9
Holy Trinity Priory, Dublin 119
honey 249
hormones 40
hospices 111
hospitals 111
House Apothecary and Family Physitian, The 142
household accounts 111, 112, 119
household recipes 140–1
household records 8
human reproduction 68
human sacrifice 276
humoral imbalance 281
humoral theory 76–7, 281, 282
humours 30, 31, 32, 33, 36, 37, 40–1, 69, 174, 175, 176, 179, 180, 183, 184, 185, 214, 276
   theory *see* humoral theory

Hundred Rolls 112, 114
    Bampton 112, 114
Hyoscyamus niger 38, 141
Hyoscyamus spp. 34
hypaconitine 278
Hypericum perforatum 250
    archaeological data 258–9
Hypericum pulchrum 258
hyssop 192, 197, 200, 203–5
Hyssopus officinalis 192, 204

ibn Ezra, Abraham 88
illustrations 47, 48, 49, 56, 59, 73
    anatomical 69–71
Imortelle 203
Inchcolm 262
Indian Moly 239
infanticide 136–7
infertility 71
Information Technology (IT) 56
Inquisitions Post Mortem
    calendars 114
insanity 261
instruction 58–9
instructions 59–61
Internal Affections 34
international trade 237–8
Internet 37, 108, 250
intestine, lower 32
Inula helenium 192, 199
inventories 9, 154, 156, 159
Ipomoea spp. 274
iris 241
Islamic ethics 281
Islamic world 23, 69
IT *see* Information Technology

jack-by-the-hedge 92
Jerningham Family Receipt Book 140
Jesuit's bark 108
John de Trevisa 120
Johnson, Thomas 91, 199, 220, 235
Jonas, Richard 67, 75, 76, 78, 79
    Birth of Mankind, The 75, 76
Journal of Herbal Medicine 291
juniper berries 94
Juniperus sabina 140

Karos 215

katastasis 30
Kew Gardens *see* Royal Botanic Gardens, Kew
Kickxia elatine 97
kitchen utensils 154–5, 159
kopos 184
kosmos 28–9
krasis 40
Kühn, Karl Gottlob 173, 174, 175, 176

labour, premature 140
Lactuca sativa 141
Ladies Companion, The 68, 75, 139
Laecanius Arius 193
Laecanius Bassus 193, 196, 197
language studies 249
Lanthony 257
laughter therapy 36
Laurus nobilis 92
Lawson, William 236
    New Orchard and Garden 236, 237
lay practitioners 11
lead monoxide 213
Ledbury Wills Group 157
Leechbook of Bald 53, 55
Leechbook, A 120
legal documents 108
legal records 107, 136–7, 149–60
Leicester 257
Leoniceno, Niccolò 191
Leonurus cardiaca 141
lepers 115
leprosarium 114
lesser houseleek 141
letters 107, 111
lettice 141
Leyel, Hilda 5
Lhuyd, Edward 262
Libellus de re herbaria 212
Liber commodorum ruralium 123
library catalogues 257–8
Lidstone 113
life habits 33
Lindley Library 108
linguistic studies 9
Linn Dean Nature Reserver 259
liquorice 123, 249
literacy 149
literary criticism 67, 72, 81

literary studies 249
Little Milton 113
Littré, M. P. E. 27
Lloyd Library and Museum 108
lluellin *see* fluellin
London Mortality Bills 135
long pepper 249
loosestrife 222
lower intestine 32
Ludlow market 117
lugos 183
lysimachia 222
Lyte, Henry 199

mace 119
Macer 258
    De viribus herbarum 259–60
Macer Floridus 258
maceration 260
magic 8, 59, 137
Maison rustique, or the Countrie Farme 236–7
malaria 271
    treatments 6
Mandragora officinarum 141
mandrake 141
mania 261
manorial records 107
Mapes, Walter 122
Marcellus of Bordeaux 53–5
    De medicamentis liber 53–4
maritime history 3
Markham, Gervase 236, 237
    English Husbandsman, The 236
Martín de la Cruz 274
Mascall, Leonard 236
massage 36
materia medica 11, 24, 27–41, 91, 118, 169–70, 282, 293
Matricaria recutita 98
Matthioli, Pietro Andrea 199, 202, 203, 204, 217, 221
Mauriceau, François 68, 75
    Diseases of Women 69
medical historians 177
medical history 8, 107, 169, 249
medical implements 155
medical knowledge
    transmission 58

medical manuals 257
medical pluralism 282
medical professions 8
Medical Writings of Anonymous Londinensis 27
Medieval Plant Survey 108
melancholie 30
melancholy 260, 261, 265
Melissa officinalis 141
Mentha pulegium 140
mesaconitine 278
Mesoamerica 272, 273, 280
    Amerindian population 280
    elite families 280
    epidemics 280
    Spanish conquest 279, 280
    Spanish population 280
mestizo 273
Methodists 32, 174
metria 30
Mexica *see* Aztec
Mexico 272, 273, 281
    diversity 272
    shamanistic tradition 281
midwifery manuals 67–81, 131, 134, 138–40, 142
midwives 69, 71, 73, 133, 134, 216
    diaries 136
    inventories 136
    licensing 133
Midwives Book, The 68, 71, 75, 80, 139
Mildmay, Lady Grace 132, 169, 216
miscarriage 133, 140
Misopates orontium 179
missionaries 281
Mnesitheus 177
Modern Herbal, A 5
monasteries 50, 114, 115
    accounts 112, 114, 119
    Augustinian 257–8
    records 114
monk's hood 222
monks 59
Montezuma 273–4
Monument of Matrones, The 133
morning glory 274, 276
motherwort 141
moxibustion 36
mugwort 140

mullein, narrow-leaved 199
mustard 92
myrrh 140, 141–3
Myrstica spp. 119

Names of Herbes, The 212, 216
Nasturtium officinale 98
Natural Faculties 185
Natural History 191, 192, 196, 198
natural history 8, 238
Natural History Museum 108
natural phenomena 29
Nature of Man, The 30, 31, 34, 174
Neckham, Alexander 107
Nero 197
nervous system 34, 141
Netherlands spice trade 117
nettle 53, 277
New Guinea 277
New Herball 89, 150
New Method of Physick, A 92
New Orchard and Garden 236, 237
Nicotiana spp. 92
Nicotiana tabacum 274
nightshade 141
Noble Boke off Cookry 122
Northnewton manor 114
Novum organum 238
nuns 59
Nutriment 30
nutrition 177, 179, 185
Nutrition 177, 183
Nymphaea alba 198

obstetrics
    textbooks 137
Odo Magdunensis 258
old age 184
Old English Herbarium, The 48, 264
olive oil 181, 196
On Antidotes 175, 178
On Diagnosis and Treatment of the Affections of the Soul 175
On Good and Bad Juices 185
On How to Avoid Distress 175
On Maintaining Good Health 173, 178, 183, 184
On Mixtures 173, 178, 179, 183, 185
On Simple Medicines 170, 173, 174–7, 179–83

    editions 174–6
    translations 175, 176–7
On the Avoidance of Grief 177
On the Elements According to Hippocrates 173, 178, 179
On the Natural Faculties 178, 179
On the Powers of Foods 173, 177, 178, 183, 184, 185
On the Properties of Foodstuffs 178
On the Therapeutic Method 178
On the Thinning Diet 176, 183, 184, 185
online dictionaries 24
Ophioglossum vulgatum 92
opium poppy 34, 214
oral history 250
oral tradition 254, 264–5
oral transmission 58, 149
Order of St Lazarus of Jerusalem 115
oregano 203, 204
Origanum dictamnus 140
Orisabius 175, 201, 202, 204
ornamental plants 240, 241
Owen, Dr 215
Oxford 118

Pamphilus of Alexandria 182–3
pan 28
Papaver somniferum 34, 214
Papaver spp. 141
Papius 88
Paracelsus 12, 92, 98, 214, 217, 262–3
Paradisi in sole 87, 95, 99, 170, 229, 230, 231, 232, 235, 238, 239, 240, 242
Paré, Ambroise 68, 138
    Works, The 139
Paris quadrifolia 215
parish records 111
Parkinson, John 24, 87, 88, 89, 91, 93–8, 170, 199, 201, 203, 204, 216, 229–42
    biography 232–5
    Paradisi in sole 87, 95, 99, 170, 229, 230, 231, 232, 235, 238, 239, 240, 242
    portrait 234
    Theatrum botanicum 87, 88, 99, 150, 170, 201, 229, 234, 235, 240, 242
parsnip 201, 202
Partliz, Simeon 92

Pastinaca sativa 201
patches 262
Patent Rolls
    Calendar 114
pathogens 40
Paul of Aegina 175
pear 180
pennyroyal 140
pennywort 141
pepper 38, 112, 114, 117, 119, 124
pepperers 117
pepsis 32
peptides 40
pessaries 138-9
Peucedanum cervaria 201
Pharmaceutical Historian 6
pharmaceutical history 249
pharmacology 38, 170, 175, 176, 177, 178, 180, 271, 291
Pharmacopoeia 235
pharmacopoeia 6, 68, 74-5
Pharmacopoeia Londinensis 88, 89, 92
pharmacy 51, 54, 57, 59
philologists 175
phlegm 30, 37, 174, 185, 279
phusai 32
phusis 28-30, 36
Physical Directory, A 88, 96
physiology 211
phytochemistry 271
phytotherapy 37
Pipe Rolls 114
Piper longum 38
Piper nigrum 35, 38, 112
plant identification 2, 39, 176, 177, 192, 194, 197-8, 218
plant names 176, 182, 212, 257-8
plant propagation 219
plant research 10
Plantago spp. 60
plantain 60
Plato 29
    Charmides 28-9
pleasure garden 240-2
Pliny 92, 96, 197, 198, 199, 201, 202, 205, 216, 219, 238
    Natural History 191, 192, 196, 198
Plutarch 201
pneuma 32, 36, 40

Pneumatists 32
Pompeii 38
Populus nigra 141
pork 185
port tax documents 112
potages 122
potatoes 237
Practical Physick 75, 80
    Culpeper's translation 76
prayers 60
Prerogative Court of Canterbury 153
Prerogative Court of York 153
preventive medicine 179, 184
primroses 241
Principal Probate Registry 151, 153
probate 150-2, 156, 157
    access to records 156-7
    accounts 111, 153
    indexes 157
    inventories 152-3
    records 157
professional training 2
Proffitable Arte of Gardening, The 236
Prunus spp. 141
Psychotis amnis 201
publishers 75-6
purgation 263
purgatives 215
Pyrus amygdaliformis 180
Pyrus communis 180
Pythagoras 29

Queens Closet 139
quit-rents 114

Raynalde, Thomas 67, 69, 72, 73, 74, 75-6, 77, 78, 79
recipe books 108, 140, 154, 160
recipe collections 5, 7, 8, 72, 107, 109, 132
record offices 154
Regimen in Acute Diseases 31, 34, 35
regulation, herbal 293
religious beliefs 132, 135
remedy books 47, 57, 61
rent payments 112
rents 112-15
reproduction, human 68
research
    transmission 56

resources 290
Rhazes 72
rheumatic disorders 6
Richard II 122
rickets 135
Rivière, Lazare 137–8
rock salt 213
Rohde, Eleanour Sinclair 90
Rose Garden, The 139
Rosegarden 78
Rösslin, Eucharius 69, 73, 75
   Rosegarden 78
Royal Botanic Gardens, Kew 108, 250
Royal College of Physicians 213, 215
   library 108
Royal Horticultural Society 108
Royal Pharmaceutical Society 6
Royal Society 240
Rubus fruticosa 141
Ruel, Jean 199, 201
Ruf, Jakub 68, 69, 73, 76, 138
   Expert Midwife, The 138–9
Ruscus aculeatus 98
Rutebeuf 118

saffron 92, 119, 140, 141
Sahagún, Bernardino de 274, 281, 282
St Bartholomew's hospital 258
St Benet Holme 121
St Bernard's Hospice 254
St Botolph's Fair, Boston 115
St Columba 262
St Gall monastery 115
St John's Hospital, Brook Street 115
St John's wort 250, 253–65
   archaeological data 258–9
St Mary of Bethlehem, hospital of 261
St Mary's Abbey, York 121
Salvia sclarea 98
salsarius 114
salt 119
saltpetre 213
Satureia graeca 204
savin 140
scammony 33
scarification 71
Schedule of Medycines 235
Schöner, Erich 31, 32
Schrader, Catherina 136

Scribonius Largus 197
Scrophularia auriculata 98
seed catalogues 4
Selby Abbey 115, 119
self-help 7
Semeiotica Uranica 88
Sempervivum spp. 141
senna 215
Sennert, Daniel 68, 76
   Practical Physick 75, 80
Sermon, William 68, 69, 76, 77
   Ladies Companion, The 68, 75
Seville 281
Sextius Niger 197
Shakespeare, William 249
shamans 276
SHARP *see* Soutra Hospital Archaeo-
   ethnopharmacological Research
   Project
Sharp, Jane 68, 72, 73, 75, 77, 79–80
   Midwives Book, The 68, 71, 80
Singer, Charles 51–2
Sinomomiae 257–8, 260
Sinonomia Bartholomei 258, 260
slender St John's wort 258
social historians 111
social history 3, 107
Social History of Medicine 52
Society of Apothecaries 232, 234, 235
   Schedule of Medycines 235
Socrates 96
Solanum nigrum 38
soporific 260, 264
sources 4–5, 9, 37–40, 107, 109, 111, 169,
   192–3, 292
   Anglo-Saxon 13
   archival 131–2
   classical 50, 54
   Greek 23
   Islamic 78
   legal 149–60
   manuscript 290
   medieval 23
   textual 23
   transmission 50
Southampton
   brokerage books 118
southernwood 218
Soutra Aisle 254

Soutra Hospital Archaeo-
    ethnopharmacological Research
    Project (SHARP) 250, 253, 265
Soutra Medieval Hospital 253–65
    drains 257, 258–9, 260
    site 254–7
Spain, Islamic 280
Spanish Pharmacopoeia 204
*Speculum Matricis; or, the Expert Midwives
    Handmaid* 68, 75
spice trade 35, 196
    internal 117–18
    Netherlands 117
spices 112, 114, 122, 123
spindle tree 222
squirting cucumber 33, 39
stillbirth 138
stills 159
stinking arrach 98
substitution 59
sugar 119
superstition 51, 60–1
Surflet, Richard 236
    Maison rustique, or the Countrie Farme
    236–7
Surrey Domestic Buildings Research
    Group 157
sweet John 234
sweet William 234
Symphytum officinale 141
symptoms 32, 36
Syzygium aromaticum 114

tacit knowledge 59
Taraxacum officinale 92, 98
temperaments 40
Tenochtitlan 273, 274, 275
    botanical gardens 276
tenures 112
Teotihuacan 273
terra sigillata 213
textual studies 9
*That the Faculties of the Soul Follow the
    Mixtures of the Body* 175–6
Theatrum botanicum 87, 88, 99, 150, 170,
    201, 229, 234, 235, 240, 242
Theobroma cacao 274
Theophrastus 177, 196, 199, 202, 203
theriac 177, 178, 180, 213, 222

Theriac to Piso 175, 178
Thornton, Alice 132, 135
Thurgaston 257
tithes 112–15
tobacco 237, 274
Toledo 281
Toltecs 273
trade accounts 108, 111–24
trade records 290
Tradescant, John 239
traditional societies 7
Tragus 91, 95, 96
training, professional 2
translation 58
travel writing 4
Treatise on Superstitions 274–5
treatises
    Hippocratic 28
Triple Alliance Empire 273
Tula 273
tulip 237, 241
Turner, William 89, 170, 201, 211–22,
    239
    contribution to medical botany
    217–22
    Herball 212, 213, 214, 215, 216, 217,
    218, 219, 220, 221, 222
    Libellus de re herbaria 212
    Names of Herbes, The 216, 218, 288
    New Herball 150
    readership 216
    twelve disciples 219
    twelve frills 219

Umbilicus rupestris 141
universities 219
Urtica dioica 53
uterus 141, 142

Vaccinium spp. 93–5
valerian 250, 253–65
    archaeological data 258–9
Valeriana officinalis 250
    archaeological data 258–9
Valley of Mexico 273, 283
Van Helmont, Jan Baptist 98
VCH Explore 157
vegetables 214
venus navil 141

Veratrum album 33, 215
Verbascum niveum var. *niveum* 199
Vespasian 194
veterinary medicine 121
Via Regia 254
Viandier de Taillevent, Le 122
Victoria County History
    website 157
Viola spp. 141
Viola tricolor 98
violet 141, 241
vis medicatrix naturae 23
vitamin deficiency 40
Vitex agnus-castus 183
vulnerary 260, 263

Waltham 257
water 30, 141
water betony 98
watercress 98
Wellcome Library 108, 140, 154
Wendy, Dr 215
Westminster Abbey 115
    Infirmarer's Rolls 121
Whalley Abbey 119
white hellbore 33
white water lily 198
wild carrot 192, 200–3
wild celery 200
wild pear 179–80

wills 111, 150–3, 154, 159
    administrators 151
    executors 151
    nuncupative 151
    published indexes 152
    statistics 152
Willughby, Percival 68, 75
witchcraft 133, 262
witches 276
wolfsbane 197
Wolveridge, James 68, 72, 76
    Speculum Matricis; or, the Expert Midwives Handmaid 68, 75
Wootton Hundred 112
workhouses 111
wormwood 92
Worshipful Society of Apothecaries 232, 234, 235
Wotton, Dr 215
wounds 260, 263
Wyke 113
Wymondham Abbey 121

yarrow 92
yeast 249
yellow bile 37, 174
York, Prerogative Court of 153
York Friars 257

Zingiber officinale 38, 117

CPSIA information can be obtained at www.ICGtesting.com
Printed in the USA
LVOW07s1746240815

451328LV00002B/50/P